DR. NANCY SNYDERMAN'S

GUIDE TO
GOOD HEALTH

DR. NANCY SNYDERMAN'S

GUIDE TO GOOD HEALTH

What Every Forty-Plus Woman Should Know About Her Changing Body

NANCY L. SNYDERMAN, M.D.

and

MARGARET BLACKSTONE

A HARVEST BOOK
HARCOURT BRACE & COMPANY
San Diego   New York   London

Requests for permission to make copies of any part of the work should be
mailed to: Permissions Department, Harcourt Brace & Company,
6277 Sea Harbor Drive, Orlando, Florida 32887-6777.

This Harvest edition published by arrangement with
William Morrow & Company.

Library of Congress Cataloging-in-Publication Data
Snyderman, Nancy L.
Dr. Nancy Snyderman's guide to good health: what every forty-plus
woman should know about her changing body / Nancy L. Snyderman
and Margaret Blackstone.—1st Harvest ed.
p. cm.—(A Harvest book)
Originally published: New York: W. Morrow, 1996.
ISBN 0-15-600471-2
1. Middle aged women—Health and hygiene. 2. Middle aged
women—Diseases.   I. Blackstone, Margaret.   II. Title.
[RA778.S634 1996b]
613'.04244—dc20 96-27108

Book design by Michael Mendelsohn of MM Design 2000, Inc.
Printed in the United States of America
First Harvest edition 1996
E G I K M N L J H F

To the women in my life: Joy and Momie, who blessed me with indefatigable spirit and resilience; and Kate and Rachel, who are everyday reminders of the rich legacy of womanhood.

ACKNOWLEDGMENTS

No project like this is possible without help from inquisitive and supportive people. I have been lucky to share so much creative time exploring, collaborating, and commiserating with my co-author, Meg Blackstone. As we have decided over the course of this past two years what information to include and what to toss, we never lost sight of the same vision: the creation of a women's medical book with a take-charge, feminist edge. A book for all women that cuts across the lines of political orientation and socioeconomic standing. A book that is intended for women over forty who want to take care of themselves and to know more about the diseases and medical problems that are particular to them.

Special thanks are also due to Tony Seidl, my literary agent, who brought me together with my very talented, fun, and insightful editor at William Morrow, Liza Dawson. Working under her guidance and getting her feedback have allowed me to stretch myself and enter this world of publishing. The task of refining my work further fell to my medical editor, Channa Taub, who assumed this job with great energy and grace. Everything that passed before her came back to me better than its original form. I would also like to acknowledge the contribution of our copy editor, Trent Duffy—if all male doctors had his sensitivity to the nuances that surround health-care issues for women, we would be better off.

Thanks are also due to three women who are invaluable in my life. Cynthia Riley, my attorney, agent, friend, and fellow Scrabble player, oversaw many of the logistics associated with this book. My assistant, Angela Bates, has protected my time, typed, edited, photocopied, mailed, faxed, and called more people on my behalf—and has always recognized that all great projects are a result of teamwork; I value her friendship and loyalty. Casandra Lenz, nanny to my children and friend to me, is my exercise partner and the one who makes sure that I get my workout done before the real part of my day begins.

Four other women have a daily influence on my life because they are responsible for supplying me with medical ideas and keeping me up-to-date on medical tidbits. Susan Wagner and Jeanne D'Agostino are the producers who run the medical unit at *Good Morning America* and are responsible for the bulk of the medical segments you see on the show. Patty Neger has produced some of my most memorable live medical interviews. I never quite know what to expect. Lisa Aliferis, my producer at KPIX-TV and *Day and Date* in San Francisco, is responsible for researching, writing, and fine-tuning much of what finally gets on the air. It is rare that we disagree about which stories are credible and which aren't.

I am also grateful to friends and patients who allowed me to interview them for this book. Their quotes are sprinkled throughout and provide various perspectives on the status of women's health care based on their individual stories. Thanks also to the experts who gave me their time during fact-finding sessions with Meg and me to make sure the information is correct and the stories straight.

Three physicians and friends who practice in my medical community in San Francisco graciously took time from very busy practices to proofread chapters and make sure that the information you get is the most up-to-date available in their fields. (Scribbled comments in the margins ranged from "Sounds like you!" to "Find another reference. I wouldn't buy a used car from this person!") Laurie Green, M.D., is a champion. She has delivered two of my children and doubles as my primary doctor and friend and cheerleader. She has been with me during my lowest lows and my highest highs. Kimberly Mulvihill, M.D., and Judy Luce, M.D., are superb physicians who have always said yes when I've asked for that last-minute favor.

Finally, my love and gratitude to my family, who allowed me to steal time that sometimes belonged to them: my husband, Doug, and our children, Kate, Rachel, and Charlie. And to my mother, Joy Snyderman, and her mother, Lillie Sandstedt, who both taught me to be strong and compassionate, and to fight for women even when others considered such feminist behavior a silly waste of time. And to a very special man, my father, Sanford C. Snyderman, M.D., who is the reason I am a doctor and who has always encouraged me to reach for the stars, even if that means falling every now and then.

CONTENTS

PART 4: THE REAL M WORD—MENOPAUSE

PART 6: AGING AND THE BODY

INTRODUCTION

*"When I turned forty, my skin started going, but
that was really okay, because my eyes started going,
too. So, I couldn't see what was happening. It was
like aging with the lights down low."*

Esther Canton (age 51)

I DON'T KNOW WHEN it happens. There is no particular day when you
wake up and say to yourself, "Mmmm . . . I'm not bouncing out of
bed quite the way I used to." But something happens somewhere
along the way from thirty to forty that gives us the first hint that we
are no longer as young as we once were. Our bodies are aging. Often
we use forty as a marker, a sort of midpoint where we have an opportunity to look at what we want to change and what we want to keep
of ourselves. We have a chance to look forward and chart a course, one
that we hope—with diligence and a lot of luck—will allow us to age
well and enjoy what can be the most fruitful decades of life.

Add to this the fact that personal health is vast and daunting to
most of us. How do I find ways to take care of myself in this relentless
modern world where time just disappears? How do I know when to go
to the doctor? And how do I know what doctor to go to? How do I
know what questions to ask, and how do I know if my questions have
been satisfactorily answered? And how can I even count on a doctor
being there for me for more than a year or two with this ever-changing
health-care scheme?

You're right to be overwhelmed. You're right to be questioning what
is good health care for you. We all need to ask the right questions, be
sensitive to the key issues in our personal health care, be aware of where
to go for help and further information, and watch out for the stumbling
blocks that age puts in our way whether we like it or not.

*"One of the greatest lessons my mother taught me
about my health was to take personal responsibility
for it. When I was a child, that meant habits like
eating right, brushing my teeth, getting enough rest,
and enjoying outdoor activities. As an adult, the
same rules apply, along with getting regular physical
examinations, maintaining personal health records,
and educating myself about things like nutrition,
medications, and stress.*

*"I have tried to pass on the lesson of personal
responsibility to my daughter, Chelsea, because
what it all adds up to is prevention. My family and
I are blessed with good health and I am grateful for
my mother's example and teaching."*

Hillary Rodham Clinton

AT THIS POINT we're old enough to be at risk for just about everything, and whether we like it our not, whether we've looked or not, our bodies are changing right before our eyes. And if we do take a look, we may think we're looking at the body of a stranger. The last time this happened to us was puberty.

Since then we've grown accustomed to ourselves, even taken ourselves for granted. Except for childbirth—and we probably felt we bounced back quickly enough from this, with all the running around we did after the kids—it's been the body familiar for a couple of decades. Now, we're starting to be surprised by our body once again. Not all at once, and not in all ways, but still surprised, startled, maybe annoyed or disappointed, or maybe just curious. For some of us, pregnancy and childbirth at a later age changed our bodies irrevocably. For others, surgery did the damage. And for still others, perhaps all of us to some degree or another, poor habits (such as too much caffeine, sun, or alcohol; poor posture, diet, or hygiene; too little exercise) have had a cumulative effect. Suddenly, our backs are killing us, our skin is dry or wrinkling. We feel some aches from arthritis in our feet and hands or worry about getting pneumonia after the flu. We don't sleep as well as we used to, and it takes us longer to get going in the morning. We're not sure if menopause is just around the corner, or if we're just having a bad day, and we do pay more visits to the doctor than we used to.

> *"The doctor of the future will give no medicine, but will interest his patients in the care of the human frame, in diet, and in the cause and prevention of disease."*
>
> Thomas Edison

THIS BOOK CAN'T make you young again, but it can help you get to know your over-forty-year-old body and help you learn to treat it like a loving friend. Sure, your body may be past whatever prime target society is focused on today, but this body of yours still has lots of great miles left. And now you have the maturity to nurture and protect it so that you ensure that the coming years are good years.

I'm a woman. I'm a doctor. I'm a medical correspondent for network and local television. I'm also a daughter and a mother. And I'm forty-three. I'm in good health and pretty good shape. But there have been times when I've been very ill and times when I've been in less than perfect shape. I've taken care of female patients and covered medical stories that affect women, and I've been a patient of both male and female doctors. I know what makes the medical system tick. Having been a part of that system for over twenty years, at this point I know its strengths and weaknesses.

When I was a medical student I was taught everything you wanted to know about anatomy, physiology, disease, and treatment. I don't remember learning anything about preventive medicine. In fact it has always been regarded by the young, eager, and brash as the most boring part of medical training. And other than routine training during two required months in obstetrics and gynecology, no differentiation was made in the disease processes affecting men and women. It took a generation of women, passing into their thirties and forties, to call attention to the inequities manifested in how we train doctors, establish research, and treat women in the medical establishment.

"We were all horrified a couple of years ago when
we found that medical journals defined 'the norm'
as an 180-pound male. That meant we [women]
were all abnormal."

Rep. Patricia Schroeder (D–Colorado)

WITHOUT A DOUBT there are grave inequities between the health care men get and the health care women get. A lot of this gross unfairness is driven by the myths that surround women's health.

One of the most common myths regarding women's health derives from the statement "Women live longer than men." Ergo, if women live longer than men, women's health care must be excellent. Women do live longer than men, but not by much, and that gap is constantly narrowing. And a woman at the end of her life is more likely to be widowed, impoverished, coping with degenerative conditions, or dependent on others. So much for the quality of life.

Another common myth is fueled by the premise that most if not all of what goes wrong with a woman's health has something to do with her reproductive tract. Yes, reproduction is one of the many things that separate the women from the men, but the three leading causes of death in women are exactly the same as for men:

1. heart disease
2. cancer
3. stroke

And one of the reasons this is a little known fact is that in general medical parlance any disease that claims more male victims than female victims is considered to be a male disease. This assumption, by the way, is one of the root causes of gender bias in the medical profession and one that has fueled the unfair treatment of women.

"If you are always treated like a third-class citizen,
you grow to expect that."

Pamela Cooper (age 39)

S O WHY HAVE WOMEN been routinely relegated to an inferior class by the medical profession?

Medicine is a male hierarchy. It's changing—but slowly. Until very recently, women had little or no voice in the arena of medical power—the inner sanctums at the teaching hospitals, the grant-bestowing institutions, and government offices.

Somewhat less obviously, the truth of the matter is that the elegant complexity of the female body has been routinely misunderstood and treated as, at best, mysterious by the medical profession. It might be said that the menstrual cycle has remained as mystifying to the male physician as the theory of relativity was to physicists before Einstein. Throughout medical history "the cycle of reproductive possibility" was considered to exist for many different reasons—"to purge," "to weaken," and so on. But it was only 100 years ago that the purpose of the menstrual cycle—to make the reproduction of human life possible—became clear. Even after this discovery, the treatment of women for pregnancy, problems with menses, and menopause yo-yoed back and forth between one "old husband's tale" and another—the consensus being that there was no consensus on how the female body functions, much less on what women want.

"Is asking for someone to listen asking for so
much?"

Caroline Davies (age 43)

W HAT WE *WANT* and what we *need* may be the same. The best place to start is with adequate, sound, and straightforward information. What women need now is:

- Medical information that will allow us to make informed decisions.
- A physician whose knowledge, compassion, and patience will en-

courage prevention of disease and foster early diagnosis when illness appears.

- The commitment from the research arm of medicine that present and future study groups on conditions and diseases will include equal numbers of women and men.
- The commitment that more studies and further research will be done on those conditions and diseases that affect primarily women.
- To have a curriculum that focuses on the medical needs of women taught in medical schools. Doctors must be educated in the particular and special concerns of women, a majority of the population that until very recently has been treated medically as a mere reflection of the male blueprint.
- When discussing the outcome of an operation or procedure, frank information not only on how long we will live, but on how we will live: What will we be able to do? How much will we be able to enjoy life? While the epidemiological data are not available as yet, it seems clear that women are also very interested in the quality of life.

> *"Knowledge is power. As women we have been raised to do what we are told. It's part of our culture. But the more information we as patients can provide our doctors, the more of a team we will be. The better the teamwork, the better the health care."*
>
> Lisa Aliferis (age 34)

WE AS WOMEN want to be connected to the process of our own health care. We want information that will allow us to enter into the dialogue of health care, treatment, and the medical future. Having the information is the first step toward interactive health care. This book is intended to give you that information and give you the ways and means to make the health decisions that will benefit you most. If we are to take care of ourselves, and teach our daughters and their daughters how to do the same, we must know how to access the health-care system, how to talk to doctors, and how to demand respect and appropriate treatment from a system that is not always kind to women. This book is a first step.

Being a doctor and a woman over forty, I've already discovered there's also a whole lot more we doctors and we women can do to make the aging experience a positive one for women. Some of what happens when we age is inevitable, but there are plenty of health issues associated with aging over which we have a lot more control than we may think we have.

"People have always thought that no one other than women would pay attention to these issues. Whether it is women's health, women's issues, or education—these are what we used to call 'soft issues.' But slowly there has been a revolution."

Lesley Stahl

THE YEAR WAS 1979. Walter Cronkite was the anchor of the CBS evening news, the highest rated network newscast. Lesley Stahl, who had just become White House correspondent, received a call one morning from the senior producer. During the morning news meeting, when the decisions were made by the men who ran the news department as to what topics would be covered that day, there was a raging debate about a story that unnecessary hysterectomies were being performed in the United States and that the numbers were extraordinarily high. The dilemma? Whether this should be the lead story on the evening news. CBS had never led with a health story—let alone a women's health story. Politics was usually the lead of the day. So Lesley got a call. The senior producer just wanted to find out what a woman had to say. You can imagine the rest. That evening CBS led with the hysterectomy story. In a quiet but evolutionary way, this was a watershed event: that single decision has had a ripple effect in news organizations and television broadcasting. Today we have grown accustomed to seeing medical reports on local and network newscasts. The revolution has taken hold.

Staying at the forefront has been a constant challenge, but there's never been any looking back since CBS took the lead in 1979. In fact, we now turn to the media as a constant source of medical information. When I first signed with ABC's *Good Morning America* I fought against being relegated to what I considered the "breast cancer and menopause circuit." I fought it because I knew it was too easy to assign the female medical correspondent to the female medical stories. I believed that, if the men could cover medical stories that affect both sexes, I could too. It was an important position to take to establish myself. Several years later I had covered most breaking medical stories that affect men, women, and children. And then I realized that many problems that affect women were still being glossed over or not being covered at all. I saw that I, as well as the medical and media establishments, had a lot of catching up to do.

In 1991 I suggested that we do a weeklong series on women's health at *Good Morning America*. The producers loved the idea, but instead of a week they wanted a month's worth of material! Although I wasn't sure at first there was enough to talk about for that many reports, I was wrong. The series was such a success and we heard from so many women all over the country that we now have a segment devoted to women's health every Friday. We have no plans for stopping.

I was always concerned that one day I would run out of medical subjects to talk about. When I started filing medical reports for KATV-TV in Little Rock, Arkansas, back in the 1980s I had no way of foreseeing the appetite that viewers would have for medical information. Now, nothing surprises me. Everywhere you turn, you can find basic medical information—in your local news, network news, newspapers, radio, and magazines. Between the basic "news you can use" and the breaking medical stories, there is no end to topics that people are interested in.

The days of state-of-the-art health care being the domain of the rich, white, male citizenry are slowly and painfully coming to an end. But it's not time yet to breathe a sigh of relief and say the battle is won. In fact, the battle is just beginning.

Most of this book is written within the context of the availability of health care, albeit not perfect health care. The truth, however, is that for many Americans access to health care is as chimerical as the happy ending in a fairy tale. Even worse, often the neediest cannot get help. Ailments such as hypothermia, ulcerative conditions, and infections often affect those who are homeless, impoverished, or otherwise disfranchised from the health-care system. Poverty and prejudice damn an ever increasing number of Americans to inferior or nonexistent health care. Not only is the system not available to them, but knowledge of how to use the system is not provided.

It will take education and accessibility to actually change this situation. At present, many minority women do not even have screening tests—such as the Pap smear or mammogram—at their disposal. Because of this, once women of color and poor women of any race do seek medical help, their disease has often progressed to an advanced stage and the death rates from cervical cancer and breast cancer are much higher among them.

Low income, lack of education, and older age are associated with not receiving Pap smears on a regular basis. And older women, who are at the greatest risk of dying from cervical cancer, are the least likely of all groups to have received screening.

The facts regarding mammography are equally unsettling. As of 1987 only 20 percent of Hispanic women forty or older, only 22 percent of low-income women forty or over, and only 28 percent of black women forty or over had received a mammogram. The target of the government for the year 2000 is to increase these percentages to at least 80 percent, still leaving 20 percent of these minority women unable to access the public health system for this routine screening. This goal is particularly ambitious in the face of drastic spending cuts for health care at local and state levels. Government budget reductions have already caused community health clinics that serve the poor in places like Los Angeles County to close.

Women have recognized that while we may not have total control over our destinies, we do have a lot of control over our quality of life and to some extent our longevity. The best way to improve quality and quantity is by being well educated and proactive. Read, listen, use common sense, and follow your gut. Use this book the same way—as a guide to getting the most out of a medical system that isn't necessarily custom designed for women and getting the most out of that difficult, powerful, and intimate relationship between physician and patient.

> *"I just want a doctor who will talk to me—who*
> *will make sense out of complicated medical matters.*
> *I don't expect answers all the time—but I want*
> *good communication. I don't feel pressure to go to*
> *a woman doctor. I just want a good doctor."*
>
> Kathy Harreld (age 45)

YOU MAY BE SAYING to yourself, the trouble with doctors is that they tell you either too much or too little—too much about scary stuff you may or may not be able to do anything about and not enough about the process of prevention and what to educate yourself about. But you may also be feeling that you do not have enough information at your disposal to correct either of these problems. This book can serve as a resource guide when you need to know more, when you need to simplify things, or when you are inundated with too much information.

As you wade through all the medical information that is available, you have to chart your own course. At the same time that you do not want to let yourself be swayed by the "voice of authority"—a dogmatic male or female physician or research done only on male subjects—you also shouldn't feel obliged to embrace radical theories or politicized advice that is not right for you.

Some questions, even when you're asking a doctor to answer them, can feel too personal. So, it's a good idea to make a list of questions and let this book answer some of them while you have the comfort of privacy and time. And in case this book can't answer your particular question, I've included other sources and references to lead you to the information you're seeking and to the help you need. And I do hope your search for answers is interesting and enlightening and that you will insist that all your doctors listen to you, answer your questions, and treat you fairly and well.

In writing this book I realized that I could help the most women most effectively if I gave enough information to help them chart and then steer their own courses in the way that's best for them. How bad is it for women when it comes to health care? Obviously that answer varies from woman to woman but I do believe the inroads that have been made are constantly improving health care for all of us. We've all gone through a time when we've been angered by how little attention is paid to women's health issues, from breast cancer to the C-section rate. And I think we've all been blue at one time or another over just how hard it is to overcome entrenched dogma, *to change the system*. But as I dug deeper and deeper into all the subjects I wanted to cover, I noticed one incontrovertible fact—change is not only in the air, it has momentum. It's happening faster and faster. I have encountered an overwhelming commitment to the issues of women's health among both women and men in the health-care profession and among you—the women who are driving this movement and making people pay attention. You are the driving force behind the changes at hand and the changes are great. Above all, writing this book has made me proud of what we've done and what we are doing, and you should be proud too. I'm encouraged. I want you to be encouraged, too.

DR. NANCY SNYDERMAN'S
GUIDE TO GOOD HEALTH

PART 1

WHOSE HEART IS IT ANYWAY?

"While a woman's lifetime risk of dying of breast cancer is a much publicized one in nine . . . her lifetime risk of dying of coronary heart disease is a startling and far less widely known one in two."

Elizabeth Barrett-Connor, M.D.

THE DILEMMA

Perhaps your male boss just had a heart attack, or your neighbor's husband, your son's track coach or (if you have exciting relatives) your grandmother's younger lover. Or perhaps you just finished reading about some male celebrity recuperating from bypass surgery after a major heart attack. You say to yourself, "Thank God, that's one thing I don't have to worry about."

Perhaps you are one of those women who is always worrying about somebody else's cholesterol level, high blood pressure, salt consumption, or lack of exercise, and *that somebody else* is always a man. You may nag *him* to get *his* blood pressure and cholesterol level checked routinely. You may even know all the signs and symptoms of an impending heart attack, and catch your breath when *he* complains of a tingling arm, chest pain, or a sudden and surprising pain in the lower back.

But the fact is you may be toting up the wrong cholesterol level, monitoring the wrong blood pressure, keeping the fat out of the wrong diet, and admonishing the wrong person to give up smoking and take up exercise. You may be pouring all your worry out on the wrong part of the couple. In short, you may be using the wrong pronoun. You may be thinking of him when you should be thinking of her—in this case, yourself—and you are probably not committing this caregiver's sin for the first time.

> *"Just thinking about it makes me mad. I knew something was wrong. But the doctor in the emergency room just said, 'There, there dear, it's just menopause.' I'm lucky I didn't die."*
>
> Rosemary Grayson (age 64)

ONE OF THE most insidious medical myths is that heart disease is a man's disease. This myth permeates the treatment of heart disease and ends up being translated into misguided reassurances such as "Oh, you'll be fine. You're a woman. You have estrogen to protect you. You don't have to worry about heart disease." Worry about heart disease? Maybe not. But *only* if you protect yourself early in the game by making prevention a mantra of your daily life. *Only* if

3

you monitor yourself as strictly as a heart specialist would monitor his male patient who's chairman of the board, who gets the royal-treatment physical and stress test every six months because he's "so important to his company" and whose cholesterol or blood pressure is consistently a little high.

Royal treatment or no royal treatment, women are at risk for heart disease, and as we age and experience menopause we are at greater risk. In fact, heart disease is the number one killer of women, just as it is for men. You need to be as concerned about your own cholesterol level and blood pressure, the fat content of your diet, and your exercise regime as you are about those of your spouse or father, brother or son. You need, first and foremost, to learn to take your own chest pain seriously and not chalk it up to indigestion or a psychosomatic condition, *even if the doctor you consult is willing to do so.* You must insist that what you are feeling may be a symptom of heart disease and that your complaint be taken seriously. You need to demand the royal treatment for yourself!

The realization that heart disease could affect women hit me square in the face years ago. I was a medical student, spending time in the emergency room. A woman came in complaining of chest pain. She was vague in her description of the pain, which didn't radiate down her left arm (as it says it's supposed to in the medical books if a heart attack is imminent). When, after waiting for a while, she was examined, nothing unusual could be found. A chest X ray was normal and an EKG was ordered just to be on the safe side. It was normal too. So the doctor talked to her about the possibility of having gallbladder disease or a small ulcer. She was given an appointment to come back in a few days to see another doctor who specializes in these areas. She thanked us and left. She never made that next appointment. She dropped dead in the parking lot—she died of a heart attack.

Her story underscores several facts about women's heart disease: women wait longer in emergency rooms to be seen than men, they are underdiagnosed when it comes to heart disease, and their disease is usually more severe at the time of diagnosis.

There is no such thing as benign neglect when dealing with heart disease. The longer heart disease goes untreated, the greater the chance of a heart attack and the more likely the chance of complications afterward.

Though heart disease is responsible for half the deaths by disease among women every year, we are only now beginning to understand how it affects women. In fact:

- Heart disease is as much a risk for women as for men.
- The risk of heart disease for women increases with age.
- Heart disease is often harder to detect and treat in women.
- Heart disease carries a more negative prognosis for women.

So, as a woman approaching menopause or having reached menopause, when you think about taking care of your health, you must put preventing heart disease at the top of your list.

Heart disease in women has remained a silent killer, the statistics largely unpublicized, for a number of reasons. Men tend to have sudden heart attacks at an earlier age than women. You've heard of or may even know a man who had a massive fatal heart attack on the tennis court or while driving. Because the circumstances were so dramatic, you've probably found the incident hard to forget. The image of a young or middle-aged man dying suddenly of a heart attack is tragic and unforgettable. A woman of sixty or seventy who has a heart attack is potentially less memorable. She is older, illness is not so uncommon, and death is by then part of the landscape. You might even find yourself saying, "Oh, well, she probably had other health complications. . . . It's all downhill from here." She falls into that great abyss of "old lady-ism" in which an elder patient is unconsciously categorized as already in the inevitable process of deterioration. Such an attitude does not encourage research on female subjects or any quest toward improved diagnostic or treatment techniques. "Has-beens" do not inspire world-class care.

Just as devastating to the quality of care for female heart patients is the insidious linkage of sexism to the medical habit of considering heart disease a male dominion. And, like a computer virus, once it's in the system it becomes ingrained and increasingly difficult to get rid of.

For example, until now there have been few studies on heart disease that have included subjects of both sexes in relatively equal numbers. A friend was attending a lecture by a male doctor and when she asked about the efficacy of this kind of research practice, the physician bullied her by saying, "You should know the answer to this. All these studies were done in VA hospitals." (As if this were an adequate response!) When early studies indicated that men were at risk for heart attack at younger ages, younger men became the target group for further examination—precisely because many early studies did not follow (or had not yet followed) subjects into the later years. In a lethally vicious circle, studies revealing that men had heart attacks at earlier ages begat studies on larger groups of men of that age; the target group was targeted ad infinitum. In short, ignoring women begat further disregard, to the detriment of fully half the victims of heart disease.

And so, for many years, the course of heart disease research resembled a process of pulling the wool over our own eyes (whether consciously or unconsciously), to maintain a conclusion that more closely resembles a well-cherished delusion. But that was then and now the news is out that studies to date have not revealed the whole truth or looked at the whole picture. Intense scrutiny of the situation that faces women with heart disease has begun.

Until recently, women with heart disease have either been treated exactly as if they were men or been ignored. Neither course of action is an acceptable solution, and both have colluded in creating a very confused picture of female heart disease. For example, women are diagnosed with heart disease when they are older and more infirm. We don't yet know whether this occurs because a woman who has in fact had heart disease for years is just diagnosed at a later age or whether the disease itself occurs later.

Because heart disease in women is frequently diagnosed at a more advanced stage, it is more often fatal for them than for men. By the time of the diagnosis, more damage has been done, and the chances of a complete recovery are not optimal. Unfortunately, we've yet to answer the question of whether this problem stems from the idiosyncratic nature of the female heart or is due to how the medical profession treats heart disease in women. But at least we are finally asking the right question.

> *"When I was in medical school we all learned that heart disease was heart disease. No differences between men and women were considered. But today, when I train young physicians, I insist that*

> *they consider symptomatology for the sexes differ-*
> *ently. At least it's a step in the right direction."*
>
> Terri Gonzalez, M.D. (age 45)

WHEN A WOMAN considers her situation vis-à-vis heart disease, the bad news is that medical protocols for heart care have routinely excluded a female model. When doctors have been trained to demand that the patient match the male model, it's no wonder that the female heart has kept many of them guessing. A great deal of this inequity of care may be attributed to a double standard and the propensity in a classically trained doctor to stereotype a woman patient in terms of "sensitivity," "mood swings," and "female hormones." The sometimes elusive nature of female heart disease is also a component in this high-stakes guessing game.

If the textbook heart is a male heart, then doctors are clearly following the wrong road map when trying to locate and diagnose a woman's heart ailment. It may well be that female heart disease is harder to predict than the male counterpart, but such a conclusion cannot be drawn until significant research and trials are conducted specifically on female heart patients. Only further research can distinguish the variable of gender bias from the variables of ignorance and misunderstanding and begin to eliminate both. The good news is, now we know what the problem is—and just how complex a problem it is at that. Identifying the problem is the first step toward the solution.

To date, the most notable gender-enlightened study is the Framingham Study, which was begun in Massachusetts in 1948. The study included roughly equal numbers of men and women (2,282 men and 2,845 women) in a town outside Boston and followed these people through the courses of their lives (in fact, it is still ongoing). The cholesterol levels of both men and women were measured and the group was monitored over the next fourteen years to see who developed coronary problems. The results were straightforward and definitive. For both men and women, the higher the cholesterol, the greater the chance of coronary disease. (Unwittingly, however, the Framingham Study helped to create the problem of considering heart disease to be a male domain: it noted extensively that men were having heart attacks early in life and thus identified them as the group at risk.)

Most other larger studies done on heart disease have excluded women as a matter of policy. Notable among them is the Physicians' Health Study, which included 22,000 subjects and demonstrated that aspirin in low doses will prevent heart attacks in healthy men. Another, the Multiple Risk Factor Intervention Trial, has an acronym, MRFIT, that devolves all too conveniently into the nickname "Mr. Fit." In the study, the cholesterol levels of 360,000 men were measured and tracked. Six years later the result was clear. A man was at least four times more likely to die of coronary disease when his total cholesterol level was above 300.

Where, you might ask, is "Mrs. Fit"? The answer is she's yet to be studied or analyzed. Does her cholesterol level put her at risk to the same degree and in the same way as a man's? Or, is she *more* at risk or *less* at risk? Does aspirin do for her what it can do for a man? The course of her future and her treatment for heart disease has yet to be documented, but new studies are in place that propose to answer these questions.

"All in Her Head"

"It seemed like I was in the emergency room for an eternity. I knew this was more than indigestion. But the doctor wasn't so convinced. I begged him to put me in the hospital and watch me overnight. I thought if I went home I would die. He finally admitted me. At three o'clock in the morning I had a massive heart attack. That doctor visited me in the intensive care unit and told me he learned something."

Mona Samuelson (age 67)

IN AN AGE in which women have gained the right to fly jets in combat missions, it is still likely that a women will be sent home by the doctor with a tranquilizer for her heart-related symptoms, while a man will be given a full battery of tests.

As a culture, we tend to trust technology more than we trust ourselves. Doctors may be particularly guilty of this affliction, depending
on where and when they were trained. All too often, a doctor may read
the test results before listening to the patient. If women tend to test
well on angiograms and still suffer the symptoms of heart disease, their
complaints may be rejected in honor of the machine, even though in
the case of women, these machines do not have a high degree of pre-
dictive accuracy. Doctors must learn to *trust the patient*—not only the
equipment.

What can you do about this? First of all, you can teach yourself to
trust yourself. If you have recurrent chest pain, you can demand your
doctor take your pain seriously, and not pooh-pooh your insistence that
this may be an indication of heart disease. If you think what you are
experiencing may be symptomatic of heart disease, keep notes, record
dates and times of your symptoms, and describe in detail what is happening to you physically. Taking your symptoms seriously is the first
step in getting your doctor to take them seriously, too. You know your
own body, and now you're aware of the high odds for a woman's having
heart disease and against her being taken seriously by the medical community regarding heart disease. You can turn the tables by insisting your
doctor pay attention to your complaint and that adequate tests be given,
and—if those test results are negative—by insisting on further testing
and a second opinion. You can remind your doctor that a negative test
result in a woman does not necessarily preclude the existence of heart
disease. And you can remind him or her that you have the facts to back
up your position. If your doctor won't listen, then find another one who
is well informed. Remember: Doctors are human. They make mistakes.
And they don't know everything.

Don't make the mistake of passively accepting a judgment you feel
justified in questioning. The aggressive heart patient gets the best treatment, and the first person you should trust as a patient is yourself.

The Catch-22 of Equality

Women are different from men. But somewhere along the way in the
battle for equality, equal began to be interpreted to mean "same as."

Nothing could be further from the truth, and nothing could be more damaging in terms of fair medical treatment for women.

Women develop differently from men. Women's hormones are different from men's. Women's hearts are different from men's hearts. Unfortunately, the only way in which women are treated differently for heart disease than men is in the wrong way. As of the writing of this book, a woman is still far more likely to have a heart attack catch her unawares and die from that heart attack than is a man. This medically sanctioned ignorance is no longer acceptable. We have a long way to go, but now that we know what questions to ask, the answers are sure to follow.

In matters of heart disease, it's clear that gender-neutral is a sexist position. Gender-specific must be the wave of the future. You can play a major role in ensuring that the future for women with heart disease is a positive one—driven by fairness, the rights of the patient, and a clear understanding that one heart is not just like another. Insist that when it comes to heart disease you have equal rights in terms of risk and demand individual and personal consideration when it comes to treatment. Remember, you don't just want to be in the front of the bus. You also want a seat.

THE AGING HEART AND HEART DISEASE

Your heart is the pump of pumps. In fact, the heart consists of two pumps and each pump contains two chambers, which are composed of muscles. Each upper chamber is called an atrium; each lower chamber, a ventricle. When these muscles contract, blood is pumped. Having been pumped out into the body on the left side of the heart via the arteries, blood returns from its journey through the body via the veins and enters the right side of the heart. From the right atrium (a low-pressure pump) to the right ventricle, the oxygen-poor blood is sent to the lungs, where it will give up carbon dioxide and receive oxygen, thereby preparing for its next journey through the body. The left atrium is the receiving chamber for the rejuvenated blood and pumps it gently into the left ventricle, which sends the blood into the aorta with a powerful, efficient pumping action. Weighing no more than a pound (and usually in women less than that), the heart does an extraordinary job. This single pound of muscle beats approximately once a second while the body is at rest and pumps 5 or more quarts of blood per minute, for a lifetime. The blood that the heart pumps provides oxygen and nutrients to all the cells of the body. The heart beats over one hundred thousand times a day, a virtual clock of life. Like a shark that must always be in motion, the heart can never stop pumping or damage will occur and a person may die. When the heart is healthy and working well, it is a biological miracle. When the heart has problems, the whole body has problems.

For the most part those problems begin to appear as you grow older and often worsen with age. While that is not the best of news, all these conditions can be easily monitored and screened for, and that gives you a head start in protecting yourself against heart disease. Nevertheless, remember, as a woman who is aging, albeit gracefully, you are at risk and you should become aware of the possible problems and warnings for coronary disease.

WHAT TO DO WHEN YOU THINK YOU ARE HAVING A HEART ATTACK

"The pain felt as if an elephant balancing on one leg had landed on my back."

Mickey Wapner (age 65)

ALTHOUGH THE HEART pumps blood to all parts of the body, it needs blood too. Providing it is the job of the coronary arteries. They supply blood, oxygen, and nutrients to the heart muscle. A heart attack happens when the flow of blood to the heart muscle ceases. There are two circumstances in which this situation occurs. Either a clot lodges in one of the coronary arteries or, in rarer cases, there is a prolonged spasm of a coronary artery itself. When the circulation of blood shuts down, at least part of the heart muscle is deprived of oxygen, which can be catastrophic. Without oxygen, the pumping mechanism can begin to fail. Then, the blood itself backs up, and this may cause you to drown, literally, in your own fluids. The heart will try

11

and try again, but as the heart's electrical activity begins to fail, so does the heart, causing it to beat erratically, flutter, fade, and finally stop.

While this is a terrible scenario, it is also an extreme case. All heart attacks do not have such bleak outcomes, and how you act in the minutes following your first suspicions of a heart attack will influence the outcome. The sooner you take action and the sooner you receive help, the better your chances of a complete recovery.

How to Recognize a Heart Attack

The most successful treatment for a heart attack is immediate and aggressive. Experts agree that the sooner treatment is administered, the better the chances that damage to the heart muscle will be minimal and recovery complete. If you hesitate in seeking help, you run the risk of causing irreparable damage to your heart. A heart attack is an emergency situation. Don't be afraid to use the word "emergency" and do call 911. The goal is to get to the hospital as soon as possible, without aggravating the situation and before permanent damage has been done.

While the same symptoms may indicate a heart attack in one situation and not in another, when the subject is heart attacks, it is always better to be safe than sorry. Here are the warning signs you should look for:

- **Pressure in the Chest.** This pressure has been described variously as a "squeezing" or "clenching" sensation, a "fullness," a "pain," a "huge weight," an "increasing weight." The pain may be differentiated from that associated with angina because it will last longer and will not be relieved by taking nitroglycerin tablets. In addition, while rest sometimes relieves the pain of angina (page 21), it will probably have no effect on the wrenching pain that is associated with a heart attack.
- **Radiating Pain.** The crushing weight or pain in the chest may radiate to the arms, shoulders, neck, or back and lower back. However, do not think that you must feel pain in your left arm to be having a heart attack. No two heart attacks are alike, nor are the early symptoms.

12

- **Nausea, Sweats, Shortness of Breath, Dizziness, Fainting.** Some people have all of these symptoms. Some have none.

If you have heart disease and your assumed angina does not respond to nitroglycerin, nor your assumed indigestion to antacids, *assume you are having a heart attack.*

When You Think You Are Having a Heart Attack

"At first I couldn't believe I was having a heart attack. But I remember when my husband had his and I remember how much he perspired. I was doing the same thing. So I called 911 and made it. That was eleven years ago."

Thelma Nishowaka (age 67)

IF YOU SUSPECT that you might be experiencing a heart attack, the first things to do are:

- Stop what you're doing.
- Sit down or lie down.
- If you have nitroglycerin tablets, take up to three at five-minute intervals and call 911 or your local emergency number.
- If you do not have nitroglycerin, call 911 or your local emergency number immediately.
- Do not drive yourself to the hospital, but if someone you know can drive you and you think you will get to the hospital faster, have that person drive you. Do not wait for an emergency vehicle if you have a faster means of transportation.
- At the hospital, *do not let anyone keep you waiting.* Repeat that this is an *emergency.* Repeat that you are having a heart attack.

If you are with someone who is having a heart attack:

- Don't let her or him convince you they are not sick.
- Administer nitroglycerin, if it is on hand.

13

- Call 911 or your local emergency number, or drive the person to the hospital yourself.
- While waiting for help, make the person as comfortable as possible.
- If you know CPR, be ready to use it if necessary until help arrives.

In general, you should remember not to minimize your symptoms or try to ignore them. Don't be passive. Don't doubt yourself. Don't equivocate. Don't say, "I'll be fine in a minute." *Don't waste time.* Remember, a heart attack can be treated. *Getting to the hospital quickly may save your life.*

At the Hospital

The present wisdom states that your best chance of full recovery from a heart attack depends on getting to the hospital within one to two hours after the first signs that you are in trouble. Once again, and at the risk of being repetitive, this is a situation in which the minutes matter. *Get to the hospital!*

At the hospital, emergency treatment is available to dissolve the clot that in most cases has caused your heart attack. There are two drugs available right now that help dissolve blood clots. and they are known in the trade as "clotbusters." At this time there is an ongoing debate regarding cost and efficacy. One, streptokinase, is older and may cause allergic reactions, but costs only $150 per dose. The other, alteplase, or t-PA, is a tissue-type plasminogen activator, and has been genetically engineered from a human protein. While it causes no allergic reaction, alteplase does costs at least ten times more than streptokinase. The debate about the two drugs revolves around the issue of whether alteplase is worth the additional cost and which drug is most effective in the long run.

Here's the real rub—for women, the debate is really about whether they are getting either drug at all.

So when you get to the hospital, remember, this time you want the drugs. Since you may not be able to speak for yourself, you will want to inform those closest to you to ask if clot-busting drugs will be used and, if so, what kind? While there is a debate at present as to whether these clotbusters are equally safe for women as for men, it is still true that many women do not even receive the drugs when they might do some good. The *Journal of the American Medical Association* stated in 1991 that these drug treatments are not given to men *or* women aggressively enough, and a more recent study stated that women receive these drugs half as often as men do.

If your heart attack is severe enough, you will spend the initial recovery period in the hospital's cardiac care unit, so that your situation may be monitored continually for further complications. The recovery process is covered in "A Patient's Guide," page 49.

ARE YOU AT RISK FOR HEART DISEASE?

*"The most encouraging feature of heart disease in women
is its tendency to develop gradually. By diagnosing and
treating the disease early, we have a good chance to stop
it before a heart attack ever strikes."*

Edward B. Diethrich, M.D., *Women and Heart Disease*

HEART DISEASE HAS one amazingly positive aspect, and that is that you can prevent and sometimes even reverse its course through diet and other lifestyle changes alone. Heart disease can be controlled most effectively if it is caught early. And heart disease *can* be caught early because there are indicators that are invariably accurate in predicting risk to the heart—these are hypertension (high blood pressure) and elevated triglyceride and cholesterol levels.

Armed with the knowledge that you may be at risk, you can lower your chances of having heart disease, and, if you have heart disease, lower your risk of a heart attack simply by making changes in how you live, what you eat, and how much exercise you get. When it comes to heart disease, you can make a very real difference in the outcome of your own treatment, but you have to know you have heart disease before you can help yourself. While being at risk for heart disease is not on anybody's wish list, there are risk factors over which you have some control and that, with guidance, you may have the power to change. Given the lack of accurate directions on the diagnostic road map for women's heart disease, it's absolutely essential to heed what accurate

15

signs there are. Make sure you know about hypertension and elevated triglyceride and cholesterol levels, because these are trusted indicators of risk.

Hypertension

Simply put, hypertension is high blood pressure. There is an inverse relationship between blood pressure and blood flow. When your blood pressure increases, the ease with which your blood flows decreases. There are basically two kinds of hypertension. *Essential hypertension,* which is the most common kind, refers to high blood pressure in which the cause cannot be readily determined. *Secondary hypertension* can be directly related to some other ailment, such as kidney problems.

If you have high blood pressure, you probably do not know it, as high blood pressure usually does not announce itself by exhibiting easily identifiable symptoms. Therefore, having your blood pressure checked routinely is essential. You must be especially diligent as you approach menopause, since a woman's risk for heart disease increases after menopause, when estrogen levels decrease dramatically.

These days, kits are available for taking your blood pressure at home. Some people suffer from what is colloquially referred to as "white coat syndrome"—that is, their blood pressure rises simply because of the stress of having a doctor take it. If that's the case, having a machine at home will be helpful in eliminating that added stress factor. You should ask your physician or health-care specialist to familiarize you with the technique so that you can monitor your blood pressure correctly. If your overall health warrants it, you should still have your pressure checked periodically by a professional.

If you find that you do have high blood pressure, you can turn a negative into a positive with some hard work. Treat your blood pressure as a warning sign and as an impetus to change your life. There is no question that high blood pressure, in both men and women, accelerates atherosclerosis, the hardening of the arteries resulting from the accumulated deposits of cholesterol along the arterial walls. The major cause of death in patients with hypertension is complications from such coronary artery disease. Hypertension is also a factor in certain types of strokes and in kidney disease. Take high blood pressure seriously and take immediate steps to lower it. This is one medical situation where you do have control.

Controlling High Blood Pressure

"At first I thought this would be impossible. I always ate everything I wanted. But then I paid the price. The interesting thing is that when I was forced to reevaluate what kinds of foods were good for me—I found all these wonderful tastes I didn't know existed."

Marie Fischer (age 47)

If you have been diagnosed with high blood pressure you will have to be vigilant in your daily life.

- Be careful about the amount of fat in your diet.
- Cut down on salt intake in your diet.
- Begin including exercise in your routine at least three times a week. (Even a half-hour walk several times a week is beneficial.)
- If you are obese or overweight, begin a weight loss program under the supervision of a doctor. (Don't beat yourself up to get overnight results. Weight goes on gradually and if you do it the right way, it comes off gradually too.)
- If these methods don't seem to be enough, your physician will want to discuss medication, though this is a last resort. (See "Drug Therapy," page 31.)

Triglycerides and Cholesterol

It's impossible to talk about heart disease without discussing the common indicators of risk—cholesterol and triglycerides. One of the most interesting differences between men and women when it comes to heart disease involves triglyceride levels. A triglyceride is a blood fat—a compound consisting of a fatty acid and glycerol and is the principal lipid in the blood. Lipids are a group of greasy compounds including fatty acids, waxes, and steroids, which are stored in the body to be burned as energy when needed. The obvious catch is that if they are not burned, they continue to collect as fatty residue. Men are considered to be at risk for coronary artery disease when their triglyceride level approaches 400, but women are at risk as soon as they show a level of 190—a startling difference. In fact, while it hasn't been proven that triglycerides act as an independent risk factor for men, they do for women, as well as for anyone with diabetes. Triglycerides are elevated immediately after eating fatty foods. They are also increased if you take birth control pills and other estrogen preparations, some diuretics, or beta blockers. While the definitive relationship between triglycerides and heart disease is a bit murky, if you have heart disease you will likely have a high triglyceride level. If you have a high triglyceride level, you will want to try to lower that level through diet, weight loss, or adjustment of your medication.

Cholesterol is a waxy, complex chemical found in all animal fats and present in the human body, particularly in bile, the brain, the blood, the adrenal glands, and nerve fiber sheaths. It is common knowledge that too much cholesterol is the scourge of a healthy heart. But some cholesterol is needed to maintain everyday body mechanics. It is necessary in the synthesis of certain hormones (notably cortisone and estrogen) and of vitamin D, and in the absorption of fatty acids. Therefore, the object here is not to eliminate cholesterol, but to *control* the cholesterol level.

On average, women have higher cholesterol counts than men. What is a dangerous cholesterol level in women is not such an easy thing to agree upon. While the Framingham Study showed that levels of 265 or higher increased the risk of heart disease in women, the Lipid Research Clinics reported that levels higher than 235 were too high.

This leads us to a discussion of those new witches in medical folklore, good cholesterol and bad cholesterol. HDL, high density lipoprotein, is the good cholesterol, which actually may help in preventing atherosclerosis. LDL, low density lipoprotein, is the bad cholesterol, which causes arterial plaque. High levels of LDL put both women and men at risk for heart disease.

The newest findings show that it is actually the ratio between these two that is the best predictor of the risk for heart disease. If you lower your overall cholesterol by lowering the HDL level, you've done nothing to improve the state of your heart's health since the LDL will be high in proportion to total cholesterol. Cholesterol levels are usually read as the ratio of HDL to the overall cholesterol level. Ideally, a woman will want to have an HDL level above 55 and an LDL level that is below 130.

Medical Risk Factors

"There's nothing like a good gene pool."

"Pick your parents wisely."

Medical folk sayings

I F YOU HAVE a family history of heart disease, you are at risk for heart disease and should take precautions. If your father had a heart attack before the age of fifty-six or if your mother had one before the age of sixty, you are considered at risk for coronary artery disease (CAD). If you have had more than five pregnancies, you are also considered at risk.

If you are a diabetic or if you have kidney disease, you are probably already aware that you are at risk and monitoring the situation with your doctor. If you are not, you should be. The Framingham Study showed that women who were diabetics had twice the risk of heart disease of nondiabetic women. And premenopausal diabetic women do not enjoy the protection from heart disease that is generally assumed in other premenopausal women.

Other medical risks include:

- *Proteinuria* (protein in the urine), which can be the result of damage to the kidneys, most commonly from hypertension.
- *An enlarged heart*, usually attributable to hypertension or obesity. An enlarged heart occurs when the left ventricle (which pumps blood from the heart to the rest of the body) is overworked and the heart wall thickens.
- *Increased fibrinogen levels*. Fibrinogen is produced by the body to aid in blood clotting after an injury. Interestingly, smokers tend to have higher fibrinogen levels than nonsmokers.

19

- A *high hematocrit level.* The hematocrit level is the percentage of blood volume attributable to red blood cells. A high hematocrit level is a sign that the blood is being deprived of oxygen and may be a warning sign of atherosclerosis or narrowing of the arteries.

Physical Risk Factors

The general rule is that the older you are, the higher your risk of heart disease. For women this risk is coupled with the increased risk after the climacteric or menopause. No matter what her age, a woman is at higher risk for heart disease once she ceases to menstruate.

And while once considered an old wives' tale, it has now been proven that body build can be an indicator of an increased risk of heart disease. If you tend to put on weight in the upper body or in the stomach or midsection, you are at greater risk than a woman who puts on weight in the hips. Therefore, you may want to discuss body type during your next visit to your physician.

Lifestyle Risk Factors

"I watched my mother smoke her way to an early death and I was not about to let that happen to me. For me cigarettes have never been a sign of sex appeal. They have symbolized an agonizingly torturous and premature ending to life."

Rue McCarthy (age 43)

HEART DISEASE IS one of the few diseases that we know is directly linked to diet and lifestyle.

The worst thing for your heart is cigarettes. A recent study from Oxford University showed that smokers in their thirties and forties suffer five times as many heart attacks as nonsmokers. The risk of heart attacks for young adult smokers is about double what was previously believed. This means that every year smoking causes 40,000 heart attacks among Americans who are still under fifty. Furthermore, it triples the risk in a fifty-year-old.

In addition, if you eat a high-fat diet and lead a sedentary lifestyle, you are just asking for trouble. It is recommended that Americans stick to a diet that is no more than 30 percent in fat. That comes out to about 50 grams of fat per day for women. But I think that is still too high. I believe you should aim to keep your total daily fat intake around 20 to 30 grams. Some experts, like Dr. Dean Ornish, believe even that is still too high and suggest a person should aim for a completely nonfat diet, knowing that some fat will creep into the diet anyway.

If you have a hard time keeping track of fat, carry a deck of cards with you. With every gram of fat you eat, deal yourself a card. Aim for dealing yourself no more than thirty cards a day—all the time remembering that you have only fifty-two cards in that deck. It won't take long for you to see how easy it is to eat fat without realizing it. That deck of cards can come in handy when it comes to the amount of red meat you should be eating too. The size of a deck of cards equals about three ounces of meat. This is your serving size and you should eat such a portion of red meat only once a week. (See "Prevention" on page 43 for a more detailed explanation.)

ANGINA

"Anyone who has anginalike symptoms should be evaluated by her doctor."

Marianne Legato, M.D., *The Female Heart*

ANGINA, OR ANGINA PECTORIS, is chest pain originating from the heart, a condition that occurs when the heart is literally not getting enough oxygen. The word "angina" is derived from the Greek *anchein*, meaning "to strangle." It's apt and terrifying. Angina is an indicator of coronary artery disease (CAD) and is a symptom that needs to be monitored very closely. And while angina pectoris is associated with heart disease, it can exist without arterial blockage.

The incidence of angina in women is said to be higher than that in men, and in 56 percent of cases of women with CAD, angina is the first symptom. (Don't assume, however, that if you don't have angina, you don't have heart disease. Many women suffer from CAD and have heart attacks without ever experiencing angina.) During an angina attack, the heart is not getting enough oxygen. But as the angina attack subsides, in most cases the heart will again receive as much oxygen as it needs. Whereas a heart attack damages parts of the heart muscle permanently, once an attack of angina passes, blood is restored to the area of the attack and the heart cells begin to function normally again. The entire attack of angina may take less than a minute. Remember that angina is a symptom, an indicator used by a doctor in the process of making a diagnosis. The diagnosis is determined by considering many factors—only one of which is the existence of angina.

If the notion of having angina makes you terrified that a heart attack will follow immediately, don't panic. In 80 percent of all angina cases involving women, a heart attack does not develop after a specific attack of angina. Angina is a warning sign of CAD, but an attack of angina does not mean that a heart attack is beginning.

As you might have expected by now, nothing about heart disease and women is easy, least of all diagnosing angina and using it as a bellwether for indicating a potential heart attack in the future. In fact, angina is often disguised and even indiscernible in women. Furthermore—and this will not be news to you—women tend to experience angina differently than men. Once again, there has been a dearth of research on women and angina. In addition, there is the unfortunate complication that women tend to be subject to innocuous and minor chest pains separate and apart from what most doctors call significant chest pain (chest pain that may indicate CAD or an impending heart attack). All this leads to confusion and at least two negative scenarios:

1. A woman who is having real, but insignificant, chest pain unwittingly compounds the stereotype of a woman as overreacting or being hysterical.
2. A woman who is suffering from angina slips through the system, either because she is not describing her symptoms in a way that is readily discernible to her physician, or because she is in the unfortunate situation of telling her symptoms to a doctor who assumes she is an "hysterical" woman.

While this is depressing news, don't let it incapacitate you. In the situation of women and heart disease, knowledge is power. The more you know, the more you can ensure that you will receive fair, accurate, and adequate treatment.

More commonly in men than in women, angina is noticeable as a dull pain directly beneath the breastbone. It may also be experienced as a band of pain across the chest. But women experience angina in at least three other ways:

1. Some women perceive their angina almost as if they were inhaling ice-cold air (as opposed to noticing a shortness of breath).
2. Angina also may be experienced as back pain.
3. Sometimes the pain may travel down the right arm (as opposed to the more common situation in which pain is experienced in the left arm).

In rare cases, even certain forms of intermittent jaw pain may be indicators of angina in women. If any of these situations sound familiar, see your doctor.

Variant Angina

> *"I wasn't sure what was happening. I had a heaviness in my chest but it didn't really radiate anywhere. At first I didn't think it was a heart attack, because I thought that pain was supposed to go down one arm or another. But when it didn't go away, I got worried and called the doctor."*
>
> Susan Williamson (age 51)

THERE IS A TYPE of angina, called variant or Prinzmetal's angina, that affects women primarily and that has now been recognized as different from what we will call ordinary angina. One difference between them is that variant angina is more likely to occur while you are at rest, whereas the ordinary angina caused by atherosclerosis is usually brought on by exertion. While heart disease in women may be a silent, undiagnosed killer, the opposite is also true—angina in women may not be a sure signal of potentially lethal heart disease. Further research is currently under way on variant angina and its impact on female heart disease.

What You Can Do About Angina

The medical situation regarding angina could be said to be a paradigm for the situation that faces a woman with heart disease. Angina is a real condition and it can indicate heart disease; however, for women, there are a great deal of "ifs," "ands," and "buts" surrounding angina, its diagnosis, and what it may indicate regarding a patient's future.

If You Are Diagnosed with Angina

- Keep nitroglycerin tablets nearby at all times—at home *and* whenever you go out.
- Have your blood pressure and cholesterol levels checked. While angina may not be an absolute predictor for heart attack risk, blood pressure and cholesterol levels are dependable indicators.
- Review your diet. If you are overweight, lose weight. If your cholesterol or blood pressure is elevated, lower the fat content of your diet, increase your intake of fiber and complex carbohydrates, and decrease your intake of red meats.
- If you have not done so already, make exercise a part of your life.
- If you smoke, give it up. If you feel that you can't, get help. Everybody needs help sometimes, and there's nothing wrong with needing help in tackling an addiction as powerful as nicotine. Start now.

DIAGNOSING HEART DISEASE

*"A male dominance in medicine has assured a male per-
spective in every facet of the profession, from medical
school classes to clinical practices and the allocation of
research funds."*

Edward B. Diethrich, M.D., Women and Heart Disease

IF YOU HAVE a high ratio of LDL cholesterol to HDL cholesterol or
if your blood pressure is consistently elevated, your doctor will probably recommend further testing to see if you have heart disease and
if there has been damage to your heart. Although we already know that
the present diagnostic tests are not always accurate for women, they are
better than the alternative, which is not being tested and allowing heart
disease to progress to the point where you may end up in need of emergency treatment.

The State-of-the-Art Tests

In men with indications such as elevated blood pressure or cholesterol
levels, an electrocardiogram (EKG) may become part of a routine
checkup. Since we know that it is less likely for a doctor to suspect
heart disease in a woman than in a man, discuss an EKG and other
possible testing with your doctor if you are experiencing symptoms that
may indicate heart disease.

Electrocardiogram and the Holter Monitor

The EKG is usually part of any comprehensive diagnostic procedure
and in most cases is the first test given to someone who complains of
chest pains or irregular heart rhythms (see "Arrhythmias," page 41).
Given the lack of accuracy of the EKG, it is usually not the only test.
It's a starting point along with routine blood and urine tests. The EKG
is noninvasive and causes no pain. A chest X ray is given in conjunction
with an EKG to screen for lung tumors and for congestion that may be
caused by heart disease.

The electrocardiogram measures the heart's electrical activity at rest. After a jellylike substance is applied to your arms, legs, and chest, electrodes are placed on these areas. Because activity is measured only while the electrodes are strapped to the patient, an EKG will register damage to the heart in only about 50 percent of cases where damage has occurred. A patient may return home and experience symptoms while going about her daily routine. In such a case, the holter monitor may be recommended.

The holter monitor is a portable EKG meant to measure the heart's activity when the patient is pursuing a normal routine, usually for twenty-four hours. The holter monitor is noninvasive and in no way uncomfortable.

Echocardiogram

The echocardiogram is an ultrasound technique that provides a three-dimensional picture of the heart using sound waves. Because the picture of the heart is three-dimensional, the doctor may observe the actual thickness of the heart, how the pump itself contracts, whether the chambers of the heart can fill with blood, and also whether there are any blood clots. It will also tell the doctor whether the valves have been damaged by infection and whether other valve disorders exist. Clearly, the echocardiogram provides a great deal more information than the EKG.

Echocardiography is usually performed when you are at rest. Again, it is a noninvasive test that will cause you no pain or discomfort. Echocardiography can be combined with moderate exercise if necessary. If you are disabled and cannot exercise, a harmless drug may be given to dilate the arteries to achieve the same effect as exercise. The drugs usually used are dipyridamole (Persantine) or adenosine (Adenocard).

Exercise Stress Test

The exercise stress tests add increasingly difficult exercise to the EKG equation. Whereas the electro- and echocardiograms examine the heart at rest, the exercise stress tests allows a doctor to observe what happens to the heart once stress in the form of exercise is placed upon it. Sometimes called a gaited exercise test, the test monitors the heart's electrical and rhythmic reactions as the demands of exercise on the heart are gradually increased. In a gaited stress test, your heart rate is measured before, during, and after a prolonged period of exercise. So, among other things, this test takes time.

During your stress test you will walk on a treadmill. As the speed of the belt increases, so will your speed. Then, the machine will begin to tilt uphill, forcing you to maintain your pace on a steeper and steeper incline. The EKG will be monitoring your heart at all times. If you develop shortness of breath or chest pain or any other sign of discomfort, the test will be stopped. So don't worry: it won't hurt and you won't be injured. And it might help by giving you and your doctor valuable information.

A caution about results: the stress test has limitations, especially for women. On the other hand, it is inexpensive and noninvasive and thus worth the effort in most cases for male and female patients. For women, if your stress test says you don't have coronary heart disease, you are probably in the clear and the relatively insignificant cost of the test has been worth it (by contrast, 40 percent of the negative results for men end up to be misleading).

However, for women, it's a *positive* stress test that has limitations. If a man tests positive during a stress test—that is, the results indicate some kind of heart disease—the result is more than 90 percent reliable. But for women there are at least four reasons a positive result can be unreliable:

1. Some women are so unaccustomed to exercise that they cannot perform the test. This is particularly true for older women who may perform only low-stress exercise and may feel no cultural imperative (the way a macho counterpart might) to "tough it out."
2. Chest pain in women can sometimes be unrelated to heart disease. This kind of unidentified pain may assert itself during such a test.
3. When a woman has high blood pressure or an enlarged left ventricle, which is common in older women, interpreting an EKG is more difficult.
4. There is a predilection among women for cardiac idiosyncrasies, including mitral valve prolapse (page 41), which may create a false response.

Thallium Exercise Stress Test

A thallium exercise stress test takes the exercise stress test one step further, adding a computerized study that reveals not only how the coronary arteries are meeting the heart's oxygen demand but also the degree of oxygen deprivation. The difference in procedure is simple. Toward the end of the stress test, you receive an intravenous injection of radioactive thallium. Once the thallium is in the bloodstream, a scanner tracks the thallium, indicating where and how well the blood has traveled. For disabled patients, drugs such as adenosine or Persantine may be used to dilate the coronary arteries, mimicking the effect of exercise. The addition of minimal doses of vasodilators is promising for those older women who cannot exercise strenuously enough for a stress test.

While more reliable than an ordinary stress test, a thallium scan is but still not perfect (see "The X Variable in Syndrome X," page 42). The test sometimes indicates disease is present when it is not. Sometimes this may happen because the arteries fail to dilate. It may also occur in patients with diabetes or significantly elevated blood pressure. In all these cases, the reasons for the occurrence are not clearly understood. The breast can occlude the picture in women, since it comes between the camera and the heart. In rarer circumstances, the test may fail to detect existing disease. For example, if the disease is so advanced that all areas of the heart are being deprived of blood in relatively the same way, the disease may not be visible.

A thallium scan, however, is a reasonably reliable diagnostic tool; in fact, it is used not only in diagnosing heart disease, but in planning the treatment as well. A thallium scan may, for example, make clear which area of the heart has been damaged and help to indicate whether a patient is a good candidate for bypass surgery.

Cardiac Catheterization and Angiography

Cardiac angiography is often referred to as cardiac catheterization, though this is not quite accurate. Essentially, cardiac catheterization is the first step of the process. In cardiac angiography, the heart and its arteries are actually visualized through the use of a constant X-ray beam, using an instrument called a fluoroscope. The image is projected on a monitor for the doctor to study.

The test is performed in a hospital under local anesthesia. The process begins with the insertion of a plastic tube (called a catheter) into the heart, via a blood vessel in the arm or thigh. The dye that the X ray will follow is injected into the catheter. As the dye mixes with blood it outlines the blood vessels of the heart.

This examination is the ultimate diagnostic test when it comes to heart disease. While all the other tests may help in determining the existence of heart disease, only cardiac angiography is conclusive. The test must be done before bypass surgery or angioplasty, but it is also advisable for any heart disease patient whose condition worsens appreciably. This invasive procedure is indicated only if one or more non-invasive tests suggest damage to the heart or if questionable data has been obtained.

Today cardiac catheterization is usually done on an outpatient basis. Only if there is a rare complication, like bleeding at the catheterization site or kidney problems from the dye, would a person be expected to stay overnight in the hospital. Although it might be considered something of an ordeal, at present it is the state-of-the-art test for diagnosing heart disease.

The Angiogram Issue

"As if to confirm the general view that women's chest pain is psychosomatic, women who are eventually given diagnostic tests are more likely than men to have arteries that look normal."

Robin Marantz Henig, medical writer,
in *The New York Times Magazine*

ONE OF THE ASPECTS of heart disease in women that is most mysterious—indeed, diabolical—is that an angiogram may fail to diagnose heart disease even when disease is present. You might say heart disease in women can outwit the greatest lie detector test the medical profession has at its disposal.

Why is it that women suffering from heart disease may still excel on the gold standard of tests, the angiogram? The answer is that we just don't know enough at this time about women and heart disease to ascertain if angiogram is the best method of detecting advanced heart disease in a female patient.

Making the Tests Work for You

A woman who survives a heart attack is more likely than a man to suffer from chronic, painful complications and a suffocating death. All the more reason for you to discover early if you are at risk for heart disease and then do something about it before the situation becomes critical.

Female heart patients are, on average, about a decade older than male heart patients. They also suffer more frequently from diabetes and hypertension, because these are conditions that increase in numbers with age. Thus, the prognosis for the female heart patient is influenced by the more advanced state of the disease and the deterioration of the patient. The attack itself is often worse, and the time of recovery can be much longer. Though this is dire, the plus side is that when female heart disease is detected early, there is a better chance of avoiding a heart attack altogether with behavior modification and treatment. It's just that *female heart disease is less likely to be detected early in the game.* Get help early. See your doctor. Discuss the relevant tests and ask to be screened if you think you are at risk. Treat your condition early. In heart disease, how you approach the situation can make all the difference.

HOW TO PREVENT A HEART ATTACK IF YOU ARE AT RISK

"Watching my mother die of heart disease when I was a teenager left an emotional imprint on my heart. I became aware of my own physical vulnerability as a woman. Vivid memories of her struggle to live serve as my urgent self-reminder to take care of myself—especially as I approach the age she was when she died."

Cynthia Riley (age 45)

MEDICATION, ANGIOPLASTY, the insertion of a pacemaker, bypass surgery, and in extreme cases heart transplantation are all in the doctor's arsenal when it comes to treating advanced heart disease. The sooner early diagnosis and prevention become the watchwords for women, the less such measures will be necessary. But until that time, it is important to understand the options.

Drug Therapy for Heart Disease

If improving your diet and exercise regimen and lowering your stress level have not made the difference in controlling your heart disease, your doctor's next line of defense will probably involve drug therapy to control your blood pressure and/or angina.

Nitrates or Nitroglycerin

Nitroglycerin, an old soldier in the treatment of heart disease, is the generic name for all the nitrates used to treat heart disease, including tablets, sprays, and ointments. To this day, nitroglycerin is one of the best ways to relieve cardiac pain and protect the heart muscle in a patient with heart disease. Nitrates work by relaxing the blood vessels, thereby increasing blood flow and oxygen to the heart muscle. Today not only can nitroglycerin be taken in time-release tablets or as a mouth

31

spray, but it can also be administered as a skin patch and in intensive care by intravenous drip.

Calcium Channel Blockers

Like nitrates, calcium channel blockers treat angina by relaxing the blood vessels. These drugs, specifically diltiazem (Cardizem), nifedipine (Procardia), and verapamil hydrochloride (Isoptin), also slow the heart rate and ease the work of the heart in other ways. Because they lower blood pressure as well, they are often prescribed specifically for that purpose. They may also slow rapid heart rhythms, such as in the case of Prinzmetal's angina. Patients tolerate these drugs reasonably well, though side effects may include constipation, headaches, and sometimes dizziness.

Beta Blockers

Beta blockers have many of the same effects that calcium channel blockers have, but they work differently and, thus, one can't be substituted for another. Common beta blockers are tartrate (Lopressor), nadolol (Corgard), and propranolol (Inderal).

Though usually beneficial to patients after a heart attack, beta blockers have been found in some cases to be poorly tolerated by women; the reasons for this are not yet clear. They have also been found to have poor results in controlling blood pressure and angina in African Americans. If you are trying to lose weight and are taking beta blockers, you may be frustrated in your efforts because these drugs slow the metabolism, inhibiting you from burning calories. Beta blockers have also been found to aggravate asthma and variant angina and they are dangerous to insulin-dependent diabetics.

Antiarrhythmics and Digitalis

Antiarrhythmics, which work to regulate the heartbeat by altering the patterns of electrical conductivity in the heart, are used to treat many arrhythmias. Antiarrhythmics include procainamide hydrochloride (Procan) and disopyramide phosphate (Norpace). Side effects may include dizziness, rash, insomnia, tremor, fatigue, loss of appetite, and indigestion. While digitalis (Lanoxin) is not classified as an antiarrhythmic, it is also used to treat arrhythmias. It is sometimes used to treat congestive heart failure as well, because it strengthens the heart's pumping action. Side effects include visual disturbances, loss of appetite, and nausea. Digitalis also can cause the heart to skip beats or cause the heartbeat to slow too much.

ACE Inhibitors and Other Drug Options

Ramipril (Altace), captopril (Capoten), and lisinopril (Prinivil) have recently provided other options for treating high blood pressure and heart failure. These drugs, called ACE inhibitors, work by preventing certain enzyme changes that would constrict the blood vessels. They also encourage fluid and sodium retention. This dual process allows a sluggish heart to pump blood more easily. ACE inhibitors cause mild side effects, including a dry cough, loss of taste and appetite, fluid retention, rash, weakness, headache, and palpitations.

Anticoagulants provide options in cases where there is a tendency for blood to clot to extreme. They decrease the stickiness of platelets and are often referred to as blood thinners. Diuretics are medications that work to flush excess fluid from the body via the kidneys. Other drugs may also be used to improve circulation.

Questions to Ask Your Doctor About Drug Therapy

"I can't tell you how many times I've left the doctor's office without having asked a few important questions. Now I always have a pad of paper and a pen in my purse and I don't miss as much."

Nancy Quentintino (age 39)

IF YOUR DOCTOR has prescribed medication for you, be sure you understand what you're taking and why. Ask questions—including what to expect. Don't be embarrassed to take notes while the doctor is talking. You'll think of more questions than these after you leave the doctor's office—so keep a pad of paper with you and jot down your questions as you think of them. Here are some questions you might ask:

- What is the name of the drug, and is there a generic preparation available that might save money?
- What is the medication supposed to do?
- What is the dosage?
- What are the side effects, physical and psychological?
- Should I take the drug with food or on an empty stomach? In the morning or evening?
- Should I alter my diet to aid in the efficiency of the drug and minimize the side effects?
- How will it effect my exercise regimen?
- Will this medication interact with any other medications I'm taking?

Many people find it helpful to write out a list of questions beforehand. If you experience side effects while taking the medication, you may also find it useful to take notes. One final caution: the most important thing that can be said about drug therapy is that if you are on a prescribed medication for a heart condition, *do not stop taking that medication without consulting your physician.*

Surgical Treatments

"I knew I was having a heart attack. My daughter drove me to the hospital and I was seen within the hour. The doctors performed an angiogram and told me that two vessels were blocked. They performed balloon angioplasty. I'm convinced the timing saved my life."

Mary Lou Witterstein (age 61)

The Angioplasty Alternative

Angioplasty is a surgical procedure in which a catheter with a balloon attached is threaded into a coronary artery and used to open up the obstruction in that artery, restoring blood flow through the blocked vessel. (In effect, this is the Roto-rooter procedure.)

34

A viable candidate for angioplasty is the patient whose angina does not respond to medication and who ideally has only one blocked artery. The benefit of angioplasty is that it is often possible to clear the blockage without the risk and complications of bypass surgery. The shortcomings of angioplasty for men and women are that often the plaque lies beyond the reach of the catheter and in some cases, even if accessible, the plaque is so hardened that the balloon is no match for such calcification. Ten percent of cases fail immediately—that is, the balloon effect is lost. Four percent of the remaining 90 percent fail within days, another third within a year.

In fact, women are less likely to be given the alternative of angioplasty instead of the more invasive open heart surgery; this is because it's only upon arriving in the emergency room after a massive heart attack, that many women *discover* they have heart disease, and by then angioplasty is usually no longer a viable choice. Furthermore, balloon angioplasty is not as effective for patients over the age of sixty-five, which may be a contributing factor in its lack of effectiveness for female patients (who are usually older). That a women's arteries are usually narrower when healthy also may have something to do with the lack of success of angioplasty in women.

At present, angioplasty is not a perfect procedure for men or women. While it may improve the quality of life, it is not clear if it increases life expectancy. It is often too late for the technique to do much good on a highly damaged artery, and there is also a good chance that plaque will recur. New techniques are being perfected to reduce the recurrence of plaque after balloon angioplasty.

There is a long way to go before angioplasty is a viable alternative for more than a few women. Since women often seem to "pass" the angiogram, the present state-of-the-art test, angioplasty is often not even a suggested alternative during the time frame when it might be successful. The use of angioplasty in treating the female heart patient will be made effective only following further research and improved diagnostic techniques for heart disease in women.

Coronary Bypass Surgery

A coronary bypass involves the grafting of a vein that is removed from another part of the body (usually the leg) to the artery in the heart that needs help. It is advised when angioplasty has been ruled out and angina is severely limiting the quality of life of the patient, or in an emergency situation after a heart attack.

More than 70 percent of coronary bypass operations are performed on men. Primarily, this occurs because women are usually older than men when the surgery is considered, and the surgery is more successful on younger patients. But a recent study at Cedars Sinai Medical Center in Los Angeles indicates that it may also be the case that doctors wait too long before referring their female patients for the surgery. The prognosis for bypass surgery is generally worse for women than for men, presumably because of the age difference and health of the patient at the time of the procedure.

Open heart surgery, such as bypass surgery, is one of the most complex of surgical procedures—yet today it is quite common. It requires cutting through the sternum and opening the chest wall. The healing process can be arduous and usually takes several months to a year. And while there is a tendency to say, "If he hadn't had bypass surgery, he'd be dead by now," this is not necessarily true. (The pronoun is specific, since more women die on the operating table than men, because the procedure is more often an emergency procedure for women than for men, and the average female patient is about a decade older.) It is important to remember that angina is not a death sentence, and bypass surgery is not a cure. Even though bypass surgery may relieve symptoms, it may not be worth the risk the surgery entails, and it is worth little or nothing without attendant lifestyle changes. The heart depends on how you treat it. If you go back to your cigarette smoking, high-fat, high-stress, low-exercise ways after bypass surgery, the plaque will return. Despite the complications and the risk of the surgery, however, in conjunction with the proper postsurgery diet and exercise regimen, bypasses have improved the quality of life for many heart patients.

Pacemakers and Miniature Defibrillators

Pacemakers were originally developed in the late 1950s with the purpose of sustaining the beat of a sluggish heart. Pacemakers have allowed at least two million people who would otherwise be disabled to pursue normal lives. Pacemakers are implanted just beneath the chest skin during a relatively minor surgical procedure, which requires only local anesthesia. When the battery wears down, the unit is changed in another minor surgical procedure.

While pacemakers monitor and improve a sluggish heart rate, there are other devices, called miniature defibrillators, to control a racing heartbeat. Because they must be installed directly on the heart, they consequently require open heart surgery. Although this means there is a risk involved and the recovery process is slower, the success rate for miniature defibrillators has been so great for patients suffering from conditions such as ventricular tachycardia or ventricular fibrillation that the procedure is often recommended.

Heart Transplants

Heart transplants are recommended only when a patient suffers irreversible heart failure or has what is termed end-stage heart disease. Because of a lack of organ donors, many patients die before they can undergo this surgery of last resort. Rejection of the new heart is also a problem, one that tends to occur more with women than with men. However, 80 to 90 percent of recipients live at least one year after a transplant and 60 to 80 percent live for five years or more, with good quality of life. Thus, as medical research continues to develop the technology to eliminate rejection, heart transplants offer more and more hope for those with end-stage heart disease.

PREPARING FOR SURGERY

Any kind of surgery is stressful—physically, emotionally, and mentally. While you can't ever be totally prepared for the unknown, the more you know about the surgery you're having beforehand, the better the chances are that you will feel at least some sense of control as you proceed with and recover from surgery.

If your doctor plans to do the surgery in the office or a surgical clinic, make sure he or she has privileges at the local hospital. In case something goes wrong, you want your doctor to be able to admit you to the hospital as a backup.

If you decide that surgery is necessary, you will want to be in the best physical shape possible before you have the surgery. You can make a difference in the success and rapidity of your recovery from surgery by preparing yourself beforehand. Just as you would prepare yourself physically and remember to pack the right supplies if you were going to run a marathon or climb a mountain, you should consider yourself in training as soon as your date for surgery has been set. Use the days or weeks before your surgery to improve your physical health as much as possible. Here are some tips:

- In consultation with your doctor, increase the dosage of vitamins that you take, especially C, A, and B vitamins to help your body cope with surgery and recovery. Keep taking extra vitamins during your recovery period.
- If you smoke, try to quit; if you can't, at least cut down on your smoking before surgery to give your lungs the opportunity to increase their intake of oxygen.
- Give up alcohol and other drugs. Do this in consultation with your doctor. If you have trouble doing so, tell your doctor.
- Be sure to tell your doctor if you take aspirin or ibuprofen regularly. These can affect the ability to clot blood. Your doctor may request that you stop taking these medicines a few days before surgery.
- If you take birth control pills, you should tell your doctor, if he or she doesn't already know.

Before your surgery, you will also want to make peace with your fears about the procedure you are about to have and plan your hospital stay in order that you maintain as much control of the situation as possible. Here's some advice to help you do this:

- Make sure your surgeon is experienced and, if possible, review the surgeon's record with another doctor you trust.
- Discuss the procedure with your surgeon and ask the following questions:
    — If I didn't have this surgery, would I survive and what would my quality of life be?
    — How long will the surgery take?
    — What are the steps of the procedure?
    — What complications should I be prepared for?
    — Will I need a blood transfusion?
    — How much pain will there be?
    — How long will my recovery take?
    — Will there be changes in my quality of life?

- If you may need a blood transfusion, ask your doctor if it is possible for you to donate your own blood for this purpose to minimize the risk of contaminated blood.
- Ask who the anesthesiologist will be and make sure he or she is board-certified.
- Discuss the procedure with others who have had the same surgery.
- Call the hospital and ask about the choices you will have in meals—if possible, choose your meals ahead of time.
- When you go to the hospital bring things from home that will make your stay more pleasant—like your own pillow. (Between you and me—there's nothing worse than a hospital pillow!) Bring a moisturizing spray for your face—hospital air tends to be extremely dry. Bring bottled water to drink or have a friend bring it for you. Bring a toothbrush, toothpaste, and hairbrush. Bring a moisturizer. Bring your own slippers and nightgown. Bring magazines and books. Bring healthy snacks—have a friend bring fresh fruit. If you are going to be there more than one night, bring a dry shampoo.

continued

- Plan for your recovery period before surgery, include a physical therapy program, if necessary, and massage. If you have surgery as an outpatient, plan to have someone take you home and stay with you at least for a day. Plan your recovery diet ahead of time, too. Freeze healthy meals and make sure your refrigerator is well stocked.
- Don't be alone for long periods of time in the first days after your surgery. Surgery is often accompanied by a letdown or period of depression afterward. Loving friends and family will make this time much easier. However, don't feel obliged to entertain well-intentioned visitors. Use the days following surgery to recuperate. Having too many people around can wear you out.

MITRAL VALVE PROLAPSE AND OTHER HEART CONDITIONS

"I've lived with a bad heart valve ever since I was a kid. It's never really held me back. I just take care of myself and take prophylactic antibiotics every time I go to the dentist."

Joanne Warner (age 34)

SOME HEART CONDITIONS are congenital, some are not. Mitral valve prolapse (MVP), for example, is a congenital condition, whereas many arrhythmias (erratic beating of the heart) may result from a heart attack or from valve damage.

About 6 to 8 babies out of every 1,000 born alive are born with some kind of heart disease. More of these babies are female than male. (Congenital heart disease is defined as a defect that occurs during the development of the heart in utero.) But many of these conditions never manifest themselves or cause only minor discomfort throughout a lifetime.

Mitral Valve Prolapse

Mitral valve prolapse is the most common of all heart defects, and twice as many women as men are born with MVP. Many women with MVP are thin and have low blood pressure and a history of occasional palpitations; however, most women with MVP lead an absolutely normal life.

If symptoms do occur, it's usually when women are in their forties. These symptoms are usually chest pain, shortness of breath, and palpitations. MVP can generally be managed by drug therapy. Patients with MVP do, however, run a greater risk of developing bacterial endocarditis, a dangerous infection of the heart lining (in the case of MVP, misshapen mitral valve leaflets can also be infected). Because of the risk of infection, you will need to take prophylactic antibiotics whenever you see a dentist or have any kind of surgical procedure. These antibiotics prevent bacteria that get into your bloodstream (even from teeth cleaning) from collecting in the heart and causing an infection. Infections like this are rare (they occur in less than 2 percent of people with MVP), and other than this slight risk, MVP is not life threatening.

Other Valve Disorders

Other valve disorders, which usually affect the aortic valve, involve calcium deposits on the valves; these occur with age and cause the valves to stiffen and not open fully. Rheumatic fever (the lingering complication of strep throat) is the most common cause of valve disease. Symptoms include mild chest pain and shortness of breath or dizziness with exertion. Abnormal valves of any kind make patients prone to endocarditis.

Arrhythmias

An elaborate electrical system controls how the heart beats. When the electrical system becomes impaired the heartbeat is erratic, resulting in an arrhythmia. A heart attack, valve disease, or excessive hormone production can be responsible for this. Sometimes this condition occurs in tandem with a congenital defect, and sometimes there is no apparent reason for the abnormality. As with most heart conditions, arrhythmias can be either imperceptible or life threatening. The good news is that arrhythmias can be controlled for years through drug therapy or, if medications fail, through the insertion of a pacemaker or miniature defibrillator.

The X Variable in Syndrome X

". . . Syndrome X is one of the most frustrating of all
heart conditions."

Edward B. Diethrich, M.D., *Women and Heart Disease*

SYNDROME X, also known as microvascular angina, has confounded doctors and defied diagnosis until recently. In this condition, the tiniest, immeasurable capillaries feeding the heart fail to dilate, thus depriving the heart of oxygen. It is the microscopic nature of these capillaries that defies detection. Since these capillaries work to feed oxygen to only a tiny portion of the heart muscle, syndrome X may be painful and disabling, but it is seldom dangerous and will not cause a heart attack or death.

Syndrome X is more prevalent among women than among men. You might say that syndrome X is the perfect symbol for the frustration women feel when searching for validation of a heart condition from a doctor who just says no. In fact, syndrome X—a documented form of heart disease—often is the condition that leaves you on the psychiatrist's couch, simply because your physician can't put a name to your condition. Nevertheless, syndrome X is also emblematic of the progress that has been made in differentiating female heart disease from the male counterpart.

In the past, when the problem was syndrome X, the scenario might go like this: A patient would complain of symptoms of angina and all early tests given would read positive for heart disease. Catheterization and angiogram would be advised. The arteries would look clear and no spasms would occur even with provocation. The conclusion would be that there was no heart disease, even though the thallium scan had been suspicious. Perhaps, the doctor might conclude, the suspicious thallium scan results stemmed from interfering breast tissue, or else ulcers, gallstones, or other conditions that could mimic the symptoms of angina were present.

But all this is changing. Via a new blood test during cardiac catheterization, the oxygen content of the blood can be measured and those areas of the heart that are not receiving enough oxygen can be identified. Thus, confirmation of syndrome X is possible, even though the capillaries are too tiny to be seen.

Although the guidelines for successful treatment have yet to be delineated regarding syndrome X, the very fact that a diagnosis for this condition is now possible is progress. At least a woman doesn't have to suffer without knowing why or with the added burden of having someone tell her nothing is wrong when she *knows* something is definitely wrong.

PREVENTION

"An ounce of prevention is worth a pound of cure."

Benjamin Franklin

Diet, Exercise, and the Healthy Heart

While the way you live might have helped you get into trouble with your heart in the first place, the way you live from now on may help you make amends. Progress in medical science is often slow and unsure, but in the case of heart disease the effect of diet and exercise is absolute and was readily recognizable as soon as the first studies were done. Once research on fat intake was refined, it became abundantly clear that high levels of fat in the diet jeopardize the health of the heart. The ideal scenario for your heart is to exercise in moderation and eat a healthy, low-fat diet from day one. But, since none of us is perfect, it is comforting to know that at any time in life you may change your diet and exercise plan and help your heart. You don't have to give up what you love to eat. You just have to moderate how much you eat and how you prepare it.

"I never really liked the idea of exercise. But after my heart attack I didn't think I had a choice. I was absolutely shocked to find out how easy it was to fit it into my life. And now I actually look forward to it."

Mary Lou Somers (age 66)

Y EARS AGO, people with heart disease were advised to basically remain sedentary and avoid vigorous activity. Now we know, nothing could be worse for you. A recent study from the Brigham and Women's Hospital and Harvard Medical School found that women who are most active have a 40 percent lower risk of heart attacks and strokes than women who are not particularly active.

Even moderate exercise can reduce the risk of these diseases. Begin with brisk walking for thirty minutes a few times a week to give yourself an edge.

If you do not have a regular exercise program, you should develop one, consulting your medical caregiver before doing so. If you have had trouble sticking to an exercise regimen in the past, read on for some more motivation.

The most important aspect of exercise is this—any exercise is better than none at all. Moderate exercise increases the heart's ability to pump blood. There is, essentially, no more important activity for the body. Exercise will also decrease the rate at which your heart beats at rest and during moderate exertion.

These two benefits of exercise are absolute. Other possible benefits include increasing the HDL and decreasing the LDL cholesterol levels, decreasing the triglyceride level, reducing weight and stress, and reducing elevated levels of blood sugar (glucose) in non-insulin-dependent diabetes. Exercise may also improve joint function, decrease the risk of osteoporosis by lessening the loss of bone mineral, keep you regular, and help maintain a sense of well-being. Who can argue with such a résumé?

Obviously, if you have a heart condition or advanced heart disease you cannot expect to get up and dance a wild tango for forty-five minutes. In most cases, however, with your doctor's okay, you can include a moderate amount of exercise, whether this be walking across a room and back a few times, walking a few blocks, or pedaling a stationary bicycle at low tension for a few minutes daily. As you build strength and endurance, you will soon be able to increase the duration of whatever form of exercise you choose. If you have had a heart attack or know that you have heart disease, you will want to discuss your exercise program with your doctor before you start, and your doctor may suggest a stress test for you before you begin to do any strenuous activity.

Smoking Your Heart to Death

If you rationalize your cigarette habit by saying that you eat healthy foods and are healthy in every other way, you're only fooling yourself. A new study, by Dr. J. Michael McGinnis and Dr. William H. Foege, ranking the top nongenetic causes of death has placed tobacco in the number one slot. As early as 1940, researchers at the Mayo Clinic documented that there was a relationship between smoking and coronary heart disease. The Office of Technology Assessment estimates one fifth of the deaths due to cardiovascular disease in 1990 were attributable to smoking.

More than 23 percent of all women smoke, and though women are quitting daily, they are not quitting in the same numbers as men. The percentage of female smokers who smoke more than 25 cigarettes per day has doubled since 1965. And a study of 119,000 nurses has confirmed the increased risk of heart disease in women. In fact, the heaviest smokers were found to have eleven times more risk of coronary heart disease than women who never smoked. Women who smoke are at higher risk for heart attack, and women who smoke become menopausal two to three years earlier than women who do not, adding to the risk of heart disease. Women who smoke are also more likely to develop severe hypertension or high blood pressure, which, again, compounds the risk of heart disease. You might say that smoking has a domino effect on the risk of heart disease in women, tumbling one defense after another in an overwhelming defeat of good health.

Even armed with the knowledge that they are systematically increasing their risk of major illness with every cigarette they smoke, many women have trouble quitting and others quit over and over, only to take up smoking again and again. If you are having trouble quitting, forgive yourself and get help. Smoking is an addiction—it's no accident that it's hard to quit, and it should not be an embarrassment. There are many new techniques and tactics available, as well as support groups. Enlist the aid and support of friends and family and try again, for the sake of your heart and your life.

Female Stress, Female Heart

There is no stress-free life. Every mother knows, for example, that being at home with the children is a stress-filled occupation. In addition to all the stress women already cope with in life, entering male-dominated professions has added new stresses to our lives without eradicating any of the old ones.

Stress has been a culprit in the deaths of many men from heart disease. Now, in order to compete in the fast, overstressed business lane, some women have embraced those old-fashioned, outmoded behavior codes that have done in so many men. Smoking, eating, drinking too much, and staying out late to prove their worth to the company have proved nothing. Partially, this self-denial of health harks back to the prototypic woman—the nurturer-caregiver who puts others first puts others first in business, too. In terms of health, none of this does anybody any good. Heart disease in women is here to prove it.

If you think this pattern may apply to you, you need to work on reducing the stress in your life. Easier said than done, you say, but resisting change will only add to the stress level in your life. We are all capable of lowering our stress levels to some degree without enormous changes in lifestyle. For example, if you work outside the home, try leaving earlier every once in a while. Walk to work. If you work inside your home, schedule time in your day for a walk by yourself. Walking is not only a good form of exercise, it is a break that allows you thinking time. It's a time to get away from everyone asking you questions, criticizing the work you've just done, demanding a favor, or begging you for chocolate milk or the family car. If you find you have trouble allowing time for yourself, consult your health-care practitioner. She or he should be able to recommend a program or a stress-reduction clinic in your area.

Estrogen Replacement Therapy—Yes or No?

Estrogen replacement therapy (ERT) has become one of *the* topics of women's health for many reasons. From osteoporosis to breast cancer, ERT invokes debate, and there is no more heated arena than that of female heart disease. The overwhelming evidence at this time is that ERT protects the female heart against heart disease.

The most important thing to keep in mind when considering ERT is that each woman's medical situation is different; there is no single answer when it comes to prescribing this therapy. First of all, you need to evaluate your overall well-being at the time of menopause and the severity of your menopausal symptoms. You will also want to discuss your personal health history and your family history, including whether anyone in your family has had breast cancer, ovarian cancer, osteoporosis, heart disease, or *especially* phlebitis or other vascular problems. All of these must be factored into the equation before you will be able to come up with the answer that is right for you. (See Part 4, "The Real M Word—Menopause.")

The Great Aspirin Debate

Every time you turn around you hear about another use for aspirin. It is truly a wonder drug. I tell my patients that if aspirin were new and presented to the Food and Drug Administration for approval today, approval would be held up for years because of this drug's many uses and noted side effects. And, if it finally did pass, aspirin would probably cost a dollar a pill!

To date, the most important study regarding aspirin and heart disease is a five-year study that included 22,000 middle-aged doctors. Guess which sex? You got it—they were all male. The results of this study were conclusive. The group of doctors who took one aspirin every other day suffered 40 percent fewer heart attacks than the group taking a placebo.

Debate over whether or not aspirin is effective in curbing heart attacks in women has ensued. Some say aspirin works only in a system where the testosterone levels are high or, conversely, doesn't work when estrogen levels are high. But the debate is one of conjecture and confusion without well-organized studies in which women are the subjects. Luckily newer studies similar to the doctors' study, but with women as the subjects, are now under way. In addition, the Harvard Nurses' Health Study, a six-year study of approximately 90,000 subjects, noted that the nurses who said they took six aspirin a week suffered 25 percent fewer heart attacks than the group that did not take aspirin. Thus, aspirin in very moderate quantities is a possible wonder drug for women as well as men.

Aggressive Is the Key Word

"When I had my heart attack, I was taken to the community hospital in a rural area near my home. My daughter insisted that I be transferred to the medical center in the city. They seemed better able to take care of me and give me definitive treatment."

Molly McElvoy (age 52)

RESEARCH SHOWS that women are far less likely to be transferred from a local hospital to a teaching hospital or an urban hospital that may specialize in a particular area. Mostly, the reason given is that women do not want to be separated from their families or cause their families too much trouble. But in the treatment of heart disease an aggressive approach is the best way a woman can aid her recovery (and thereby her family).

Additionally, while type A personalities are certainly at high risk for heart disease, the interesting factor in female heart patients is that it is the less competitive, less aggressive, less ambitious women who often suffer the most in every way from heart disease. In other words, the woman who is the caregiver to all others and not to herself may put herself last in terms of diet, exercise, and general self-care and may feel the stress of such self-denial.

A PATIENT'S GUIDE

"Worrying is like paying interest on a debt you may never owe."

Mark Twain

ONCE YOU HAVE SURVIVED a heart attack, the most important time in your life will be the recovery period. You will have a great deal of concern regarding the state of your heart, and you will probably spend some time feeling very fragile. The best way to counteract the natural tendency to worry about how you will do and whether you will have another attack is to follow a recovery plan into which you can invest your energy positively.

You must tell yourself that you are willing to put yourself first for six months, and then to keep putting yourself first at least part of the time for the rest of your life. This is not to say that life will not intervene—it always does. But when you can, you must get what you need. Let me explain. Many women who are used to being the ones who give the care have a hard time relinquishing duties on the home front when they first return from the hospital. You must let others cook for you; you must let others clean the house and care for you; in sum, *you must let others help*. If you are a social butterfly you must be careful not to overschedule yourself, leaving adequate time for your heart to rest. As much as it is important that you get out of bed and begin to embrace exercise and your own way of life again, it is also vital to rest. Heart patients who do not use their recovery period to truly recover often have bleaker prospects than those who do. If your family resists your need to do less at home, allow your doctor to intervene. Make it clear that if you do not get help, you will have to hire help. In most cases, your doctor will second this. In the long run, there is no choice. The better your recovery period, the better your chances of resuming a full and normal life.

Possible Complications After a Heart Attack

If you have had a heart attack, you will want to be well-informed regarding what possible complications may follow. Speak to your doctor regarding a recommended reading list, and note the suggested reading in the Directory of Health Resources. You are obviously at risk for another heart attack and if you have habits you need to change, now is the time to change them. The patients who do the best after a heart attack are those who use the experience as a marker—not a tragic one, but a marker indicating that it is time to make a change in lifestyle and attitude—and proceed to take the appropriate steps.

Clot formation and congestive heart failure are two possible complications after a heart attack. You will also be watched closely during the recovery period for rhythm abnormalities, pericarditis, and other complications. This is a time when you need to stay in close touch with your doctor and her or his staff. You will want to follow your medical plan carefully and to take note of any peculiar sensations or symptoms, alerting your doctor to them at once. Caution and taking things one step at a time are most important right now.

Having a Week-by-Week Plan

If you are hospitalized for a heart attack, in all probability, you will not be going home the next day. *The Mayo Clinic Heart Book* recommends a program of rehabilitation that lasts about six months and is divided into four stages: hospitalization, early recovery, late recovery, and maintenance.

The length of stay in the hospital will vary, depending on the severity of your heart attack and what treatment you receive, including angioplasty or bypass surgery. In the hospital, you will begin adding nonstrenuous activity to your daily routine and work with your doctor to establish an increasing level of physical activity, including walking and some limited stair climbing.

Early recovery lasts between two to twelve weeks and refers to your first weeks at home after the hospital. During this time you will likely begin an exercise routine, which may include walking slowly for ten minutes or pedaling an exercise bicycle. You will also begin to resume your social life. By weeks three or four, you may expect to resume driving (though not alone at first), as well as gardening, shopping, and walking up to thirty minutes at a time. Remember that during this time you will want help at home from family and friends. At this point in your life, being a martyr can literally kill you.

Late recovery begins about three months after your hospitalization. Your goals, by now, include continuing to modify the behaviors that put you at risk for heart disease in the first place, such as smoking, obesity, a high-fat diet, or stress.

Maintenance refers to keeping those habits out of your life and returning to your doctor for periodic checkups for the rest of your life.

Coming to Grips Psychologically

*"I had a real talk with myself. I knew I wasn't ready to
die—so I made peace with this heart attack and decided
to use it to change my life for the better."*

Arlene Saunders (age 55)

BOTH THE PATIENT and the patient's family go through a similar series of emotional responses to a heart attack. From anger, shock, and fear, to denial and a period of adjustment or bargaining, you will start to make your peace with this major event in your life. If you are a patient who has settled into denial, and you are continuing unhealthy habits that helped get you into trouble in the first place, you will have a struggle on your hands. No amount of therapeutic care or heart surgery can protect a damaged heart from further physical abuse— and cigarette smoking and a high-fat diet constitute abuse. If you are having trouble moderating your intake of fat, starting an exercise regime, or giving up cigarettes, you must seek help. If your anger at the situation is directed at your loved ones, you may also want to get some help in resolving your feelings, in order to protect yourself and your family from unnecessary added stresses during this already difficult time.

Depression is a common aftereffect. It is natural to feel vulnerable and be depressed about the loss of physical ability and to be frightened by such a clear reminder of mortality as a heart attack. Most depression, but not all, passes. Cardiac rehabilitation programs take into account the emotional price of heart disease, and you may take advantage of the counseling that is offered. If you find that you can't stop thinking about your heart attack or you live in constant fear of having another attack, ask your doctor for advice regarding therapeutic counseling.

Just as every heart attack is different, so is each recovery process. The most important thing is to find ways of using your experience to make constructive changes in your life.

From Sex to Mah-jongg, or Resuming Your Own Life

Besides the myth that women do not get heart disease, there are two other myths associated with this disease. One is that you will have to stop living an active life after a heart attack, and the other is that you will have to curtail your sex life. While it is true that sexual activity raises your risk of a heart attack slightly, so does the mere act of living. In fact, studies have shown that bedrest without activity ages you; certainly, bedrest has been proven to cause more complications than it helps to avoid.

As soon as you are able to walk up two flights of stairs without pain, severe shortness of breath, feeling light-headed, or feeling your heart skip, it is generally assumed that you are ready to resume the enjoyment of sex. This usually (though not always) occurs within a month of the heart attack. As with all other areas of your life, use common sense. Just as you would not resume driving alone immediately, without the aid of another driver, you will want to go slowly in the bedroom too. Talk to your partner, stop and rest if you need to, try again, talk about it again, build back the connection step by step.

Having an orgasm does not in itself increase your risk of heart disease, though how you proceed in the bedroom may or may not stress your heart. For example, if your sex life with your partner was fraught with tension or if your favorite foreplay was a heated argument, then you may have to rethink how you now approach sex. If your lovemaking depended on advanced calisthenic techniques, you will also have to modify your approach. You may discover that the drugs you are taking or your exhaustion has taken a toll on your libido. This, too, is normal. Give yourself time. On the other hand, you don't want to begin to use your heart attack as an excuse to never enjoy the sexual limelight again. Some women begin to associate their heart attacks with their graying hair, their added wrinkles, their sagging breasts or thighs—in other words, to equate it with the end of the era of sexual desirability. Nothing could be further from the truth. Consider yourself desirable, and if you don't, take the steps you need to make yourself feel this way, whether it be a new haircut, a new perfume, or a new exercise and diet plan. The better you feel about yourself, the better your partner will feel about you, and the more you will want to make the sexual connection.

Most important in all of this, discuss sex after a heart attack with your doctor. If you or your doctor feels uncomfortable with this, ask for a referral, so that you can explore, medically and personally, regaining this part of your life.

Fear is not an aphrodisiac. Your fear—as well as your partner's fear of hurting you—can impede your progress in the bedroom. The more you can talk about your fears and work them through with your partner, the easier it will be to resume an enjoyable sex life.

The enjoyment of life depends on the quality of life. If you like sex and it has always been a part of your life, you can and should have sex after your heart attack. Approach the resumption of your sex life just as you would approach exercise, humor, or anything else that makes life robust.

If you have heart disease or have had a heart attack, you will be most successful if you allow your experience to *change* your life rather than consider that your life has been *limited*. One of the best ways to take control of your life is to find out more about women and heart disease and use your knowledge accordingly.

A woman's greatest enemy in the battle against heart disease is ignorance. While knowledge won't suddenly eradicate your risk of heart disease and heart attack, it is the first step toward making the changes in your life that will. Until now, heart disease has too often accosted women like an unseen vehicle speeding out of a blind alley. But all that is changing. Because of what you now know, you can take the necessary steps to make sure heart disease doesn't sneak up on you. The first step in this process is examining how you live day by day.

PART 2

WOMEN AND CANCER

"There are times when I feel like I can't get away from it. 'Do this and you'll get cancer. Eat that and you won't get cancer.' It's enough to drive a sane woman absolutely crazy!"

Naomi Brande (age 37)

EVERY TIME I see a patient in my office with a new diagnosis of cancer, I can see the fear in her eyes. While I talk, her eyes glaze over and very little information is being retained. It will take two or three conversations before I feel that she is really prepared to make informed decisions about what path to take in her treatment.

The patient whom I deal with is not different from you or me in the same situation. We all know people who have been diagnosed with cancer. We have known people who have died from their disease. And we know people who have won—for whom the diagnosis of cancer is a distant memory.

Cancer is on the rise, whether the result of our living longer, living in an industrialized world, succumbing to poisons in cigarettes, or simply because we have improved methods of early detection. But the situation is not hopeless. The treatments that are available for most cancers offer the possibility of remission and, sometimes, a period of remission that is long enough to be equated with a cure. Cancer does not always have the dreadful consequences it once had. Even though treatment for cancer is often trial by fire, many patients do emerge safely and with excellent life expectancies. In the diagnosis and treatment of cancer, modern medicine has made great progress, from the improvement in chemotherapeutic techniques to the possibilities for genetic screening. New advances are being made every day. This is an exciting time in the area of cancer research and cancer treatment.

In order to approach cancer with informed expectations rather than fear, we need to understand what cancer is, what it does, and how we can fight it.

CARCINOGENESIS

Every day cells in our body die and are replaced by new ones. As cells multiply to keep our bodies in a steady state, they undergo a very regulated series of division and multiplication. *Mitosis* is the process by which normal cells divide and multiply. *Carcinogenesis*, the development of cancer, is mitosis gone awry. Havoc develops in the cell as it replicates. In layperson's terms, chaos overcomes order. This chaos leads inevitably to trouble.

Cancer proceeds when cells multiply wildly out of order. The process begins at the most elemental level, with our DNA, life's building blocks; it involves proto-oncogenes (growth-promoting genes) and tumor-suppressor genes (growth-retarding genes). Carcinogenesis begins with alterations in the genes contained in the DNA of a single cell. Cancer is such a powerful disease precisely because it alters life at its most fundamental level.

DNA directs the synthesis of the proteins that orchestrate the functions of all living things. DNA replicates itself exactly and continually, producing two daughter cells from a parent cell again and again. Healthy cells are constantly bombarded by unhealthy substances that may alter the gene structure. In a healthy cell, repairs are made by an intricate mechanism whose sole function is to eliminate or prevent chaos in the cell. But if this mechanism is damaged and the cell alteration persists—as it does in carcinogenesis—multiplication of the cell will also go haywire. The mutant cell will begin to replicate rapidly, eventually turning into a tumor with the possibility of invading neighboring tissues and spreading.

An "All-American" Disease

Cancer is also an increasingly common disease: more than one quarter of the population of the United States will suffer from cancer at some time in life. Like it or not, cancer is part of the culture. In 1990 more than one million new cases of cancer were diagnosed in the United States, and over half a million people died from it. In 1960, the five-year survival rate for white patients was 39 percent, and for black patients, 27 percent. This rate has improved—in 1990 the overall five-year survival rate was 52 percent (the rate of survival for black patients still lagged behind, but was also improving). The numbers of those affected by cancer are staggering and increasing, despite the enormous sums spent in the search for more effective treatments and a cure.

The ten most common types of cancers in the United States in order of the number of cases are:

1. lung
2. colon and rectum

3. breast
4. prostate
5. bladder
6. non-Hodgkin's lymphoma
7. genitourinary system
8. the oral cavity and upper respiratory tract (including the lip and pharynx)
9. pancreas
10. leukemia

In this part, breast, colon, gynecological, and lung cancers will be covered individually, in alphabetical order, to focus on those cancers that have an impact on the greatest number of women. Some of the other most common cancers will be covered in the last section of this part, "Other Cancers."

At present, early detection is the best weapon we have in the case of any cancer. That so many cancers may be silent, in terms of symptoms, early in the course of the disease makes screening more difficult and that much more important. Symptoms and screening options will be covered in each section.

BREAST CANCER

"Breast cancer is not a logical disease."

Daniel Hayes, M.D., Dana-Farber Cancer Institute

BREAST CANCER is the third most common cancer in the United States, but it is the first cancer on most women's minds. Breast cancer has become a haunting subject for women, partly because a concerted effort to focus attention and research dollars on the issue has made us aware of just how common and life-threatening this disease is. This push also reminds us that at this time there is no cure.

Breast cancer is a personal topic, striking women in an anatomical and psychological place that so clearly defines them as female and so intimately connects them to their sexuality and the nurturing of their children. With breast cancer in the news all the time, you may fear for

A DIAGNOSIS OF CANCER—
PREPARATION FOR HEARING
THE NEWS

If you have discovered a suspicious lump in your breast or blood in your stool and your doctor has recommended further tests, you may have discussed possible causes with your doctor, which include cancer. If you haven't, and there are many of us who were brought up not to question the doctor, you'll want to familiarize yourself with the topic now. It makes sense to prepare yourself for hearing the results of the biopsy and other tests, so you can make the situation as comfortable as possible for yourself. Some doctors schedule an office visit and wait until then to give you the news, good or bad. Nowadays, many physicians deliver the news over the phone because they've learned that the less time spent waiting in apprehension, the better, and that bad news is often tolerated more easily at home. When you have your biopsy, discuss with your doctor how she or he will give you the news and request your preference. Many patients report that once they have heard a positive diagnosis, they find it hard to listen and to focus their attention on the information that is given to them regarding the type of tumor, the spread of the disease, and the suggested treatment. Therefore, it is important to take notes or have a friend or family member do this for you, so that you will not miss important information.

Questions You Will Want to Ask Your Doctor

- What is the size of the tumor?
- What course of treatment is recommended?
- What will be the duration of the treatment?
- If surgery is part of the treatment, how long is the recovery period from surgery?
- What are the side effects of the treatment? Will I be too tired to work? Will I need help in the home?
- What can I do to prepare for this?
- What is my prognosis?

- I may want to get a second opinion. How much time do I have before I must decide?
- What quality-of-life changes can I expect with each treatment choice?

Unless you immediately agree with your doctor and feel ready to proceed, you will want to get a second opinion. The best choice is to consult a doctor who has trained at and who practices at a different hospital or health-care center than the doctor who is treating you. You will want this distinction to be clear because doctors who train together and work together often (but not always) have less variance of opinion regarding treatment options and prognosis.

When you are diagnosed, you must ask for help from friends and family. Whether or not you get the support you need from your loved ones, you will also want to consider support groups, as well as seeking help from a therapist, counselor, or religious mentor. Consider the help you get now to be an investment in your future. In the next few months, you will be going through a lot, and you will want to have the structure in place to get the help you need when you need it.

your breasts and wonder what to do about that fear. You probably know just enough about odds and risk factors to scare you, and you probably don't have enough data to reassure yourself and to separate the facts from the fiction. Finally, you know that not only does breast cancer kill, it also can come back. A woman may have had breast cancer five, ten, or more years ago and then get it again. And no one can really tell you why, except that breast cancer seems to go away, but may really be just hiding in tiny, even undetectable malignancies that won't be noticed for years. Breast cancer is mysterious because it may exist undetected and because it does not always respond to treatment in the same way. In confronting breast cancer medically, treatment is varied and individualized, which in itself is confusing. A lumpectomy may suffice in one case, and yet in another a mastectomy may not be able to eradicate the disease. While high levels of estrogen, such as those in premenopausal women, might encourage the growth of tumors, treatments that are estrogen based may work to suppress tumor growth. It doesn't always make sense. There is possibly nothing so frightening and frustrating as being told no matter what you do, we can't predict whether or not you will beat this. And breast cancer seems to be everywhere.

AIDS has claimed an alarming number of lives, yet this number is less than half the number of lives that have been lost to breast cancer during the same period. Since 1980, approximately 205,000 Americans have died of AIDS while approximately 450,000 have died of breast cancer. The facts have finally become part of the culture. For too long, they were not. This staggering number of deaths has turned breast cancer patients into activists. In the past year, awareness of the epidemic proportions of the disease has grown logarithmically. Statistics have been used to shock, horrify, and basically awaken a somnolent system to the facts, the truth, the need for funding, research, early diagnosis, and extensive treatment options.

As a result, at the present time, the health topic the American woman is probably the most confused about is breast cancer. A woman may whisper the words ". . . breast cancer . . ." to a friend about some other friend. She may begin examining her own breasts, saying the terrifying mantra to herself, because she has been lax in her regimen of self-examination. She may be appalled by the statistics and dread approaching her forties or fifties, knowing that the risk is higher as she ages. She may fear, most of all, the knowledge of how little knowledge there really is—85 percent of all breast cancers diagnosed have no known cause and are diagnosed in women who are not considered to be "at risk"—either by heredity, age group, early menses, or late menopause. She fears the unknown, and all she knows is the unknown.

You may know that your lifetime risk of getting breast cancer is one in nine, but you may not be aware that the five-year survival rate for breast cancer is 80 percent. Compare that to a 15 percent five-year survival rate for lung cancer, and you will begin to see that a diagnosis of breast cancer is not a death sentence.

But while cure rates can be talked about optimistically, the straight facts need to be addressed. For example, women have been made aware of the famous one-in-nine ratio, but few of us know that this ratio is based on an average life expectancy of eighty years (therefore, in a population of women who all live to be eighty, one in nine will contract breast cancer). A more realistic prediction would be to estimate that in a population of women who all live to be only fifty, one in fifty will get breast cancer.

Furthermore, just to put risk in perspective, while one in nine may sound like frightening odds, a woman has a one in two chance of dying from heart disease. In addition, lung cancer has surpassed breast cancer as the number one cancer killer of women. Breast cancer is not the only issue facing women when it comes to demanding and receiving fair medical treatment and adequate funding for medical research.

Breast cancer may or may not be the prime example of inadequate treatment of women by the medical profession. There is, however, an interesting silver lining to the situation. Breast cancer became a national issue because it was a woman's disease that was being ignored, but it is this very problem that enhances the efficiency of research and treatment of the disease in the end. In other words, the fact that breast cancer is for the most part a female disease automatically ensures that all research performed is applicable to women and that the effects and side effects of all treatments have necessarily taken women into account. As breasts were once cut off cadavers by doctors who decided there was nothing to be learned from them, now breasts are studied because of the knowledge that breast cancer is unique unto itself. Even though it may spread to other organs, the cancer maintains the characteristics of breast cancer. To investigate breast cancer, the subject, trial, or study group must comprise women. In other diseases, this is not the case, and often results of studies done on male subjects are wrongly assumed to apply to women as well. While breast cancer is still a mysterious disease, at least there can be no mistake in whom we are talking about when we talk about breast cancer.

Breast Self-Examination

"Early detection is not prevention, but it's the closest thing we've got."

Judy Garber, M.D., Dana-Farber Cancer Institute

ONE OF THE GREAT PLUSES when it comes to breast cancer is that it's not only possible, but easy to physically examine the breasts. One of the most important things a woman can do for herself is to examine her own breasts regularly. When it comes to breast cancer, vigilance (but not obsession) in terms of regular examination is key. As scary as it may be, the sooner you know something, the better.

So, what's so difficult about touching your own breasts? Nothing, right? And yet some of the most sensually expressive, liberated women still cringe at the idea and end up avoiding the process entirely. What is gained in the process of self-examination, and in getting to know your body and the many changes it goes through, is a sense of control and the pursuant confidence that the power for self-care is quite literally in your hands. Next to fighting relentlessly for further research on all fronts in the battle with breast cancer, a woman can do no greater service to her healthy self than take the matter of self-examination and monitoring into her own hands.

I must tell you that not everyone agrees with that. To Dr. Susan Love, for instance, the idea that examining your breasts every month can save your life is wishful thinking. Her belief is bolstered by the fact that these "search and destroy" missions do not yet have any scientific data to support their efficacy. Some women find these exams anxiety-provoking and yet feel guilty if they don't do them. Therefore, if the guidelines that follow don't fit for you, talk to your doctor to settle on a schedule where she or he can perform the exam for you.

Practical Tips

"I've never felt comfortable examining my breasts. I get queasy . . . maybe it's the fear that I'll find something. Anyway, I know I should do it but it seems that months slide by and I haven't checked."

Anna Simonson (age 34)

- Examine your breasts during a quiet time when you won't be interrupted.
- Examine your breasts lying down so you can relax and be comfortable.
- Use liberal amounts of lotion or a pleasant smelling, healthy massage oil while examining your breasts.
- Have your mate examine your breasts for you.

- If you don't examine your own breasts regularly, make your gynecologist or family doctor aware of this so that she or he will be
extracautious during checkups.
- Examine your breasts three days after the last day of your period.
- If you no longer menstruate, pick a day on the calendar (for example
the first of each month, or the fifteenth) and stick with that schedule.

Women often do not examine their breasts on a regular basis or
they go to the other extreme and examine their breasts every day. Neither strategy is helpful.

What deters women from this simple procedure? Fear and sometimes squeamishness—particularly if you are a woman whose breasts are
lumpy. If you are one of the many women who do have lumpy breasts,
you may be afraid of every lump and you may be afraid you won't be
able to tell anything through your self-examination. But you don't have
to be. There is no link between lumpy breasts and breast cancer. And
you can get to know your own lumpy breasts better than your doctor,
making you the best authority on changes and abnormalities.

Self-Examination, Fear, and the Truth About Fibrocystic Disease

*"Fibrocystic disease is . . . a wastebasket into which
doctors throw every breast problem that isn't cancerous."*

Susan Love, M.D.

B REASTS MAY BE lumpy. Breasts may swell. Breasts may be painful
or tender when touched. Until recently, any and all of these
conditions were labeled by most doctors as fibrocystic disease. A
woman goes to the doctor complaining of breast pain, swelling, or tenderness, and she is quickly diagnosed as having "fibrocystic disease."
She might as well be diagnosed as having a myth. The clinician may
then send a woman with a lumpy breast for a biopsy, and a piece of the
telltale tissue will be examined by a pathologist under a microscope.
Then the pathologist gets to create yet a second definition of that non-
disease fibrocystic disease, because he or she may indeed find something.
The truth is there are approximately fifteen microscopic conditions ex-

isting in most women's breasts that have nothing to do with cancer. They're part of the aging process, like benign sun spots or wrinkles. The third version or definition of fibrocystic disease is the creation of the radiologist who gives a woman a mammogram, finds nothing indicative of malignancy, but does find dense or lumpy tissue. Ironically, this form of fibrocystic disease relies on the youth rather than the age of the patient. The younger you are, the more breast tissue and less fatty tissue you have in your breasts and the denser the tissue is.

Thus, the same catchall phrase is used to define a very normal condition in young breasts and a very normal condition in aging breasts, and in all cases the word "disease" is used to refer to what may best be called just a variety of normal breast conditions. The most important thing to remember is that these variations are *not* associated with an increased risk of breast cancer.

There is no connection between the discovery of a breast cyst and a cancerous growth, except possibly chance—the chance that a woman who does examine her breasts regularly finds a lump, goes to the doctor and is told the lump's a cyst, but in the course of the examination *another* smaller lump is discovered. Certain studies years ago hypothesized from such sheer coincidence that the cyst had something to do with the cancer and the cyst was the culprit. Nothing could be further from the truth. In the case of the discovery of the smaller lump at the time of examination, the cyst is more of a detective's assistant—allowing for the discovery of information that otherwise would have been impossible to retrieve.

Caffeine, Salt, Cheese, and Vitamin E

"I was diagnosed with cystic breasts and told to get a mammogram at thirty-two. The lumps were benign. I had fibrocystic disease. My doctor told me to give up coffee, cheese, and tuna fish—because of the salt, I guess. A few years later, I had a baby and nursed him for a year and a half. I haven't had a lump since. Maybe the breast-feeding helped. Who knows? I'm older, too."

Caroline Gleason (age 44)

UNTIL RECENTLY, many doctors advised their patients with lumpy breasts to abstain from caffeine. Some also claimed that salt was a culprit. And then there's fat—which lately has been blamed for everything. The truth is, if a younger woman is diagnosed with benign lumps (which may often be particularly dense breast tissue), the best advice is simply to get a little older—a prescription you can't help but fill. Vitamin E has recently been in the limelight as the savior that may counteract fat's villainy across the board. But there is no evidence that shows that vitamin E prevents cysts or lumps in the breast or, for that matter, guards against breast cancer.

Classifying Noncancerous Breast Symptoms

Under the ugly and useless umbrella of "fibrocystic disease," there are at least six categories of breast problems that affect women.

1. Tenderness or pain before menstruation
2. Severe breast pain that may inhibit the patient's quality of life and may or may not be associated with the menstrual cycle
3. Nipple discharge and other nipple problems
4. Extreme lumpiness (more than would be considered normal)
5. Inflammation or infection (often associated with nursing, but not necessarily)
6. Cysts and fibroadenomas, referred to collectively as dominant lumps

Because this is a general book on women's health, it is impossible to go into as much detail as I would like to in many important areas—one of which is the many noncancerous conditions that may affect a woman's breasts. A great source for a sensitive and thorough treatment of the subject and for information on the female breast in general is *Dr. Susan Love's Breast Book.*

When You Are Diagnosed with Breast Cancer

"In the three minutes that will elapse at the beginning of this talk, another American woman will be diagnosed with breast cancer."

President Bill Clinton

THE NIGHT MY MOTHER called to tell me that she had breast cancer, I remember not being surprised. Over the years she had had repeated biopsies. And while they had been benign and I knew that there is no correlation between lumpy breasts and cancer, somehow going through all those biopsies helped prepare me for the day when one of those biopsies would bring bad news. The bad news came to my mother when she was sixty-four years of age. Today, after she underwent a mastectomy, I consider my mother cured. Nonetheless the "one-in-nine" statistic is now part of my family tree.

All of us live with the knowledge that having breast cancer is a possibility—and more of one as we get older. But it's still a shock when it happens. All your fears are suddenly focused. You say to yourself: How could this happen to me? What could I have done to prevent this? That there are no good answers will make you angry. That this has happened will make you cry. Anger and grief are normal and necessary. You'll need time to work through your emotions, which will be many and varied.

Although most women's breasts are important to their sense of iden-tity, one common response after a diagnosis of breast cancer is to want to be rid of that part of your body that betrayed you. It's not uncommon for a woman to say, "Cut it off. Get rid of it." This is an emotional response to shocking news. You must beware of the patronizing doctor who takes advantage of the situation by having you sign a mastectomy consent form immediately. While some form of mastectomy may indeed be the right course of treatment for you, *no decision needs to be made at the moment of diagnosis.* What you want from this meeting with your doctor is information, not snap decisions. You need all the facts so that you can weigh your options and so that you will be comfortable with the decision you and your doctor make regarding the course of treatment. Removing your breast immediately will not restore your life to the way it was before your diagnosis.

There is no denying that your life has been changed and you need to find the most constructive ways to deal with that change. After the support of friends and family, what will help you most during this process of acceptance will be to plot your strategy for handling your disease.

Types of Biopsy

If you or your doctor has discovered a lump, and it is suspicious, it is likely that a biopsy will be recommended. Biopsy refers to five different procedures. Except for a fine-needle biopsy, a breast biopsy is performed by a surgeon. Don't be alarmed that you are seeing a surgeon. A breast surgeon is best qualified to diagnose breast cancer, and in this case "surgeon" is not synonymous with "operation."

The five biopsy techniques are:

1. Fine-needle aspiration
2. Tru-cut needle biopsy
3. Incisional biopsy
4. Excisional biopsy
5. Stereotactic core needle breast biopsy

Fine-needle aspiration biopsy is the least invasive of the five procedures. The physician holds the lump in his or her fingers. Then a needle is passed in and out of the lump a few times to obtain cells that will then be analyzed. This is not a surgical procedure. Fine-needle aspiration is most accurate when the results are positive—that is, if you have cancer. If the result of this test is negative, that may be the end of it. In other cases, if your physician believes that the needle may have missed getting enough tissue, you may want to go ahead and have a surgical biopsy to confirm that this result is accurate.

The tru-cut needle biopsy removes a core from the tumor, not just a group of cells. Although, like fine-needle aspiration, the tru-cut is a nonsurgical procedure, it's more uncomfortable because the surgeon has to push much harder with the needle to get the core. Still, it can be done in the office under local anesthesia, and there is normally enough tissue to obtain an accurate diagnosis.

An incisional biopsy requires a local anesthetic. After a small incision is made in the skin, the surgeon goes into the tumor to remove a wedge of tissue, which is then sent to a pathologist for evaluation. This procedure is indicated only if repeated needle biopsies fail to make the diagnosis. Incisional biopsy is being supplanted by fine-needle biopsies now that fine-needle biopsies can be used to test for hormone receptivity—that is, whether or not the tumor is receptive to hormone treatment.

An excisional biopsy involves removing the entire lump. Usually, a local anesthetic is used for the procedure, though in some cases a general anesthetic may be used. If the lump is so tiny that you can't feel it, but it has been seen on a mammogram, this is the procedure that must be used. That's because at the present time, a sizable lump is required to perform a fine-needle biopsy.

A relatively new method of diagnosing breast cancer is stereotactic core needle breast biopsy. It is minimally invasive, leaving the patient with a small scar (about 3 millimeters, or less than 1¼ inches) and no deformity. This procedure is also highly accurate—it has a miss rate of 0.32 percent—and is less expensive than open surgical needle biopsy.

Technical Terms Your Doctor May Use

The breast is composed of fifteen to twenty sections, which are called *lobes*. Each lobe is composed of smaller sections, called *lobules*. Tiny tubes known as *ducts* connect the lobules and lobes; both lobules and ducts are glands. Approximately 86 percent of all breast cancers begin in the ducts, so they are referred to as *ductal cancers*. Twelve percent originate in the lobules and are referred to as *lobular cancers*. The last 2 percent of breast cancers are found in the surrounding tissues, and these are referred to as *adenocarcinomas* (*adeno* means related to a gland).

Here is some other medical terminology you may hear:

ER Negative and ER Positive: ER stands for estrogen receptor—a protein normally made by breast cells that helps the hormone estrogen work in cells. An ER positive tumor may respond to hormone therapies, whereas an ER negative tumor usually will not. Tamoxifen is one of the hormone therapies that is effective on ER positive tumors. An ER negative tumor is considered to be more dangerous than one that is ER positive. Tumors that are ER positive are generally considered to grow more slowly and have a better prognosis. In general, postmenopausal women are more likely to have ER positive tumors, while premenopausal women tend to have ER negative tumors. You may also hear the terms HR positive and negative, which means hormone receptor, and this includes progesterone as well.

In Situ: This Latin term literally means "in its original place" or "at the place of origin." Carcinoma in situ is a cancer that has not spread. If this term is used in your diagnostic report, it's good news: The chances of complete recovery are very good. Intraductal carcinoma in situ, ductal carcinoma in situ, and lobular carcinoma in situ all refer to noninvasive cancers, which are sometimes called *precancers*.

Infiltrating Ductal Carcinoma with an Intraductal Component:
This refers to a situation in which precancer and cancer are present in the same lump.

Lobular: Indicates a small lobe or part of a lobe.

Lymph Node: A glandlike mass of tissue that contains cells that will become lymphocytes, part of the immune system.

Lymphocyte: A nongranular white blood cell important to the production of antibodies.

Metastasis: The spread of a tumor from its site of origin to distant sites.

Necrosis: This refers to cancerous cells that are dead. It's a sign that the cancer has outgrown its blood supply, which means it is growing rapidly.

Nuclear Grade: A term referring to how quickly cancerous cells are dividing. Less aggressive cancers have fewer cells dividing. A higher nuclear grade means the cancer cells are dividing with greater frequency and the tumor is, therefore, growing rapidly.

Vascular Invasion: A term used to define a cancer that has infiltrated a blood vessel or a lymphatic vessel. This situation may also be referred to as lymphatic invasion and suggests that the cancer is potentially more dangerous.

Stages

The stage ascribed to a cancerous tumor in the breast and often in cancers found in other organs will depend upon the following:

1.   The size of the tumor and whether or not it has spread to any other organs of the body
2.   Whether or not any nodes are involved
3.   Whether the tumor is in situ or invasive

THE FIVE STAGES

Stage 0. Stage 0 is often referred to as precancer. In situ, intraductal, and the in situ lobular carcinoma are all stage 0 cancers. So is Paget's disease of the nipple, which does not involve a tumor at all. A stage 0 cancer is also referred to simply as in situ.

Stage 1. The tumor is no larger than 2 centimeters (¾ inch) in diameter. The tumor has not spread outside the breast.

Stage 2. Stage 2 breast cancer refers to three distinct situations:

A tumor no larger than 2 centimeters that has spread to lymph nodes under the arm.

A tumor between 2 and 5 centimeters that may or may not have spread to the lymph nodes under the arm.

A tumor that is larger than 5 centimeters, but which has not spread to the lymph nodes under the arm.

Stage 3. Stage 3 cancers are divided into stage 3A and stage 3B.

Stage 3A refers to either of the following: a tumor smaller than 5 centimeters that has spread to multiple lymph nodes under the arm, which have grown into one another or into other structures; or a tumor that is bigger than 5 centimeters and has spread to lymph nodes under the arm but no farther.

Stage 3B refers to either of the following: the cancer has spread to tissue near the breast, such as the chest wall and muscles in the chest; or the cancer has spread to lymph nodes near the collarbone.

Stage 4. The cancer has spread to other organs of the body (most often, the bones, lungs, or liver, which are the organs breast cancer spreads to most readily).

RECURRENT BREAST CANCER

Recurrent breast cancer means the cancer has come back after being treated. It may return in the breast itself, or in other parts of the body.

Rare Cancers and Rare Situations

Sometimes a woman is diagnosed with cancer in each of her breasts— a condition known as bilateral breast cancers. Each cancer is called a primary cancer. In other words, each is a new cancer. One is not a result of the metastasis of the other. In this case, the prognosis that you receive will be the one that pertains to the cancer that has progressed farther.

In certain cancers, it's the situation—as opposed to the cancer it- self—that makes the cancer unusual. One such situation is to be diag- nosed with breast cancer while you are pregnant or while you are nursing.

When I was pregnant with my son, I was forty-two years old. My breasts had already undergone normal changes in texture over the years. I nursed him for six months and during that time they changed again. They became not only larger, but also lumpier. One evening I felt a hard, tender mass about an inch across. It was rock hard and I imme- diately assumed the worst. Fortunately this turned out to be a clogged milk duct, which is usually the case when a lactating woman discovers a breast mass. But until I figured it out, my heart raced because I knew that the possibility of cancer always has to be considered. If, while you are breast-feeding, you are diagnosed with breast cancer, you will have to stop breast-feeding if you are going to undergo chemotherapy or radiation.

The situation in pregnancy is more complicated. In the first trimester, a therapeutic abortion is an option, depending on a woman's beliefs and what the pregnancy means to her. A mastectomy is usually possible in the second trimester, though the option of chemotherapy or radiation is not considered a safe one for the fetus at this point in a pregnancy. In the third trimester, a lumpectomy or mastectomy is possible, and your doctor will probably recommend waiting until the birth of your baby to begin chemotherapy or radiation. Another possibility is to remove the baby by cesarean section as soon as it is safe to do so and then begin treatment.

Inflammatory breast cancer is another rare form of the disease. The breast appears to be inflamed and is warm to the touch. The skin may also appear to be pitted, or it may be marked by ridges and wheals. This cancer spreads very quickly.

Other rare cancers include metastasis to the breast from another site in the body, primary lymphoma or sarcoma of the breast, and cystosarcoma phylloides—a rare and usually benign tumor of the breast that can occur in women even in their teens.

The Great Mammography Debate

"In women over fifty, mammography reduces the mortality rate from breast cancer by 30 percent."

Susan Love, M.D. (*Today*, NBC News, October 18, 1993)

SUSAN LOVE DOES not stand alone in her endorsement of mammography. There are now eight randomized trials, conducted in various parts of the world, that underscore the significance and benefits of this screening procedure.

At the same time, we are engaged in a nationwide effort to cut medical costs. In the process of examining what we spend on tests and procedures, we must make sure, however, that we do not allow ourselves to succumb to the double standard of care so long in place in the medical hierarchy (that is—women get less). On October 19, 1993, the Na-

A BILL OF RIGHTS FOR THE BREAST CANCER PATIENT

"I went in expecting a fight. My biopsy had already come back positive and I wanted more from my doctor than just a dismissive pat on the head. I was surprised when my doctor invited dialogue and told me he wanted me to be a part of the decision-making process."

Suzanne Emerson (age 52)

- Do not sign a mastectomy consent form immediately.
- When you have a biopsy, decide with your physician if you want to receive the results immediately over the phone or in the physician's office. Then decide whom you want to have with you when you hear the results and make sure that person is available to you at that time.
- Obtain a written report of the results of your biopsy.
- When you meet with your physician to discuss the course of treatment and prognosis, bring someone you trust to the appointment. No matter how intelligent, independent, and well educated you may be, you are confronting too many issues—from losing your life to losing your breast to fear itself—to be expected to recall or take notes on everything that is being said. You are entitled to the help of loved ones and friends.

tional Cancer Institute announced that mammography did not significantly decrease the mortality rate for breast cancer in women under the age of fifty. This raised all kinds of questions about whether it therefore makes sense to spend money on mammograms for women under fifty when the expenditure cannot be equated with lives saved. The issues at hand are complex: mammography is not a perfect test, and women under fifty (approximately) have fattier breast tissue, which is harder to examine. But many of the studies that have been done to date have involved older equipment and inexact testing procedures. It is important to keep in mind that what is being debated is whether standard screening mammography should be paid for by insurance, *not* whether a woman under fifty should undergo mammography if her doctor recommends the test.

The question everyone is asking is whether or not mammography is worth it. But "worth it" to whom? I believe mammography is worth it until something better comes along. What is also not in question is whether a woman over fifty should get the test. She should—although the sad news is not enough women over fifty do. Only approximately 40 percent of women over fifty get a mammogram at least every other year. Clearly the age of fifty is an arbitrary cut-off point in terms of the efficacy of the test. But, if you are over fifty, you should take advantage of health-care coverage and have the test. If you are under fifty, you should prepare yourself to add this to your health regimen and make it a habit on or before your forty-ninth birthday. While we need to find a way to end the confusion for women under fifty, we must also find a way to encourage our friends and family members who are women over fifty to get their mammograms. *Every single test and piece of evidence says yes for mammograms for women over fifty.*

Mammography for Women in Their Forties

"Isn't it ironic that breast cancer is suddenly the disease where cost consciousness is an issue? What we're really talking about is cutting health-care costs off the fronts of women."

Cokie Roberts (age 52)

THE DEBATE BETWEEN cost effectiveness and lives saved is not an inconsequential one. Each year 40,000 women under the age of fifty are diagnosed with breast cancer. Each year 10,000 women who developed breast cancer between the ages of forty and forty-nine will die of their disease. Only one in five of those women will have had a family history of breast cancer. While the number of diagnosed cases is certainly higher in the over-fifty age group, consider the years of life saved when a forty-two-year-old is diagnosed early, treated, and saved.

> *"If we disenfranchise women in their forties by say-*
> *ing don't bother with mammography, it's not for*
> *you, and then tell them at fifty this is the perfect*
> *test for you . . . what are they going to think?"*
>
> Judy Garber, M.D., Dana-Farber Cancer Institute

MAMMOGRAPHY IS NOT a perfect screening test for breast cancer in younger women, but this is not to say that there are no benefits. The lack of success in statistically reducing mortality from breast cancer in younger women may be due to the lack of benefit of the test itself on younger breast tissue. But it could also be due to the state of today's technology or inadequate screening frequency in the decade between forty and fifty. At this point, there are no research trials that have included sufficient numbers of women between ages forty and forty-nine to provide such information. This is because breast cancer is a much less common disease in women under fifty. Twenty-five percent or less of all new cancers occur in women under fifty. And many of the studies being used in evaluating mammography as a viable test for women under fifty are at least seven to ten years old.

The data that the National Cancer Institute (NCI) used in redrawing its guidelines for mammography screening come from the eight randomized trials mentioned earlier. None of these trials has been proven to be properly designed to evaluate women in their forties. Five of the trials do show a benefit in mortality reduction that varies from 14 to 49 percent.

The three trials that did not show a benefit have met with consistent criticism. The National Breast Screening Study of Canada included more women with incurable cancer in the screened group than in the control group, an obvious flaw in a study designed to demonstrate a test's effectiveness in lowering mortality rates. The Ostergötland trial in Sweden included, among women screened, those who were in the screening group but had refused to be screened—a decided shortcoming.

Lastly, the Stockholm trial was conducted with too long a time between screening tests.

> *"Women ages forty to forty-nine should not be denied access to screening simply because analysts are unwilling to admit that the trials that have been performed have not been designed or performed properly."*
>
> Daniel B. Kopans, M.D., Director of Breast Imaging,
> Massachusetts General Hospital

MANY BREAST SPECIALISTS and oncologists fear that the NCI's decision not to recommend mammography for women between forty and forty-nine years old will serve to heighten confusion on the issue and keep women from utilizing the only available test. Dr. David Bragg, for example, a member of the National Cancer Advisory Board who actually worked on the resolution asking that the NCI "defer action" regarding the policy change, stated: "The statistical data derived from the multinational trial program is difficult to interpret for women under age fifty as the studies were not designed to assess this age group. . . . The NCI statement does little to clarify an area of scientific confusion and will add further uncertainty to the role of screening mammography at all ages." In the meantime, I personally get a mammogram.

If you want to be autonomous and aggressive regarding your own health care, the door isn't shut regarding the benefits of mammograms at younger ages when you and your physician agree there is a need. For example, if your mother or sister (or both) has had breast cancer, you will want to have regular mammograms starting at an earlier age. Occasionally, a doctor may suggest that a woman have a first mammogram at age thirty-five if she has a family history of breast cancer in young women. But the sensitivity of this test in the younger population is decidedly less and should be made on a case-by-case basis.

MAMMOGRAM SCREENING RECOMMENDATIONS

Women with No Special Risk Factors

Age 20–39

Monthly breast self-exam

Clinical breast exam every three years

Baseline mammogram beginning at age 40

Age 40–49

Monthly breast self-exam

Annual clinical breast exam

Mammogram every one to two years

Age 50 and Older

Monthly breast self-exam

Annual clinical breast exam

Annual mammogram

Women with Family History Risk Factor

The staff at Memorial Sloan-Kettering Cancer Center in New York recommends a more aggressive approach for those women who have had a mother or a sister with breast cancer, because their family history puts them at increased risk.

Monthly breast self-exam

Annual clinical breast exam

continued

Annual mammography, beginning ten years earlier than the relative's age at the time of diagnosis. (If the mother was diagnosed at the age of 40, for example, the woman should begin mammograms at 30. However, annual mammograms should not begin at an age younger than 25.)

Etiology and Prevention

Etiology, or the study of cause, is at the core of how we will figure out treatment and possible prevention. The most promising areas of etiological research right now are genetics, premalignant and tumor markers, hormones, and, to a lesser degree, risk factors in diet, physical activity, and environment. For prevention of a recurrence of breast cancer, understanding the metastatic process is also essential.

There is some good news about diet as a risk factor. A recent report in the *Journal of the National Cancer Institute* found that women who consume olive oil at more than one meal daily have a 25 percent lower risk of breast cancer than those who ingest it once a day or less. The study also found protective effects from a high consumption of fruits and vegetables. These findings reinforce the belief of some scientists that the traditional Mediterranean diet is healthier than the average American diet.

The etiological goals in the areas of genetics and tumor markers include:

- Identifying genetic changes during the transformation of normal tissue to premalignant or malignant tissue
- Identifying markers that are present in the interval from initial breast abnormalities to the detection of actual breast cancer
- The study of cell proliferation and how this is controlled via hormones in the normal breast during all stages of female development
- The identification of genes in the normal breast and then in cancerous tissue that are regulated by hormones in contraceptives, hormone replacement therapy, and endogenous (growing within the cells) hormone activity

DIGITAL MAMMOGRAPHY AND OTHER NEW TACTICS FOR THE FUTURE

Digital mammography may be the most promising new technology in breast imaging. This new technique has the potential to improve accuracy and image interpretation, as well as image storage and retrieval. It may also facilitate the transmission of images to expert mammography interpreters in other locations.

The Mammography Quality Standards Act was passed in 1992. The Food and Drug Administration is responsible for implementing the law but at present is in the process of modifying it. The law will ensure that all women receive acceptable quality mammography and will eliminate conflicting standards.

The National Cancer Institute also recommends the promotion of mammography and breast examination for groups of women who are rarely screened at present. This group includes African American, Native American, Latina, Asian American, and other ethnic populations, as well as rural women, older women, and women of lower socioeconomic status.

• Research on "low-dose" hormonal contraceptives, comparing estrogen and progesterone combination therapies

Hope for the Future

In 1994 a genetic marker for breast cancer was located; a second will follow. Soon the gene for breast cancer will be isolated. These advances will allow us to target women at risk and, it's hoped, perform "gene surgery" to prevent this disease.

Progress for women suffering from breast cancer is inevitable. We must all work toward the solution and never give up hope as we go through the day-to-day horror of what our family and friends suffer.

How We Now Wage War

If you have just been diagnosed with breast cancer, the cancer has most likely been with you, beginning in microscopic stages, for at least several years. By the time a mass is one centimeter in diameter, it contains one billion cells and can be seen on a mammogram.

Oncologists are the front line in cancer research and cancer diagnosis. Cancer, however, is not a simple foe. Its adversarial capacity is multifold and multidimensional. As we begin to understand just how remarkably diverse and unique breast cancer cells and breast cancer progression can be, debates have made oncology more complicated. Opinions and theories within the discipline are understandably diverse and there is not always complete agreement among specialists.

Thus, a woman approaching the long haul of breast cancer treatment may encounter, along with her fear, a sense of muddled confusion that will only add to her unease and trepidation regarding the decision-making process. The flip side of this, though, is that in the war against breast cancer, a second opinion is always valuable.

There are many approaches to the treatment of breast cancer. What follows are the procedures and options that you and your physician will be choosing from. You will need to be familiar with them, especially when seeking a second opinion and then making an informed choice regarding your course of treatment.

Radical Mastectomy

The radical mastectomy was first developed by William Stewart Halsted at Johns Hopkins University in the 1890s, though a similar procedure had been done in England by Charles Moore. At the time, doctors thought that breast cancer spread lymph node by lymph node, and when it had occupied the last lymph node, then spread rapidly through the rest of the body. Therefore, removal of the lymph nodes seemed of paramount importance. The Halsted mastectomy removed the breast, all lymph nodes, and also the chest wall muscle. A similarly radical surgery was practiced in London by a surgeon named Sampson Handley. Though neither procedure was ever shown to prolong life, both became popular. Any doubts about the surgery's effectiveness attributed lack of success to the surgery not being radical enough.

In the old days a radical mastectomy was a woman's only option. Today it is a rare occurrence. In this procedure, all breast tissue and overlying skin are removed. So are the lymph nodes fanning out from the breast under the armpit. So are the pectoralis major and minor muscles. The loss of muscle means your arm will be weakened. Movement is limited and women often experience chronic pain after the surgery.

In most hospitals, the *modified radical mastectomy* has replaced the radical mastectomy because it is less disfiguring and does not impede mobility. The modified radical mastectomy removes only the breast tissue and some of the lymph nodes. The muscle is left behind. However, even modified mastectomy has not been shown to increase survival rate.

COMPLICATIONS AFTER RADICAL AND MODIFIED RADICAL MASTECTOMY

There is a component of risk to any surgical operation. During radical and modified radical mastectomies a number of blood vessels are severed. In some cases, when the blood supply is insufficient to the healing tissue, an area of skin may die and form a scab. This is usually not a serious complication, unless the area of skin is a large one or there is an infection.

A second complication involves the collection of fluid under the scar once the drains have been removed. If fluid is collecting, you will notice a swelling at the incision. This is also not a serious complication, though it may be annoying. If you notice swelling or hear a sloshing sound when you are walking, you should consult your physician.

The risks from the removal of lymph nodes include phlebitis, lymphedema, winged scapula, and damage to the thoracodorsal nerve. Phlebitis is generally an early problem, showing up approximately three days after surgery. Symptoms include a worsening of postsurgical pain and swelling of the arm. The best treatment is aspirin and ice packs. Phlebitis usually subsides within a week.

Lymphedema, the swelling that is the major complication in removal of the lymph nodes, is rare (occuring only in 3 percent of cases) and can be temporary or permanent. It may be very slight so that you are only aware of the condition because of a swelling in your fingers or it may be so severe that your entire arm swells. Another complication after lymph node surgery is commonly referred to as winged scapula. Such cases are extremely rare and occur when the long thoracic nerve is injured during surgery. Damage to this nerve causes your shoulder blade to stick out instead of lying flat. The effect is similar to a wing, hence the name "winged scapula." If the condition is temporary, it will go away within a few weeks or months, but sometimes it is permanent. If you are not athletic, it will hardly hamper you in your daily activities. However, if it does bother you, exercises may help overcome the problem, and in severe cases an orthopedic surgeon can perform corrective surgery. The other motor nerve that may be damaged during surgery is the thoracodorsal nerve, which goes to the latissimus dorsi muscle. Damage to this nerve is rare and may give you a sensation of tiredness in the arm and a little less mobility, but these problems are generally quite minor.

Partial Mastectomy

The alternative to radical and modified radical mastectomy is the partial mastectomy, or lumpectomy. This type of surgery removes the cancerous lump and some of the surrounding normal tissue. There are many terms for this surgery that are used virtually interchangeably; besides partial mastectomy and lumpectomy, these terms are wide excision, segmental mastectomy, and quadrantectomy. What is meant by any one of these terms is somewhat dependent upon the doctor and should be clarified by patient and doctor.

Among other advantages, a partial mastectomy is a less extensive surgery than a radical. It leaves the chest musculature and arm mobility intact, and the patient faces a somewhat easier recovery. Depending on the type of partial, a quadrant or less or more of the breast tissue is removed, along with the lymph nodes if this is indicated. The pectoral muscles are left intact.

COMPLICATIONS IN PARTIAL MASTECTOMY

If a large lump was removed during a partial mastectomy, you may have a permanent numb spot, but not the same total numbness that occurs after a radical mastectomy. Your breast will obviously be smaller in size and different in shape. However, it is the complications of lymph node surgery that may be the most serious. As with radical mastecomy, these complications are phlebitis, lymphedema, and winged scapula (see page 83).

Breast Conservation Surgery—Lumpectomy

If your cancer is small enough to be removed without sacrificing too much surrounding breast tissue and has not spread, then a lumpectomy will probably be your treatment of choice. A lumpectomy is a type of partial mastectomy that will leave your breast intact, if sometimes markedly or slightly dimpled at the site of the surgery. In most (if not all) cases, an axillary dissection is performed at the same time; this removes some or most of the lymph nodes in the armpit, where most breast cancers spread first. Once the lymph nodes are removed they can be checked under the microscope to see if any of the tumor cells have spread. You may be encouraged to undergo radiotherapy to the breast area to ensure that the tumor won't come back.

THE CONTROVERSY OVER LUMPECTOMY RESEARCH

The National Surgical Breast and Bowel Project, which has conducted many of the largest and longest-lasting cancer studies in the nation (some dating from 1958), sponsored a research project under the supervision of Dr. Roger Poisson. Dr. Poisson and a team of University of Pittsburgh researchers were studying the efficacy of lumpectomy in the treatment of breast cancer. Early reports suggested that lumpectomy was just as effective as mastectomy in terms of how long women lived free of the disease after surgery. In 1992, Dr. Poisson was suspended from the work because it was found that he had falsified reports in order to place more women in the study. By the spring of 1994, when the National Cancer Institute stepped in to suspend the clinical trials, what had by then become known as the "Poisson affair" had frightened many women.

However, a team at the University of Pennsylvania reexamined the study's data and has since determined that the results are still the same. Women who have breast conservation surgery—in this case, lumpectomy—enjoy the same amount of time recurrence-free as those who have had more extensive surgeries. In other words, the allegedly suspect methodology used by Poisson and his team did not alter the results. It is thus still safe and wise to consider lumpectomy as a possibility if this course of treatment has been suggested to you.

Radiation, Chemotherapy, and the Human Cost

In all surgical treatments of breast cancer, it is important to remember that surgery can take care only of the tumor visible to the surgeon. Any spread of the tumor must be treated systemically. Chemotherapy in conjunction with surgery is referred to as adjuvant treatment—that is, two forms of treatment working in tandem. If your cancer has spread, your doctor will probably recommend chemotherapy in order to treat any microscopic disease that might have spread to other parts of the body. Radiotherapy is used following surgery to take care of any residual local disease in the breast or chest wall. (See page 92 for further information on chemotherapy treatment.)

Tamoxifen is now considered the first line of hormone therapy for postmenopausal women. In premenopausal women, chemotherapy is the first line of treatment—the most common agents being cytoxan, methotrexate, and fluorouracil; another common treatment regimen includes doxorubicin and cytoxan. In premenopausal women the major side effects of chemotherapy include low blood counts, early menopause, ulcerations of the lining of the mouth, and increased tearing. At this time there are some experimental trials looking at higher doses of doxorubicin and cytoxan in women where the tumor has spread to lymph nodes.

Many report that it takes six months to recuperate from a full course of chemotherapy. It can be an ordeal but it's an ordeal that's worth it. Nonetheless, it takes some preparation. Before undergoing chemotherapy, a patient is advised to organize her life very well. Cut back on the hours that you work, get help at home, and inform family members that you will need their support in very real ways, both physically and emotionally. Those patients who endure the process most successfully do so by realistically altering their routine to accommodate this grueling endeavor, rather than by attempting to live up to a "macho" image.

Postsurgical Hormone Therapy—Tamoxifen

There may not yet be a way to prevent breast cancer. But in postmenopausal women who have had breast cancer, the anti-estrogen drug tamoxifen has been proven to lower the recurrence of cancer by up to 30 percent overall and reduce the appearance of new breast cancers in the opposite breast by 30 to 40 percent. For reasons not even the most respected specialists understand, conventional chemotherapy tends not to be as effective in most postmenopausal women, which is one reason that tamoxifen is so attractive. Tamoxifen has both estrogen and anti-estrogen properties and in the breast acts like an anti-estrogen. Hormone therapy, which like chemotherapy is a systemic treatment, is clearly effective in postmenopausal women. Tamoxifen works as an estrogen blocker, minimizing the negative effects of estrogen, while providing many of the same positive effects that estrogen provides.

Tamoxifen cannot be called a wonder drug. It also has side effects. The most common complaint is the development of hot flashes. There is also a low risk of blood clots and of endometrial cancer. But tamoxifen does seem to have progress written all over it. Among other things, tamoxifen apparently has the ability to provide the same benefits that we associate with estrogen, including lowering the risk of both heart disease and osteoporosis.

Because of tamoxifen's promising nature in lowering the incidence of recurrent and new breast cancer in already diagnosed women, it is now being investigated as a drug that might be able to prevent this disease altogether. In a multi-institutional study, tamoxifen is being given to selected women in the hopes of preventing breast cancer. Investigators have been very excited about this project because it's really the first well-thought-out study aimed specifically at preventing breast cancer.

However, there is controversy regarding the use of tamoxifen. The National Cancer Institute has alerted physicians that twenty-five women taking tamoxifen in a clinical trial for women already diagnosed with breast cancer developed endometrial (uterine) cancer. The Cancer Therapy Evaluation Program of the NCI advised that all patients be notified of the risk and that consent forms be revised to include the information. The risk for the development of endometrial cancer is very low but it exists nonetheless. The risk exists for women taking tamoxifen after mastectomy and for those taking the drug in the hopes of preventing breast cancer. Most investigators stress, though, that the risk of developing endometrial cancer is less than the risk of developing breast cancer.

After Breast Cancer

"Of course I was scared. I was afraid I wouldn't live to see my grandchildren grow. I was afraid this meant the end of my sex life. I was afraid I would be going through this alone. Lucky for me, I was wrong on all counts."

Margie Gersmire (age 58)

THE DIAGNOSIS OF breast cancer does not have to be a death sentence. Once you have been diagnosed and treated, you play a very important role in making sure that you are a patient who will prove that it is possible to recover from breast cancer. You must continue to see your doctor. Many women find this difficult to do, and put off appointments because of the very natural fears they have regarding a recurrence. Put your fears on hold and keep your appointments.

You will also want to continue to get help when you need it, whether this means keeping in touch with your support group, finding your own therapist, or simply continuing to modify your business schedule or to have help around the house. You may be fine, but you're going to want to stay that way. Although some might call it pampering, you might prefer to think that getting help when and where you need it is being in charge of your recovery process.

On a Positive Note

"I will not go silently. I will go shouting into that dark night; enough is enough."

Sherry Kohlenberg, *The New York Times Magazine*, August 15, 1993

WHEN DISCUSSING breast cancer, I've noticed that the un-initiated—those who do not have breast cancer but think about having it—tend to panic. There is, perhaps, no health concern affecting women that is more able to bring fear to a voice and panic into the eyes of a woman approaching midlife than breast cancer. But fear and panic serve no use. Instead, we need to use statistics to help us win the research battle and not let the numbers scare us. We need to arm ourselves with the knowledge that we have a lot of catching up to do with regard to useful information and research and funding. But we also know much more about how to care for ourselves, what to look for, and what to do.

We owe it to ourselves to stay vigilant regarding self-examination and checkups and to help those friends whose fear may overcome their better judgment, by urging them to keep their necessary appointments. We also owe it to ourselves to remember and remind others of how much progress has been made.

The history of breast cancer and its treatment breakthroughs presents a mirror for the progress women have made socially and politically. When breast cancer was first discovered, women almost always died of the disease and they had no say in their own treatment. Times changed. Corsets and stays were abandoned. Bras were invented. Women went to work. Women voted. Women found their voice in many ways. Women began to have their say. Though the progress they were making had actually taken centuries to realize, the results seemed fierce and fast and certainly were profound. In much the same way, it seems to have taken a very long time to recognize the devastating magnitude of the breast cancer epidemic in this country. Progress has been hard won and slow, but the attendant results regarding identifying and treating the disease seem to be gaining momentum every day.

COLON AND RECTAL CANCERS

My grandfather died from cancer of the colon. At the age of sixty-three, my father was diagnosed with the same disease. I believe that I am destined to get it too. It doesn't scare me. In some ways I'm relieved because I know what my demon is and I am working hard to catch it before it gets me.

MANAGING RADIATION THERAPY

While the notion of radiation is frightening, so much progress has been made in the area of radiation therapy that the process is less frightening than you might think. Precisely because radiation seems like something out of science fiction, a brief grounding in the facts of radiation is probably helpful.

In 1895, Wilhelm Conrad Roentgen published a paper entitled "On a New Kind of Ray." He named his new ray the X ray. Roentgen received the first Nobel Prize in physics in 1901, and the scientific discipline of radiation became extraordinarily popular. About the same time a French scientist, Antoine-Henri Becquerel, discovered that the radiation given off by uranium was similar to X rays. Marie Sklodowska, a student at the Sorbonne, and her future husband, Pierre Curie, continued the work Becquerel had started and found a substance in the ore containing uranium with at least two million times as much radiation as uranium; they called it radium. In 1903 the Nobel Prize in physics was shared by Becquerel and the Curies.

Almost immediately, it was discovered that X rays and radium damaged body tissues and the application of radiation to treat cancer was begun. Now, varying forms of radiation treatment are used on approximately half of all cancer patients. External-beam radiation, radiotherapy, is a combination of gamma radiation and X rays, forms of electromagnetic radiation. (X rays are produced by X-ray machines, while gamma rays are produced by the decay of radioactive isotopes such as cobalt.) The treatments are divided into ranges or voltages of electromagnetic radiation. Superficial radiation is the lowest range, orthovoltage is the medium range, and supervoltage is highest. Two techniques are used in the application of external-beam therapy. Brachytherapy is localized—given within or very close to the target organ. Teletherapy is given from a distance of several feet or more and uses only an orthovoltage or supervoltage machine.

Internal radiation is the second type of radiation treatment; it relies upon the injection or insertion of radioactive material directly into the tumor. The doses of radiation therapy are carefully adjusted to kill cancer cells while minimally affecting the adjacent normal cells.

Radiation therapy may be used in combination with surgery and/or chemotherapy as adjuvant treatment or as the sole form of therapy. It may also be used as a palliative treatment in advanced cancer.

Side Effects

Side effects of radiation treatment vary widely, ranging from none to severe. One of the most common reactions to external-beam radiation is weariness and lethargy. If you are fatigued, you will have to adjust your activity level and get more rest. Other reactions include hair loss and changes to the skin. Your skin may become dry, red, and itchy, and you may also notice it is darker. Applying vitamin E to the area may help. Some women also experience nausea and vomiting, which can be controlled with antinausea drugs.

My father had an intuition that he would get cancer of the colon. He has always watched what he eats and goes to aerobics every day; every year *he* insisted that he get a proctoscopy. When he was sixty-three, he told his doctor that he wanted a colonoscopy instead, since this exam examines more of the colon. Just beyond what the proctoscope would have seen was a polyp that turned out to be cancer. He underwent a colon resection. That was nine years ago.

With this kind of family history I decided when I turned forty that it was the time for me to be vigilant. I talked to my father's surgeon about what screening tests were appropriate for me. I checked my stools for occult blood with a hemoccult test, even though now we know that this is a very nonspecific test and will miss cancers many times. I knew I had to get really serious about the early detection of this disease once I turned forty. So for my fortieth birthday I gave myself a colonoscopy. Why not? I value my life and how better to celebrate it than to figure out a way to maintain my quality of life and have some influence on my longevity. The test was easy. And what do you know . . . my doctor found an abnormal polyp and removed it. It wasn't cancer—but I believe it was a small time bomb. This was the best birthday present I could have ever given myself.

To this day I schedule important medical tests around my birthday. It's an easy way to remember to get them done. I get my pelvic and

LIVING WITH CHEMOTHERAPY

Chemotherapy is a systemic treatment that affects the entire body—not one particular area—and therein lies its blessing and its curse. While this systemic effect is necessary to fight a cancer that has spread, the treatment will also affect the entire body and not just the cancer. Chemotherapy refers to the use of cytotoxic chemicals—chemicals that kill cells—and such chemicals are lethal not only to cancerous cells but to some normal cells as well.

The term "chemotherapy" is attributed to Paul Erhlich, a German scientist who tested the usefulness of certain chemicals and antibiotics as treatments for diseases in animals. The strategy was applied to cancer in animals by George Clowes in the United States in the early 1900s. It was during World War II that the strategy of using chemicals to combat cancer in humans took shape; nitrogen mustard gas, a secret of the chemical warfare program, provided the clue that chemicals might be able to kill cancer cells without killing the patient. In 1943 at Yale–New Haven Medical Center, work was begun on applying the techniques of chemical warfare to patients with Hodgkin's disease and other lymphomas. By 1948, nitrogen-mustard compounds were shown to be effective in human leukemia. That year Dr. Sidney Farber applied a technique using a compound that inhibits normal cell metabolism, called an antimetabolite, on children with leukemia. The antimetabolite, called aminopterin, was startlingly effective. Such results spurred further research efforts. By the 1950s it was observed that the combination of certain treatments could effectively cure tuberculosis in children and the notion of combining therapies in cancer treatment was born. In children with leukemia, aminopterin, which caused dramatic but temporary remission of the cancer, was combined with other antileukemic agents (to attack the cancer cells that had become resistant) and given for a year or more of maintenance therapy. Many children were cured and the lives of many others were extended.

Chemotherapy was first thought to be effective in treating leukemia, a cancer of the blood, since the chemicals moved through the system via the blood, as did the cancer. Eventually it was used for any cancer that had metastasized, or spread to other organs. There were two problems with chemotherapy in the early stages: there were so many cancer cells that the drug could not attack them all, and some cells became resistant to the chemicals. Hence, adjuvant chemotherapy was born. Because the results of adjuvant therapy have been so positive, such systemic treatment is now given for many different types of cancers.

Despite the extraordinary progress that has been made in the application of chemotherapy, the public tends to view chemotherapy negatively, possibly because in the early development of chemotherapy the treatment itself caused such severe side effects. While side effects are still part of the picture, they are not nearly as severe today and there are drugs to alleviate them.

Treatments

Chemotherapy treatments are given in cycles. The cycles vary, usually from 21 to 28 days. In a 21-day cycle, you would receive an injection every 21 days. In a 28-day cycle, you would receive an injection every 28 days. The cycle and the duration of treatment depend on the type of tumor, the severity of the cancer, and the drugs that are chosen. These are all points you should discuss with your physician before your treatment starts.

Side Effects of Adjuvant Chemotherapy

Because a woman undergoing systemic treatment for breast cancer usually has no symptoms caused by the cancer, she almost always feels worse when undergoing chemotherapy. In other words, there is no way to go but down. However, if the cancer has metastasized, she probably already has felt certain symptoms as a result, and because of this, chemotherapy may even make the patient feel better.

The side effects of chemotherapy, which vary according to the treatment and the individual, commonly include nausea, vomiting, loss of appetite, and, in certain cases, hair loss. Some women also experience sexual problems, such as vaginal dryness or soreness. If you have an IUD, certain chemotherapies may interact negatively with it, causing irregular bleeding or an infection. If the diaphragm is your birth control method, you may also find that you begin to have problems with it. Mouth sores, conjunctivitis, runny nose and eyes, and diarrhea or constipation are other side effects; headaches or bleeding gums may also occur. Extreme side effects include chronic bone marrow suppression and secondary cancers.

continued

While all this sounds bleak, you may not encounter all or any of these side effects. And they are temporary. When your chemotherapy is completed, you will probably not bounce back immediately, because your body has just undergone an extraordinary and rigorous treatment, but you *will* bounce back. It may take up to six months to feel like your normal self. During this time it is important not to push yourself too hard, or you may become depressed at what seems like slow progress. Consider that you have just undergone a battle in which survival itself is a victory, and reward yourself with the necessary rest and recuperation you not only deserve, but need in order to make as healthy a recovery as possible.

breast exams and my colonoscopy and mammogram every March. This way there's no excuse for missing them.

Now I know there will be those who will say that the colonoscopy isn't necessary that often. But I have made this a personal choice for *me*—and I believe that that's what matters for most women. We gather information, look at our own lives, and then make individual choices about how best to take care of ourselves with guidance from our physicians. I feel very comfortable with the screening procedures I have outlined for myself and I believe you have to be just as comfortable with whatever you establish for you.

Colon cancer doesn't just spring up overnight out of nowhere. This cancer develops slowly, usually as a polyp, which undergoes malignant degeneration. Because of this genesis, a doctor will usually remove any polyp that is found on an examination.

A great deal of progress has been made recently in understanding and diagnosing colon and rectal cancer, including the recent discovery of two genes that work as markers for colon cancer. Colorectal cancers are often curable if caught early. More than 20 percent of colon cancers are hereditary. Colon cancer is linked to ovarian cancer, so that if your mother had ovarian cancer, you are at risk not only for ovarian cancer, but also for colon cancer. Thus, if you have a family history of colon or ovarian cancer and if you are forty or over, regular screening for colon cancer is imperative.

It is conceivable that in the near future you will be able to get a blood test for the colon cancer genetic marker. Then you will know if

MINORITY WOMEN AND CANCER—THE ACCESS ISSUE

"The U.S. medical system prides itself as being the best in the world, yet millions of its citizens are unable to get access to health care. It makes no sense to have technological advances and preventive services that are not available to all persons."

Byllye Y. Avery (age 57)

The news when it comes to black women getting equal and sufficient health care is not good. In fact, it's downright bad. African American women are more likely than white women to be diagnosed with breast cancer when the cancer is already in an advanced stage. That is to say that while 53 percent of diagnosed white women are in stage 1 (in situ or contained tumor growths), only 42 percent of African American women are diagnosed with stage 1 disease. In 1992 the National Cancer Institute (NCI) noted that 80 percent of white women survive for five years or more, but only 62 percent of African American women do. The same poor survival is true for cervical cancer and the other gynecological cancers.

Alarmingly, the gap seems to be widening. The NCI recently announced that the death rate from breast cancer for white women fell 5.5 percent between 1989 and 1992 while black women experienced a 2.6 percent rise. Although figures aren't available yet for Hispanic and Asian American women, overall Asian American women have the lowest incidence of breast cancer and Hispanic women mirror their African American counterparts more closely.

Is there an easy explanation for the disparity? Yes and no. While access to good health care is one important issue, studies looking at why some women undergo screening tests and others do not have been insufficient. One might easily project that poverty has a great deal to do with this skew, but this is not the only factor: education, family background, health-care coverage, environment, diet, genetics, and other fac-

continued

tors need to be analyzed in an effort to motivate all women to take advantage of screening tests for breast and cervical cancer and to benefit from early detection.

However, that is easier said than done. The public hospitals in cities and counties around the country are in fiscal crisis. They are scrambling in these tough economic times, trying to figure out what services they can afford to continue to offer and which ones must go. And one aspect of local health care that will likely die are the neighborhood clinics that serve as outreach posts for the hospitals. These clinics are the hands and fingers that reach out to people in the community who—because of fear, intimidation, cost, or inconvenience—might never make it to the larger medical centers. As many of these clinics shut their doors, I believe many of the city and county hospitals that have for decades provided care to minorities will cut back in draconian fashion or be forced to close their doors. The bottom line, I fear, is that even more women and their children will be cut off from the health-care system. That will translate into more women delaying diagnoses and more women dying.

While there may not be easy and fast solutions to the fiscal problems in today's health-care climate, as a physician I believe we can't afford to turn our backs on this huge segment of our population. We need to look at the whole picture and find ways to absorb everyone into the health-care scheme.

you are at particular risk for developing this cancer and you and your doctor can be vigilant in your screenings. However, at the present time, no such test is available. There are three or four genes involved in these tumors and figuring out which ones will prove useful is not yet clear. Only the gene for familial colonic polyposis is close to being usable for testing. This marker may be present in a member of a family who has inherited this gene and may herald the risk of developing this cancer. Despite the current lack of usable and reliable tests, genetics marks one of the most exciting areas of development in cancer research.

Symptoms, Screening, and Diagnosis

"I started having fresh blood in my stools. I chalked it up to hemorrhoids for a while. But then it just didn't go away. I was lucky. This was the first sign I had of my tumor."

Heraldine Hannon (age 63)

THE MOST COMMON early symptom of colon cancer is a change in bowel habits, like blood in the stool or sudden constipation, though a change in bowel habits does not necessarily indicate cancer. Other gastrointestinal (GI) symptoms include abdominal cramping, alternating constipation and diarrhea, loss of appetite, weight loss, and weakness. The most serious and critical symptom is rectal bleeding. While most rectal bleeding is the result of hemorrhoids or a fissure you should contact your doctor if the symptoms last more than a few days. Depending on the severity of your symptoms, your physician will perform some or all of the following tests:

1. A physical examination. Your complete physical exam will include a digital rectal exam. Your physician will wear a thin latex glove and insert a finger into the rectum to feel for growths.
2. Laboratory tests. Your physician may want to take a stool sample to test for occult (invisible to the human eye) blood. A routine blood test may be taken to check for anemia that can result from persistent internal bleeding from a tumor, and you may receive a blood test to check for CEA (carcinoembryonic antigen)—a tumor marker that is elevated in about 28 percent of early colon and rectal cancers.
3. Special diagnostic tests. Your doctor may recommend a scoping— a look inside the bowel with a special telescopelike instrument. In one of these tests, a proctoscope, sigmoidoscope, or colonoscope is inserted into the rectum and colon to view the colon and tumor mass directly. Most of the time, these examinations don't require any type of anesthesia. However, some doctors prefer to give their patients undergoing a colonoscopy a little intravenous sedation to

take the edge off. During the exam the doctor is able to snare a small polyp (a premalignant growth) and remove it or obtain a biopsy of a larger tumor. The tissue is then examined by a pathologist to determine whether it is benign or malignant. In some cases a barium enema is useful. After a barium solution is introduced into the colon via an enema, X rays are taken of the patient's abdomen over a one-hour period. Masses in the colon and rectal area will show up on the X ray as dark shadows.

Stages

Colon and rectal cancer are divided into stages, from 0 through 5.

Stage 0. Stage 0, also called in situ, is a very early cancer usually found in a polyp. It's sometimes called Dukes stage A colon cancer, after Dr. C. E. Dukes, who created a staging system for colon cancer in 1932.

Stage 1. The cancer has spread inside the wall of the colon, through the first and second layers of the lining, but not to the muscular wall or outside of the colon. (Also known as Dukes stage A and B.)

Stage 2. The cancer has spread deeper into the wall of the colon or even through the wall to nearby tissues, but not to any lymph nodes. (Also known as Dukes stage B.)

Stage 3. The cancer has spread to surrounding lymph nodes. (Also known as Dukes stage C.)

Stage 4. The cancer has spread to other parts of the body. (Also known as Dukes stage D.)

Recurrent Colon Cancer or Stage 5

The cancer has come back after being treated, either in the colon or another part of the body. (Recurrent colon cancer often reappears in the liver and/or lungs.)

Treatment

If colon or rectal cancer is caught early, either can be cured with current available therapy. There are few cancers of which this can be said. Current therapy involves surgery either with or without follow-up chemotherapy. If the cancer is diagnosed early enough, it may be removed without even cutting into the abdomen. If a microscopic portion of a polyp has become malignant, the surgeon may be quite comfortable with just locally excising the mass, in an operation is called a polypectomy. The surgeon inserts a scope into the rectum or colon. The abnormal polyp is snared and removed at its base.

If the tumor is larger, the tumor and some of the adjacent healthy bowel will be removed. This procedure involves abdominal surgery. If a very small amount of tissue is removed, the procedure is called a wedge resection. If more of the colon must be removed, the procedure is called a bowel resection. Usually it is possible to sew the edges of the bowel back together, obviating the need for a colostomy. If this is impossible due to the extent of the tumor, an obstruction, or contamination, the surgeon will make a colostomy opening or stoma on the outside of the body for waste to pass through. A disposable bag is glued to the abdomen to gather the waste. In some cases, the colostomy may be necessary only while the colon is healing. In other cases, when there is not enough colon available to be sewn together, it is permanent. The colostomy bag does not show under clothing, and most people can maintain their colostomy without any special help. Radiation therapy and chemotherapy may be used in conjunction with surgery.

As with other cancers, treatment for colon cancer depends upon the stage at which the cancer is diagnosed. I'd like to stress that when diagnosed early, colon cancer is completely curable. In addition to the excellent screening tests available today, a strong family history should be enough reason for you to see your doctor. There is also a correlation between this disease and cigarette smoking (yet another reason to quit). A low-fiber, high-fat diet may also play a role.

It should also be noted that the incidence of colon cancer increases remarkably with age; it occurs ten times more often in those over sixty-five than in forty-five-year-olds. All the more reason to be watchful and conscientious about screening for this common cancer as you age—especially since the chances are, if you catch it early, you'll live through it and live through it well. Once you turn fifty, you should undergo a colonoscopy. If it is normal you may be told to get checkups every two to three years after that. During your forties a yearly rectal exam as part of your pelvic exam should be done, and depending on your risk factors, a colonoscopy may be indicated every two to three years.

Hemoccult tests that check for occult blood in the stool are very sensitive but not very specific. And while this test can be a good companion test, you shouldn't rely on it as the only screening tool. If you have hemorrhoids or an anal fissure, blood from these areas may give you a false positive test. On the other hand a colon cancer may bleed intermittently and a hemoccult test may miss the time when the tumor is bleeding. Because of these shortcomings, experts suggest that the hemoccult test be combined with one of the invasive procedures.

THE GYNECOLOGICAL CANCERS

Cancer can occur in any of the female reproductive organs—the vulva, vagina, cervix, uterus (including the body of the uterus and its lining, the endometrium), ovaries, and fallopian tubes. The different cancers have different symptoms, screening methods, and treatment. Fortunately, most of theses cancers are easy to detect in their early stages and afford excellent cure rates early on.

Cervical Cancer

"I was a child of the sixties and have had a very colorful, diversified, and active sexual life. How many sexual partners have I had? I'm not sure. But I do know that the life I lived then puts me at risk for cancer of the cervix now."

Patricia Geller (age 52)

CERVICAL CANCER IS a common cancer of the female reproductive organs. The highest rate of incidence is between the ages of thirty-five and fifty-five. The cancer is slow growing, and when it is caught at the precancerous stage (cervical dysplasia), it is almost 100 percent curable.

Thanks to the Pap smear (or Papanicolaou test), cervical cancer can be caught at the dysplasia stage or early on and eradicated before it advances from the cervix. The incidence of and mortality from invasive cervical cancer in the United States has decreased dramatically as a result of the Pap smear. In fact, the test serves as a model for effective screening techniques for the early diagnosis of other cancers. Because it can detect abnormal cells even before they become cancerous, the Pap smear allows for effective treatment before major surgery is necessary.

Its effectiveness depends very much on how the smear is performed and where it is read. A single smear is 50 to 90 percent reliable, depending on the technique and the experience of the lab. This is an area where it might be wise to ask questions up front about the accuracy of your health-care provider and the lab that interprets the specimens. To do this, simply ask what the lab's percentage of accuracy is. Anything under 98 percent should be questioned. In good hands, the Pap smear is very effective in diagnosing cervical cancer. The newest innovation is a computer program called Auto Pap that allows the lab to double-check Pap smears that appear negative. It improves the accuracy rate of the Pap smear to about 98 percent.

A yearly Pap smear is recommended. It's particularly important for women who are sexually active and/or whose partners do not use condoms; this is because cervical cancer is more likely to develop if you've had a sexually transmitted disease, such as herpes or genital warts. Your chance of developing cervical cancer also increases if you began having sex before you were eighteen or if you have had many pregnancies, beginning at an early age.

Cervical cancer grows unnoticed, without symptoms, so the Pap smear is essential for early diagnosis and successful treatment. Almost every woman with cervical cancer who is diagnosed and treated early is cured.

A Pap test should be performed in conjunction with a pelvic exam. Most gynecologists recommend annual exams and Pap smears after forty. Once a woman approaches her fortieth birthday she should have a conversation with her physician about risk factors, any possible symptoms, and a plan for screening tests that is individualized and sensible.

The risk of carcinoma of the cervix peaks at age forty. Women are at a higher risk of developing invasive cervical cancer if they have stopped having regular Pap smears, which many women do after having their children.

If you do not have regular Pap smears, you should begin to do so. If you notice any vaginal bleeding between periods or after menopause (if you're not taking ERT), or bloody or watery discharge from the vagina that is smelly and sometimes heavy, or if you have bleeding after intercourse, you should inform your doctor and make an appointment for a pelvic exam and Pap smear. In advanced stages, a dull backache and generally poor health may also be symptoms.

Treatment

If the cancer is diagnosed in situ, it can be destroyed by laser surgery, cauterization, or freezing. The five-year cure rate for the cancer when discovered in situ is almost 100 percent. In the type of surgery most often used, called a cone biopsy, a cone-shaped wedge of the cervix is removed. If the cells at the border of the wedge are normal, then the biopsy is considered to have removed all of the cancerous cells. If they are not, another biopsy is performed. If the cancer is invasive—that is, if it has spread into the uterus—a hysterectomy is required. If a biopsy reveals that the cancer has spread to other organs, chemotherapy will also be required.

Radiation therapy is a treatment option for early invasive cervical cancer. In fact, the cure rates among women with early invasive cancer are almost identical for surgical and radiation therapy treatment. (See "Managing Radiation Therapy," page 90.)

Uterine or Endometrial Cancer

Women with few or no children are at higher risk for endometrial cancer. Other risk factors include obesity, hypertension, diabetes, and being on estrogen replacement therapy (when this therapy does *not* include progesterone).

Symptoms, Screening, and Diagnosis

There is no screening test for endometrial cancer that is as straightforward as the Pap smear is for cervical cancer. Although the Pap smear itself is used in screening, it does not usually detect endometrial cancer precisely because the cancer begins within the uterus. Presently, an endometrial biopsy is the best test and can diagnose this cancer in its earliest stages. It is being explored as a screening test in high-risk women.

Early symptoms of uterine cancer include abnormal vaginal bleeding. The blood is red or brown in premenopausal women and a watery, bloody discharge in postmenopausal women. More than 75 percent of the cases of uterine cancer occur in postmenopausal women, so a bloody discharge is alarming. If you are postmenopausal and have bloody discharge, you should consult your physician immediately. Only a definitive evaluation and diagnosis can ascertain the cause.

After a routine examination that will include a pelvic exam and taking a complete health history, your doctor will do a Pap smear, even though they are less than 50 percent effective in diagnosing uterine cancer. Special laboratory tests are necessary to specifically diagnose uterine cancer and the stage of the cancer. These include:

- *Aspiration Sampling of the Endometrium.* Tissue is taken from the endometrium, the lining of the uterine cavity, via a syringe inserted through the cervical opening, and then analyzed for cancer cells. Fifteen percent of cancers are not detected by this method.
- *Dilation and Curettage of the Endometrium.* The patient is anesthetized. The uterine lining is scraped out with an instrument called a curette and any growths are removed. Fragments of the recovered tissue are then checked for cancer. Cancers are rarely missed when this method is used.

Other tests may be required depending on the individual situation, but these two tests are done in the majority of cases.

Treatment

For cancer of the endometrium, surgery is the most common treatment. When surgery is the treatment of choice, one of two operations will be used. The first operation is a total abdominal hysterectomy and bilateral salpingo-oophorectomy. The surgery involves removal of the uterus, fallopian tubes, and ovaries via an incision in the abdomen. In some cases, lymph nodes in the pelvic area may also be removed.

The second operation is a radical hysterectomy, which involves removal of the uterus, fallopian tubes, ovaries, and part of the vagina.

Once again, lymph nodes in the surrounding area will be removed.

Radiation and chemotherapy are used in combination with surgery to kill remaining cancerous cells. External-beam or internal radiation may be used (see page 90). Chemotherapy may be administered orally, in pill form, or intravenously. Hormone therapy may also be used and is usually administered in pill form.

Tamoxifen and Endometrial Cancer

In early clinical trials, the results using tamoxifen as an adjuvant therapy for women with breast cancer were very positive. In 1989 early results of the trials headed by Dr. Bernard Fisher for the National Surgical Breast and Bowel Project (NSBBP) found that women treated with tamoxifen had a 40 percent reduction in new breast cancers. There were side benefits, too. It seems that tamoxifen works much as estrogen does to regulate the balance in serum lipids in postmenopausal women. In other words, tamoxifen was found to lower cholesterol and possibly to lower the risk of coronary artery disease. In addition, tamoxifen was found to prevent bone loss and thus potentially lower the risk of osteoporosis and hip fractures among the elderly.

But treatment with tamoxifen was also found to pose certain serious risks, most notable among them an increased risk in incidence of endometrial cancer. Endometrial cancer was three times more common in women taking tamoxifen. But NSBBP statisticians have found that the benefits still outweigh the risks, since the chances of developing breast cancer are much higher than developing endometrial cancer. So tamoxifen remains a beneficial treatment for breast cancer in most cases. The most important thing regarding trials involving tamoxifen is that women who participate should be warned of the risk of uterine cancer. Then the choice of whether to proceed should be the individual's.

Ovarian Cancer

"Ovarian cancer scares the hell out of me. It may not be very common, but it's all we read about."

Suzana York (age 40)

The comedian Gilda Radner's death in 1989 from ovarian cancer made the cancer a household word, even though it is not one of the most common cancers. Women who were not at risk began to worry about it, and suddenly it seemed to be everywhere. It should be remembered that even though ovarian cancer is the fifth most common cancer in women, it is still relatively rare, occurring in approximately 2 percent of women. At age seventy, the incidence peaks at 4 percent.

While the public paranoia regarding ovarian cancer probably took its toll on many women's peace of mind, it has also served to increase the funding for important research.

About 22,000 women are diagnosed annually in the United States, and 70 percent of those are diagnosed with advanced disease. There is approximately a 70 percent mortality rate within the first five years. Ovarian cancer is a silent cancer with very few early symptoms. Ironically, when caught early, it has one of the highest cure rates of any cancer that afflicts women. But that's the problem: it is rarely caught early. Because so many women are diagnosed with advanced disease, it is often difficult or impossible to remove all the cancer surgically and the mortality rate is high. But current research is moving toward better diagnostic techniques and improved adjuvant chemotherapy.

Screening, Symptoms, and Diagnosis

Unfortunately, there really aren't any early warning signs for ovarian cancer. By the time a woman even complains of satiety and bloating, there may already be advanced disease. And these symptoms could also indicate a host of other ailments, from fibroid tumors to ulcers. But if you notice that you seem to be full soon after eating or that you are bloated for no apparent reason, see your doctor. Abnormal periods are not a sign of ovarian cancer.

Early detection is often a matter of chance. A woman may experience pelvic pain that is the result of a twisting ovarian mass. Or, during a routine pelvic exam a suspicious mass may be discovered on the ovary. In fact, the best screening test to date is a good pelvic examination with bi-manual palpation. This means that one of the doctor's fingers should be in your vagina and another in your rectum while the other hand presses on your abdomen. This way the ovaries can be felt between the two hands.

There are problems with some of the present screening tests, the most important of which involves screening for high levels of a compound called CA 125, which is found in the blood serum. The majority of women with ovarian cancer do show elevated levels of CA 125. Thus, for those who have been diagnosed, CA 125 is a good marker. But one problem with CA 125 as a general screening procedure is that it is not specific for ovarian cancer and is often found to be elevated in benign conditions such as pregnancy, and in endometriosis, pelvic inflammatory disease (PID), and even other cancers. In addition, in terms of early detection, CA 125 is elevated in only approximately half the cases. These major drawbacks indicate that CA 125 used alone will probably never achieve the rate of reliability in screening that the Pap smear has for cervical cancer. For high-risk patients (those with two or more first-degree relatives with ovarian cancer), some doctors suggest a combined screening that includes a pelvic exam, a vaginal sonogram, and testing for elevated levels of CA 125.

While there is no adequate screening procedure as yet, ovarian cancer is sometimes detected in a routine pelvic examination, particularly in women who have been through menopause. The woman who does not go for an annual pelvic is without an ally when it comes to detecting such a stealthy foe as ovarian cancer. Many women cease to keep up the yearly routine of pelvic examinations after menopause. Since the median age for ovarian cancer is over sixty, it makes sense to remain vigilant regarding yearly examinations. After menopause a woman's ovaries shrink and should not be palpable. If you are past menopause and your doctor says she or he can feel your ovaries, there is a cause for concern. Since early detection is key to a successful prognosis, the yearly pelvic exam is an essential for postmenopausal women. In addition, it can find other problems, such as sexually transmitted diseases (the rate of STDs in older people is on the rise in this country). Go get checked.

Treatment

The surgery for a woman diagnosed with ovarian cancer is a complete hysterectomy and oophorectomy (removal of the uterus and ovaries and removal of the omentum, which contains the lymph nodes), depending on the stage of the disease. (See "Endometrial Cancer," above, for surgical procedures.) She will then be treated with adjuvant chemotherapy in order to destroy as many residual cancer cells as possible. It is worthwhile to note that if you are facing this diagnosis, it's a good idea to find a gynecologist with oncology training.

TAXOL

A great deal of progress has been made recently in treating ovarian cancer patients with taxol. Research on taxol as a chemotherapeutic agent began in the late 1970s. The drug is only now being used in clinical trials, but the results are already significant. A recent study of 48 women with advanced, previously treated ovarian cancer showed that there was a regression of the tumor in 16 of the women and one woman's cancer disappeared completely. One of the most exciting advances has recently been announced by the National Cancer Institute. In a phase 3 clinical trial involving 200 women with advanced ovarian cancer, taxol in combination with cisplatin has increased median survival time by 50 percent.

Taxol is made from the bark of the Pacific yew tree, and it takes 38,000 trees to make 55 pounds of taxol, which is only enough to treat about 1,200 patients. The recent synthesis of taxol has been heralded by conservationists as well as doctors and patients.

Between advancements in chemotherapeutic treatment—most important, the advent of taxol—and continued efforts at improved diagnostic techniques, the future for those at risk for ovarian cancer looks better and better.

LUNG CANCER

> *"Something is out of whack when women who smoke are more terrified of breast cancer, about which they can do little, than of lung cancer, which they can effectively prevent—and when one of the main reasons they continue to puff away is that they fear the modest weight gain often attendant on quitting."*
>
> Katha Pollitt

WE HAVE COME a long way, as the cigarette ad would have us believe. But along the way we've picked up some rather stupid habits. The worst is smoking, which the ad in question and others promote, flagrantly targeting the female market. In the last decade of the twentieth century, we are seeing a disastrous increase in the occurrence of lung cancer in women. And women are not kicking the habit in the same numbers as men. Men have been successfully warned not only regarding the connection between smoking and lung disease, but also regarding the connection between smoking and heart disease. Women are not quitting as much as men because:

- It is hard to quit and smoking is an addiction.
- The fact that women die of heart disease as often as men do is only now becoming public knowledge. Women have not been sufficiently warned about the correlation between smoking and heart disease.
- Society still sanctions thinness as an important goal for women, often to the exclusion of considering the health of women. Sadly, many women don't quit because they don't want to gain weight, even though the consequences of smoking are so much more dire than those of any moderate weight gain.

We need to stress that the rate at which women die from smoking will increase into the twenty-first century. In 1900 there were fewer than 50,000 deaths attributable to cancer in the United States. Now, more than half a million deaths per year are caused by cancer. This is due to three factors, the simplest being that the population of the United States has risen so dramatically. In addition, a greater proportion of the population is aging. The third factor is the one that provokes both investigation and fear: that is, that the risk per individual has risen over time.

The risk per individual is debated, analyzed, and sometimes used to instill fear—that our water is contaminated, our food is killing us because of the pesticide content, our air is poisoned by pollution. But the truth behind the statistic is told in the history of tobacco. The single factor driving up the risk of cancer in the population is smoking.

Eighty-five percent of the cases of lung cancer are attributable to smoking. Smoking is the largest preventable cause of premature death and disability in the United States. Although lung cancer is still more common in men, the rate of death and disability for women is steadily increasing and will continue to do so for years to come.

If you smoke more than a pack a day your risk of lung cancer increases twentyfold. If you quit smoking, your risk of lung cancer will decrease, although never to the level of a person who has never smoked. However, the sooner you quit smoking, the sooner your lungs will begin to recover. Unfortunately, many people do not quit smoking until they get a wake-up call—a major heart attack, cancer, or crippling pulmonary disease.

Cigarette smoking is a powerful addiction, and it can be tremendously difficult to quit. If you want to try to quit, you may very well need help to do so. Also keep these tips in mind:

1. Set a date when you will go "cold turkey."
2. Before that date, switch to a milder brand of cigarette and begin to smoke only half of your cigarette.
3. Tell your friends and family of your plans, asking for their support.
4. Change your daily routine as much as is possible to avoid situations that encourage you to smoke.
5. Don't frequent places that encourage you to smoke, such as bars and parties.
6. Plan activities that you can engage in when the urge to smoke hits.
7. If you have trouble quitting—and many people do—consult your doctor regarding the nicotine patch or nicotine gum, either of which can help you kick the chemical addiction.
8. Find a support group and keep trying.
9. Don't assume it's hopeless if you go back to smoking after quitting once. The odds are actually better that you will quit for good if you have quit once or twice before.
10. Most important—never give up!

In the late 1980s, lung cancer surpassed breast cancer as the leading cause of death in women, and as stated before, the mortality rate for lung cancer in women has not plateaued and will not do so until sometime early in the next century. While there is a higher incidence now of lung cancer among African American men than white men, the numbers for women of both races are the same. After World War II, women took up smoking in greater numbers than ever before and women have been slower to quit than men. Whereas in the past men have been encouraged to give up smoking (because it is definitely linked to the increased risk of a heart attack), no such targeting of women has been done. In fact in recent years women have been preferentially targeted by the tobacco industry. The industry has shamelessly gone after young and minority women and seduced them with images of liberation and sexiness. They neglect to show how sexy a woman is after years of smoking when she's prematurely wrinkled, gasping for breath, and coughing up thick phlegm.

Smoking also puts women at risk for a greater number of health problems than it does men, including increased bladder infections, cervical and colon cancer, and osteoporosis. In addition, even though 85 percent of the cases of lung cancer are found in smokers, a substantial fraction of the cases found in nonsmokers are attributable to second-hand smoke.

In many industrial countries, lung cancer accounts for nearly 40 percent of all cancer deaths in men and 30 percent of all cancer deaths in women. This data is staggering and yet smoking remains appealing to many people. Perhaps this is most easily explained by the addictive nature of cigarette smoking, in particular, a fact that even in 1994 the national tobacco industry vehemently denied.

While we as women are justifiably concerned about breast cancer and the lack of attention this disease claimed until recently, we must now sound the alarm and warn women who smoke that they have a greater chance of dying of heart disease and lung cancer than they do of dying of breast or ovarian cancer.

Types of Lung Cancer

There are two types of lung cancer, small-cell and non-small-cell lung cancer. Both are associated with a history of cigarette smoking. Small-cell lung cancer, which is less common, is also referred to as oat-cell lung cancer, because the cells are round and small—only about one half the size of the cells in non-small-cell. The cancer is found in the spongy tissues of the lungs. Like almost all cancer, small-cell lung cancer has a greater success rate of treatment when it is diagnosed early.

Non-small-cell lung cancer is also associated with passive or secondhand smoking and radon exposure. It is highly malignant, and the

110

sooner it is diagnosed, the better the chances that treatment will be successful. There are three main kinds of non-small-cell lung cancer, named for the types of cells found in the carcinoma itself:

1. Squamous-cell carcinoma—flat cells that are like skin cells
2. Adenocarcinoma—cells that form glandlike tumors in the lung
3. Large cell undifferentiated carcinoma

Prognosis and treatment depend on the stage of the cancer at the time of diagnosis.

Symptoms, Screening, and Diagnosis

Periodic chest X rays taken of smokers' lungs have not proven to be a useful screening technique, because X rays do not often detect the cancer early on.

The most common symptom of lung cancer is the chronic cough that many call "smoker's cough." Such a cough may persist for months or even years. If you are a smoker and you have anything like a smoker's cough, your automatic response may be one of denial—"I've had a cold." "The air is so dry." "Oh, my sinuses." If you do smoke and have a cough, see your doctor An ache in the chest is also common, as is increased sputum, which sometimes contains blood. If you have any of these symptoms, you should see your doctor. But the sobering truth is that by the time most lung cancer patients have symptoms, their cancers are usually advanced.

During the physical examination, your doctor will look for—and possibly find—fluid or congestion in the lung. Enlarged lymph nodes in the neck may indicate metastasis. Laboratory tests may include liver function tests and a chest X ray. Additional laboratory tests may include:

*   A sputum examination to check for cancer cells.
*   A bronchoscopy to retrieve cells from the walls of the bronchial tubes or a small piece of tissue (biopsy), in either case to check for cancer cells.
*   Thoracentesis, where a needle is inserted between the ribs to withdraw fluid that is then checked for cancer cells.

- Aspiration biopsy: a needle pierces the skin and tumor and a piece of tissue is taken and checked for cancer cells.

There are other tests that may be used, including a complete metastatic workup, which is done to check other organs for the presence of cancer cells.

Non-Small-Cell Lung Cancer

Stages

The stages of non-small-cell lung cancer are labeled occult, 1 through 4, and recurrent.

Occult. Cancer cells are found in the sputum but no tumor is found in the lung.

Stage 0. Cancer is found locally in the lung, but has not penetrated the outside lining of the lung. This type of cancer is also labeled in situ.

Stage 1. Cancer is in the lung, including the lining.

Stage 2. Cancer has spread to the lymph nodes adjacent to the affected lung.

Stage 3. Cancer has spread to the diaphragm or chest wall or to the lymph nodes in the center of the chest.

Stage 4. Cancer has spread to other organs.

Recurrent. Cancer has recurred after treatment.

Treatment

As with other cancers, the stage at which non-small-cell lung cancer is diagnosed will determine the course of treatment. Patients with this cancer are divided into three groups, with a different course of treatment for each. The first group has been diagnosed as Stage 0 or 1 in the cancer's progression and can be treated with surgery or radiotherapy. If the surgery involves the removal of only a small part of the lung, it's called a wedge resection. In some cases, a whole section or lobe must be removed, in which surgery is called a lobectomy. If the entire lung must be removed, the surgery is called a pneumonectomy. If a patient in this group has other medical complications that make surgery impossible, the patient will be treated with radiation therapy. This is still referred to as local treatment because it works only on the cells in the area where the cancer has occurred.

The second group of patients has lung cancer that has spread to the surrounding tissue. Treatment involves surgery and radiation, or radiation alone, if the patient cannot have surgery. The third group has lung cancer that has spread to other parts of the body. In this case, radiation therapy is used to relieve pain, reduce discomfort, and shrink the cancer, but it is not considered to improve the chances of recovery. Surgery is not performed because the cancer is too advanced.

Small-Cell Lung Cancer

Stages

Limited Stage. The cancer is found in one lung and nearby lymph nodes.

Extensive Stage. The cancer has spread to other tissues of the chest and/or to other parts of the body.

Recurrent Stage. The cancer comes back after having been treated. At this point, it may be found in the lungs or other parts of the body.

Treatment

There are three choices of treatment for limited stage small-cell lung cancer. The first is chemotherapy and then radiation therapy to the chest as well as to the brain (to prevent the spread of the cancer there). This latter kind of radiotherapy is called prophylactic cranial irradiation. The second is chemotherapy with or without prophylactic cranial irradiation. The third is surgery in combination with chemotherapy and, possibly, prophylactic cranial irradiation.

The treatment for extensive stage small-cell lung cancer may involve chemotherapy combined with radiation therapy to the chest, or chemotherapy alone. In either case, prophylactic cranial radiation may be included in the treatment. The third treatment option is radiation to the parts of the body where the cancer has spread, such as the spine or the bones, to relieve symptoms.

If the cancer is recurrent, radiation therapy may be used to reduce discomfort and pain, or new drugs may be used in the course of a clinical trial.

In all of the above cases, clinical trials are under way to test new drugs and also new ways of administering surgery, chemotherapy, and radiation therapy in combination.

National Health Care Crisis: Whether We Blame the Victim or Not

According to Barrett Rollins, M.D., of the Dana-Farber Cancer Institute, a great deal of apathy regarding improved treatment for lung cancer victims has developed because we, as a nation, have come to blame the victim for this disease. And there are few lobbyists on Capitol Hill because most of them are dead. There is no voice demanding treatment and cure for this disease, which has now surpassed breast cancer as the cancer that kills the most women every year. To blame the victim when it comes to lung cancer victimizes the nation as a whole in the end. Like it or not, lung cancer is the number one cancer killer now and will continue to be in the first quarter of the twenty-first century.

Secondary Smoke Is Not a Rumor

"I was stunned when I was diagnosed with lung cancer. I have never smoked a day in my life. But my husband did. He died of a heart attack four years ago. I never put two and two together, but my doctor said his smoking may have caused my cancer."

Mildred Thomas (age 67)

THE DANGER TO health that smoking presents is not limited to the person who is smoking. It is also dangerous to those who inhale secondary or sidestream smoke. While exactly how dangerous secondary smoke may be is still being debated, that it is harmful is clear. There have been studies that clearly connect secondary smoke to an increased risk of lung cancer and lung disease, particularly for women and children. In an article published in the *Journal of the American Medical Association* environmental tobacco smoke (ETS) was found to increase the lifetime risk of lung cancer in nonsmokers, particularly in children and in women who had been exposed to it. Secondhand smoke also contributes to allergies, bronchitis, premature wrinkling, emphysema, asthma, and some ear infections.

So, if you live with a smoker, it is in your best interest to encourage and help him or her to quit smoking for the sake of everyone's health.

Advertising Abstinence

While the debate regarding cigarettes and health was settled thirty years ago, the Tobacco Institute still attempts to foster doubt about the health risks of smoking. Despite such statements as "eminent scientists believe that questions relating to smoking and health are unresolved," in Tobacco Institute publications, there is no longer scientific debate on the subject. Cigarette smoking causes lethal disease in humans. If you smoke and continue to smoke, smoking will have a deleterious effect on your health. At this point in time, it is women, young people, and minority groups that are being targeted by advertisers for the tobacco industry.

In February 1994, results of a study directed by Dr. John P. Pierce of the University of California–San Diego Cancer Center were published in the *Journal of the American Medical Association*; the study demonstrated the link between the advertising promotion meant to attract women smokers in the late 1960s and early 1970s and the record number of teenage girls who took up smoking at that time. From 1967 to 1973, there was a 110 percent increase in the number of twelve-year-old girls who started to smoke. The study focused on advertising campaigns launched by Virginia Slims, Silva Thins, and Eve cigarettes—all brands that targeted women exclusively.

The data show that mostly highly educated, affluent women are quitting smoking. It is possible to extrapolate from present studies that black women—particularly young black women—will continue to be at high risk for lung cancer if advertisers continue to encourage smoking in these groups.

While teenage, adult, and most minority women are a major target group for cigarette advertising, they are not a major target group for clinical trials to explore improved treatments for lung cancer. Although new chemotherapeutic techniques are being tested, the mortality rate from lung cancer has not significantly improved—any new smoker has the same old death sentence.

Teach Your Children

The targeting of young people in cigarette advertising might be termed a form of passive child abuse. Smoking is an addiction, no matter how young the smoker. The younger you start, the longer you smoke and the harder it is to quit.

If you smoke, and you need inspiration in making the decision to quit, consider your children's health. If you have children, a smoke-free environment is the healthiest gift you can give them and the greatest encouragement you can provide them not to start smoking themselves.

OTHER CANCERS

Some of the other most common cancers that affect women which we will discuss in the next few pages, are bladder cancer, non-Hodgkin's lymphoma, cancer of the oral cavity (including lip and pharynx), pancreatic cancer, and skin cancer, including malignant melanoma.

Bladder Cancer

Since as early as 1895, bladder cancer has been linked with exposure to certain chemicals. It has also been linked to the residue of tobacco tar present in the urine of smokers. The incidence of bladder cancer increased by almost 12 percent from 1973 to 1987, but the mortality rate has decreased by almost 23 percent. The cancer is usually diagnosed in women and men between the ages of fifty and seventy. Men are three times more likely to develop bladder cancer than women.

The most common types of bladder cancer are papillary and transitional-cell cancers; these are also the most easily cured. Squamous cell cancer is more invasive, less common, and harder to cure.

Symptoms, Screening, and Diagnosis

Pain or a burning sensation upon urination and blood in the urine are generally the first symptoms of bladder cancer. Frequent urination and feeling the need to urinate and being unable to do so are also symptoms.

A routine urinalysis that detects even a small amount of blood may indicate bladder cancer. Blood in the urine will make the urine appear rust colored or even bright red. A physical examination, health history, and routine laboratory tests will also be part of any screening procedure for bladder cancer. Special tests will include:

- Examination of the urine for cancer cells.
- Intravenous pyelogram to detect a tumor or tumors in the bladder. A special dye containing iodine is given intravenously to make the bladder easier to observe on an X ray.
- Cystoscopy—a cystoscope is inserted into the bladder through the urethra. If abnormal tissue is visible, the physician will take a biopsy to examine under a microscope.

Stages

The stages of bladder cancer are 0 to 4 and recurrent.

Stage 0. Carcinoma in situ (found only in the lining of the bladder). This stage is divided into two forms: Tis (flat in situ carcinoma) and Ta (papillary cancer).

Stage 1. Cancer cells have spread through the inner lining but not to the wall of the bladder.

Stage 2. Cancer cells have spread to the wall of the bladder.

Stage 3. Cancer cells have spread throughout the wall of the bladder and sometimes to the tissue surrounding the bladder.

Stage 4. Cancer cells have spread to nearby pelvic organs and/or to the lymph nodes or to distant sites.

Recurrent. Cancer cells have reappeared after treatment either in the bladder or in other parts of the body.

Treatment

Traditional ways of treating bladder cancer include surgery, radiation therapy, and chemotherapy. Surgical treatment can range from destroying a single tumor to removing part of the bladder (segmental cystectomy) and removal of the bladder (cystectomy or radical cystectomy).

Non-Hodgkin's Lymphoma

The sixth most common cancer in the United States, non-Hodgkin's lymphoma is slightly more common in men than in women and in white individuals than in black. Although the risk for non-Hodgkin's lymphoma increases with age, it also tends to strike people in the prime of life (around forty).

The cancer cells in non-Hodgkin's lymphoma are found in the lymph system. The lymph vessels are thin, veinlike strands that carry lymph, which contains white blood cells called lymphocytes, throughout the system. Lymph nodes are strung along the lymph vessels and produce and store cells that fight infection; they are clustered in the pelvis, neck, and abdomen and under the arms. The spleen, thymus, and tonsils are also part of the lymph system. Non-Hodgkin's lymphoma may start almost anywhere in the body because the lymph system is so far-reaching—and it can spread to almost any organ.

Symptoms, Screening, and Diagnosis

Symptoms include pain or swelling in the lymph nodes of the neck, underarm, and groin, fever, fatigue, skin rashes, dramatic weight loss, lumps in the skin, bone pain, and swelling of the abdomen.

There are no screening tests available at present for non-Hodgkin's lymphoma. After a physical examination and routine laboratory tests, these special tests may be required:

- Staging CT scan or MRI, to assess the presence of lymph nodes in the chest and abdominal cavities
- A bone marrow examination

- A lymphangiogram of lymph glands in the abdomen, which may be filled with cancer cells
- Biopsy of lymph node or liver
- Serum studies of immune globulins

Stages

The stages of non-Hodgkin's lymphoma are 1 to 4 and relapsed.

Stage 1. Cancer cells are found in only one lymph node or one organ outside the lymph nodes.

Stage 2. Cancer is found on one side of the diaphragm, but in two or more lymph node areas.

Stage 3. Cancer is found on both sides of the diaphragm in the lymph node areas. Cancer may also have spread to a nearby organ or to the spleen.

Stage 4. Cancer is found on both sides of the diaphragm in the lymph node areas and has spread to an organ or organs outside the lymph node system, or it has spread to only one organ outside the lymph node system but has also spread to lymph nodes far away from the organ. Bone marrow and liver involvement constitute stage 4 lymphoma.

Relapsed. Cancer has returned after treatment.

Treatment

Prognosis and treatment for non-Hodgkin's lymphoma depend upon what type of cancer cell is found. T-cell or lymphoblastic lymphomas are hard to cure and the prognosis is unfavorable. B-cell and nodular lymphomas have a more favorable prognosis. Surgery, radiation therapy, and chemotherapy are all sometimes used in the treatment of non-Hodgkin's lymphoma.

Non-Hodgkin's lymphoma is on the rise among older adults. No one really knows why, although it is clear that this cancer is related to the weakening of the immune system that occurs naturally as we age. It is also a common cancer in people who have been diagnosed with HIV. Exposure to high doses of radiation, such as radiation fallout or the extensive X rays sometimes used as treatment for arthritic spinal conditions, also puts people at risk for the disease.

Cancer of the Oral Cavity

There are three things we take for granted every day—eating, breathing, and speaking. If you get a cancer of the oral cavity or upper respiratory tract, the likelihood is that at least one of these functions will be altered, perhaps forever. Sadly, most of these cancers are preventable: just don't smoke. Any tobacco product puts you at risk, including chewing tobacco, snuff, pipes, and cigars.

Cancer of the tongue or mouth may present itself as a small sore that doesn't go away. Most of us have had canker sores, but after about a week the pain goes away and the tissue returns to normal. However, with a tumor the pain gets worse as the ulcer gets larger and deeper. Sometimes the area will appear white or red. If the problem doesn't go away in a few weeks, see your doctor. The area will need to be biopsied. If the biopsy is positive, the usual treatment is surgery, radiotherapy, or both. As with most tumors, early diagnosis and treatment means a better cure rate.

The other common tumor in this area is cancer of the vocal cord. This tumor is associated with smoking and with gastroesophageal reflux. The most common symptom is persistent hoarseness. If the quality of your voice has changed and you are at risk for this cancer, see an ear, nose, and throat doctor who knows how to examine the vocal cords. If something suspicious is seen, a biopsy will be necessary; this procedure is usually done as an outpatient under general anesthesia. Early cancers can be treated with the laser or radiotherapy and the cure rates are excellent. More advanced cases involve removing part or all of the larynx. Radiotherapy after surgery is very common.

Cancer of the Pancreas

Cancer of the pancreas is highly malignant; unfortunately, by the time of diagnosis, the cancer has usually advanced beyond the point of curative treatment. Long-term exposure to industrial chemicals and tobacco are both known causes of cancer of the pancreas. The five-year survival rate for all stages of cancer of the pancreas is only 3 percent. This is the lowest of any cancer.

The signature symptoms are sudden, unexplained weight loss and abdominal pain. Loss of appetite, jaundice, and an intolerance for fatty foods are also symptoms. There are no screening tests for pancreatic cancer, though a possible screening procedure that uses monoclonal antibodies to detect the antigens on cancer cells is on the horizon.

Skin Cancer

Skin cancer is common, but it need not be fatal. The key to catching skin cancer in time is self-maintenance and self-observation—neglect is the factor that kills. If you notice a new growth on your skin that ulcerates and does not heal, you should see your doctor.

Exposure to ultraviolet radiation (contained in sunlight) is considered to be the chief cause of skin cancer, and fully 90 percent of skin cancers occur on areas of the skin regularly exposed to the sun. Other factors include chemical pollution, X-ray radiation, inorganic arsenics used in medicines before 1970 (and still used today in herbicides), and genetic predisposition.

Basal Cell Cancer

The most common form of skin cancer, basal cell cancer accounts for 75 percent of all cases of skin cancer. If you find a waxy bump on your face, neck, or ear, or if you find a flat brown or flesh-colored lesion on your chest or back, see your doctor. Basal cell cancer almost always occurs on areas of the skin that have been regularly exposed to the sun, and it usually occurs after the age of forty. This cancer almost never spreads to other areas of the body.

Treatment, which depends on the size of the cancer, may include scraping, cauterization, or surgical excision. Another possibility for treatment is Mohs' surgery, a series of shaved excisions. When diagnosed early, the cure rate is more than 95 percent.

Squamous Cell Cancer

More aggressive than basal cell cancer, squamous cell cancer may spread to other parts of the body. It usually appears on the face, ears, neck, hands, or arms. If you notice a hard, red nodule or a scaly or crusted lesion that doesn't heal, see your physician.

Treatment may involve surgical removal of the tumor and a skin graft to replace the excised, surrounding skin tissue. If the cancer recurs, Mohs' surgery may be the method of treatment. With early treatment, the cure rate is over 95 percent.

Malignant Melanoma

Malignant melanoma is the most dangerous skin cancer. Although it is, thankfully, also the least common, it is increasing in epidemic proportions in this country. Melanoma is directly related to a person's history of exposure to the sun. The more sunburns in your life—especially sunburns where you burn and peel—the greater your risk for developing this cancer. In fact, the incidence has doubled in the last twenty years among Americans.

Malignant melanoma arises from the cells that produce the skin's pigment—melanin. About 70 percent of cases appear as growths on normal skin, while about 30 percent arise on a preexisting mole that undergoes sudden changes in color and size and may begin to itch, bleed, or swell. The condition usually develops between the ages of twenty and sixty. Men have a higher mortality rate than women, and this is generally believed to be because men avoid taking a skin condition seriously and seeing a doctor for treatment.

The easiest way to determine if your should see your doctor for a possible skin cancer is to remember ABCD:

A is for asymmetry of any mole. If the borders of a mole change shape, you should notify your doctor.

B is for bleeding. Any skin lesion that starts to bleed should be checked.

C stands for color. Be sure to note if a mole or freckle has changed color.

D is for diameter. If a mole is getting larger, you should see your doctor.

The usual course of treatment is surgical removal of the tumor and surrounding tissue. Nearby lymph nodes may also be removed, and a skin graft may be necessary. Immunotherapy may be used as a follow-up treatment. In this case, a vaccine is injected in an effort to stimulate the immune system to destroy the cancer cells. When treated in the early stages, the cure rate for melanoma is 85 percent. If the tumor has spread to the lymph nodes or grown into the deep tissues the five-year survival rate is 30 percent. Monitoring through periodic medical checkups is necessary once you've had malignant melanoma in order to avoid recurrence.

But the cardinal goal is prevention! Make sure you cover up before going into the sun and always wear a sunscreen—even on overcast days. A public service campaign in Australia uses the motto "Slip, slap, slop"—meaning slip into clothing, slap on a hat, and slop on the sunscreen.

While we still have a long way to go in the war against cancer, what we do know now is that early detection in dealing with all cancers is key. When it comes to early detection, no one is more important to the process than you yourself. Get regular checkups and, after turning forty, make sure you receive the screening tests that are recommended for the individual cancers. The risk for cancer, in general, increases with age. Watch for warning signs and don't be afraid to call your doctor or health-care practitioner about that suspicious bump or lump. You have more control than you may think. Being responsible about warning signs is the first step toward early diagnosis, and early diagnosis is the first step toward successful treatment.

PART 3

PREGNANCY, CHILDBIRTH, SEXUALITY, AND GYNECOLOGICAL ISSUES IN THE MIDDLE YEARS

"The biological mismeasurement of women's bodies poses many emotional and intellectual conflicts for women, who are caught between defending their reproductive differences from men and asserting their intellectual equality and competence."

Carol Tavris, *The Mismeasure of Woman*

PREGNANCY

Having a baby when you're a little older and wiser can be one of the greatest pleasures of life. I know. I just had a baby at the age of forty-two. Notice I did *not* say it was easier (the weight hasn't come off as easily!), but it really wasn't any harder. This time I knew what to expect and I also had the bittersweet knowledge that this would be my last pregnancy. So I really paid attention to the changes in my body and life and relished every moment. I have less difficulty at this stage in life in sorting out the important stuff from the not-so-important. I remember my mother telling me not to sweat the small stuff a couple of years ago, when I was getting after one of my girls for something. Her statement echoed in my head for the nine months I carried this little boy. The missed lunches, the occasional cocktail, the loss of a waistline—none of it held any importance. The only things of importance were to have a healthy pregnancy and to enjoy myself.

I knew from my previous pregnancy (Rachel; my older daughter, Kate, is adopted) that exercise would be difficult at the end (I became very short of breath), so I tried to plan ahead this time. I exercised five or six times a week, knowing that being in shape at this stage would make things easier later on. My diet was already different—in fact, it was much better than it had been five years earlier. So I felt I was off to a good start and I was determined that my age would not be a deterrent.

I checked in with my gynecologist as soon as I knew I was pregnant just to talk things over. She's a straight shooter and I wanted to know up front the special concerns that would face me as an older mother. Nothing she said scared me or made me believe I wasn't up to this challenge.

Another advantage of having forty-two years of living under my belt was that I was able to approach this next stage of motherhood with realistic expectations. I was more relaxed. I had a great time sharing every incremental change with my daughters and laughing about my huge belly. It was fun experiencing this pregnancy through their eyes.

Some advice a friend gave me also made a difference. Lesley Stahl told me that when you try to juggle things—and we all do—think in terms of juggling balls. Some are rubber and some are glass. The rubber balls represent things like dinner dates, hair appointments, some career moves. If you drop them, chances are they'll come bouncing back to you. Consider the family, birthdays, children's school programs, and anniversaries the glass balls. If you drop them too often, they'll break and you might never get them back. I think this is a good metaphor— not only for enjoying a pregnancy but for living life to the fullest. It also underscores that none of us has to try to be a superwoman. For those of us who love our families and our work, a sense of humor is the best tool for smoothing out rough spots. It's a valuable weapon.

Planning a Prime-of-Life Pregnancy

"Of course there are certain health concerns for women over forty who want to have a baby. Getting pregnant is the primary stumbling block. But that aside, if you go to a doctor who understands the risks for this age group, you should be able to carry to term. You don't want to be handled with kid gloves. You are not breakable. You just want to be prepared to have good physical and mental health. After all, you want to enjoy this pregnancy."

Laurie Green, M.D. (age 45)

GETTING PREGNANT is the first hurdle for the older mother-to-be. We are born with all the eggs we have for the rest of our lives. And by this time those eggs are older and have been exposed to more substances in our environment that may have a deleterious effect on the ability to reproduce. So, if you have been trying to get pregnant and thought it would be easier at this stage in life, since everything else has always gone your way, there may be a genuine medical reason for the delay. Interestingly, one aspect of fertility at this stage provides a paradox. Because women in their late thirties ovulate earlier in the menstrual cycle, some women will produce two eggs at a time. Consequently, the peak age for having fraternal twins is thirty-seven!

Carrying a pregnancy to term and then enduring labor and delivery are not light work and can present an added challenge for a woman in her forties. You'll want to do all you can to meet this challenge in the most prepared manner possible. Many women purposefully wait until this stage in life to have a baby, as they get their careers going in the earlier years. For others it's the result of years of treatment for infertility. And for others it's a delightful "accident."

If you do decide that having a baby a little later in life is right for you, you should go ahead and get to work. No matter how healthy you are at forty, your eggs are a little older and getting pregnant does not always happen as quickly as you might want. If you are debating this decision, it's a good idea to involve your gynecologist in the process from the beginning, so that you can enlist her or his support and advice regarding preparation for pregnancy. There are things a woman can do before she becomes pregnant to help assure her of a successful outcome. For example, if you have never had German measles, your doctor will want you to be inoculated. In addition, you may decide to begin to take prenatal vitamins prior to becoming pregnant; since the first few weeks of gestation involve a great deal of growth in the fetus, additional vitamins and minerals help to ensure healthy development in these early stages.

Taking Healthy Steps Before and During Pregnancy

In many cases women blossom and are even rejuvenated by their pregnancies. I felt great all the way through mine, and I'm not alone—a lot of older moms report the same thing. So much of enjoying the pregnancy has to do with the preparation. Try to get in shape before you get pregnant. Stop drinking alcohol, limit your caffeine, eat nutritious foods, exercise, and stay away from cigarettes.

However, regardless of whether you had the time to prepare, pregnancy takes a toll on the body. The body gains weight, loses weight, and forever changes shape. It's all worth it. But the more prepared and informed you are, the better you and your baby will fare.

Getting Enough Folic Acid

Even if you aren't contemplating getting pregnant at this time but you are still in childbearing years, you need to take folic acid every day. This B vitamin can be found in many multivitamin tablets. Deficiencies in folic acid have been linked to spina bifida and anencephaly (the absence of a portion of the skull or brain) in infants. Supplementing your diet with folic acid can minimize the risk of these birth defects.

Again, even before you are pregnant, you should discuss vitamins with your doctor. The doctor may advise you to take a maternal vitamin during the time that you are trying to conceive. Maternal vitamins contain sufficient quantities for you and your baby's needs in the very early stages of pregnancy, during pregnancy, and afterward. If you are not taking maternal vitamins, you should begin to take a multivitamin that contains 100 percent of the RDA (Recommended Dietary Allowance) of folic acid and continue to do so through the time that you are nursing, and even beyond. Recent studies have shown that most Americans, pregnant or not, do not get enough folic acid.

Getting Enough Calcium

Calcium should already be a part of your daily routine. If you can't get enough calcium in your diet (and few of us can), use supplements. Aim for 1500 milligrams (mg) of elemental calcium per day. Calcium carbonate and calcium citrate are the best combinations. Read the labels of your supplement carefully because the dosage combinations can be confusing. For instance, 1000 mg of calcium carbonate contains 400 mg of elemental calcium. So you'll have to do a little arithmetic to make sure you are getting enough.

If you are contemplating pregnancy or are pregnant and haven't been taking calcium, start now. This will help your future child, and it will also help you. You need calcium almost as much as your baby does at this point in your life. Three to four glasses of skim milk or the equivalent of low-fat yogurt and low-fat cheese should be a daily goal. But again, if you are having trouble meeting these goals, discuss an additional supplement with your doctor.

Getting in Shape Before You Need to Stay in Shape

Exercise should be an important part of life at any age, including the times when you are pregnant. But if you haven't been gung ho on the exercise front before your pregnancy, you won't want to decide to run a marathon in your first trimester. In other words, don't take on too much too quickly.

If you have already established a reasonable exercise routine before becoming pregnant, you will be a lot better off. If you are planning a pregnancy, establish an exercise program that's manageable for you. Don't shoot for something unrealistic. If you do not go to a gym, walking and swimming are both excellent forms of exercise. If you are a walker, you will probably be able to maintain your walking schedule through your pregnancy. If you swim and are having an easy pregnancy you should be able to swim until the very last month of your pregnancy. Some women enjoy the buoyancy of the water, but others find it uncomfortable to swim while pregnant. You may need to experiment a little to find the exercise program that's right for you. But do something! Exercising now will make your pregnancy more fun and will make your recovery easier.

Whether you carry your baby high or low will affect which exercises you enjoy. I became short of breath around the seventh month and reduced my regimen by about 30 percent. Talk to your doctor about what is best for you. Remember, you don't have to aim for a marathon every day—but aim for something.

Sex and Pregnancy

In most cases, when a woman and her pregnancy are both healthy, it's possible for sex to remain a pleasurable part of life throughout most of the pregnancy. In the last month, however, some women feel too uncomfortable to even consider sex. Other women want to take advantage of every opportunity to have sex before the baby comes. Either of these choices is perfectly normal.

Some women complain of cramping after an orgasm. This is just a tightening of the muscles of the uterus—a normal reaction to sexual intercourse. This is usually transient and does not progress. Nonetheless, if this happens to you and you find it frightening, check with your doctor. Mild spotting may also occur if the penis touches the cervix, which is engorged with blood. Again, if spotting persists, this is also a reason to check with your doctor.

Embracing Bedtime and Rest

When you're pregnant, you can't wait for your baby to get here. Your excitement knows no bounds. You can't wait to hold her, bathe him, read her stories, rock him to sleep in your arms. Ah, sleep . . . that's the key word. When most of us are pregnant with our first baby, our mothers and friends go along with our enthusiasm, becoming almost as excited as we are. Few, if any of them, tell us the dreadful truth. Sleep? Forget it! Get ready for sleep deprivation. The first year is a desert of sleeplessness. But the silver lining is that you will have many a wonderful midnight conversation with your little one—stolen time when the rest of the world is slumbering. Those middle-of-the-night sessions disappear so quickly that they are worth relishing.

As far as sleep and rest go, plan ahead, just like you should with other aspects of the pregnancy. Get as much rest as you can before the baby comes. Whenever possible, lie down with a good book, elevate your legs on a couple of pillows (to guard against varicose veins), and enjoy the last few moments of peace before the baby comes. And don't feel guilty. Soon enough you won't have a moment to yourself.

If Your Pregnancy Is a Happy Surprise

We can plan and plan and plan and still fate and chance will win in the end. You may have been trying for years to get pregnant and finally given up. You may have already had your family and not have been trying at all. If you are caught by surprise—and happily so—you may worry that you are not in the best of shape. Even if you were not taking as good care of yourself as you could have been—and no one usually is—it's never too late to make those improvements. So don't be depressed about not having done everything perfectly prior to conception; nobody does. Just begin to follow all of the advice in this section as soon as you find out that you are pregnant.

Common Conditions During Pregnancy in the Older Mother

If you are an older woman planning a pregnancy, take extra care in choosing your obstetrician/gynecologist or midwife. Some physicians cater to older mothers and have centered their practices around this select group. Start thinking now about how you will give birth and where. Find out which problems your doctor will be watching for. Ask questions and keep notes. Although some problems are more common in older women, most can be successfully managed with knowledge and patience.

Hypertension

Hypertension, or high blood pressure, is more common in pregnant women over forty. However, if you begin your pregnancy with a normal blood pressure, eat healthy foods and exercise throughout your pregnancy, you can avoid hypertension and its complications in most cases. Your physician will monitor your blood pressure in any case, since many cases of hypertension have no symptoms at all.

You may find that your blood pressure runs a little lower during the first trimester of your pregnancy, say 100/70. In normal cases, the blood pressure will then rise to about 110 or 120/70. If your blood pressure begins to exceed 130/80, your doctor will monitor you carefully and try to control it with diet, salt restriction, and exercise. There are many medications that can help control blood pressure, but most women feel uneasy using them during pregnancy, except in very serious situations. This is all the more reason to start your pregnancy healthy, and maintain a healthy diet and exercise routine throughout this period.

If you have already been diagnosed with hypertension and are planning to conceive, you must talk to your doctor before getting pregnant. Your doctor will set up a careful diet and exercise regimen for you to follow and will monitor you especially closely during your pregnancy.

Preeclampsia and Eclampsia

Preeclampsia, which is also known as toxemia, is manifested by hypertension; edema or swelling of the hands, ankles, and face due to water retention; rapid weight gain (two pounds a week in the second trimester, three pounds a week in the third trimester); and the spilling of protein in the urine. Protein in the urine is determined by a simple "dipstick" test your doctor will perform on your urine in the office. It is important that preeclampsia be diagnosed early to avoid complications. If diagnosed early, there is usually no harm to mother or child—but diagnosis is key! This condition usually occurs during the last six weeks of the pregnancy. This is why your doctor will want to check you weekly as your pregnancy draws to a close.

Preeclampsia can lead to a far more serious condition called eclampsia, which may be characterized by extremely high blood pressure, blurred vision, severe abdominal pain, and headaches. Convulsions may follow and this condition is sometimes fatal.

Preeclampsia is treated in various ways, depending on the severity of the hypertension, the stage of gestation at which it is diagnosed, and the condition of the baby. Women with mild preeclampsia are often allowed by their doctors to stay at home on bed rest. However, in some cases hospitalization might be necessary. In a hospital setting, it is easy to monitor both the mother's blood pressure and the baby's condition. A test called a non-stress test (NST) measures the baby's heart rate after it kicks or moves; the test helps determine whether the baby is continuing to grow and develop normally. If your doctor decides that the baby's activity level is changing and that the baby may be in jeopardy, she or he may advise that the baby be delivered ahead of schedule. In fact, delivery of the baby is the definitive treatment for preeclampsia and eclampsia. Interestingly, labor in these situations is usually quite swift, as if the body knows that separating the fetus from the mother is imperative.

The best treatment for preeclampsia is prevention, which means that if you have hypertension you will want to plan your pregnancy carefully with your doctor, stick to your dietary and exercise regimens, and have your blood pressure checked frequently. Also, don't skip any prenatal checkups, especially during the last two months. This is when little problems can be diagnosed and solved.

Gestational Diabetes

Gestational diabetes, also referred to as maternal diabetes, is usually diagnosed at the beginning of the third trimester. If your doctor informs you that you have maternal diabetes, this does not mean that you or your baby will have diabetes after your baby is born. (However, older mothers who have had maternal diabetes are more likely to develop adult diabetes later in life.) Gestational diabetes generally does not cause birth defects, which usually occur in the first trimester.

Gestational diabetes does not occur until approximately the twenty-fourth week of pregnancy. Although your doctor will be checking for glucose in your urine, she or he will also suggest that you get a one-hour glucose tolerance test at this time. It's an easy test: you just drink a thick cola solution and have your blood drawn one hour later to make sure that the sugar levels rise and fall normally. If diagnosed and then monitored, maternal diabetes will not harm your baby or you. Because of this condition, however, your doctor will probably discuss with you the possibility of a C-section delivery if your baby is very large or induction of labor if you reach your due date without going into labor.

In the United States, 3 to 5 percent of all pregnant women are diagnosed with gestational diabetes. Although any woman may develop gestational diabetes, there are certain risk factors that increase the chances. These are being overweight before conception; a family history of diabetes; a previous birth to a very large infant, a stillbirth, or a child with a birth defect; too much amniotic fluid; or being more than twenty-five.

Gestational diabetes occurs because during pregnancy the placenta produces a number of hormones that, while helping to preserve the pregnancy, may block the production of insulin. This contra-insulin effect usually begins soon after the midway point of the pregnancy (twenty to twenty-four weeks). As the placenta grows larger, the production of these hormones increases. Usually, the pancreas is able to counteract the effect of these hormones by increasing the production of insulin, but sometimes this is not the case. When there is not enough insulin to do the job of overcoming the contra-insulin effect of this hormone production, gestational diabetes occurs. When the placenta's hormones are removed from the mother's blood after delivery, gestational diabetes usually disappears.

The American College of Obstetrics and Gynecology recommends the one-hour glucose tolerance test for all pregnant women. This is the best way to accurately diagnose gestational diabetes early in your pregnancy. The glucose tolerance test is in addition to the "dipstick" urine test for protein and sugar that your doctor will request during your office visits.

If gestational diabetes is not severe, it can be monitored and treated with diet. The key to preventing complications is controlling blood sugar levels as soon as the diagnosis is made. Your physician will probably ask you to make more frequent prenatal visits so that she or he can monitor the size of the baby more closely and check your blood sugar levels weekly. When the mother's sugar level is too high, the sugar passes through the placenta and affects the fetus. The fetus converts the extra glucose from the mother's blood into fat. This is a condition called macrosomia, which, simply put, means "large body," and in this case, large baby. A large baby is one of the major reasons for C-section delivery. Your baby may also be at risk for hypoglycemia (low blood sugar) following delivery. So if you deliver a baby that weighs over ten pounds and you have not been previously evaluated, your doctor will check you for diabetes. Your baby's blood sugar will also be checked frequently in the first few days of life.

Gestational diabetes is one of the more common conditions that develop in pregnancies of older women, but if treated quickly and appropriately it need not cause any serious complications.

Common Tests

Ultrasound

Ultrasound, also known as a sonogram, is used to determine the position and size of the fetus and the approximate number of weeks of pregnancy; it can also detect the position and size of the placenta and the position and growth of fibroid tumors. Ultrasound is noninvasive, and it is not painful. The greatest discomfort you will probably endure is being asked to drink three or more glasses of water and avoid urinating until after the test. The full bladder serves as a refernce point in the lower abdomen. To perform the test, a jelly will be applied to your abdomen, and a device much like a microphone will be rubbed over your now well-lubricated belly. Sound waves will bounce off solid tissue and pass through other areas, thus recording pictures of your uterus. You will see the fetus on a screen. It's usually easy to watch the developing baby move and observe the heart beating. I have always found this part of pregnancy to be a real thrill. Many test centers will allow you to bring in a VHS tape so you can leave with your own copy of the ultrasound.

Fetal measurements taken during the ultrasound can determine the age of the fetus. Measurements of the skull and the length from the crown to the rump are taken and the data is fed into the computer which then calculates your due date. The date you are expecting to deliver is based on a forty-week pregnancy. Doctors worldwide consider a pregnancy forty weeks long (gestational age) even though we only carry for thirty-eight weeks (fetal age). Although it seems confusing that by your doctor's calculation you are two weeks pregnant when you conceive, these are terms you will hear and should be familiar with.

This test is also a wonderful way to establish a baseline. Sometimes it is overused to reassure mothers and may often be unnecessary. However, it is very comforting to ascertain that all is well with the baby and most women report that it is delightful to watch the fetus curling, uncurling, and performing somersaults on the screen.

Amniocentesis

Amniocentesis is usually done between the fourteenth and eighteenth weeks of pregnancy. Many conditions can be predicted by the test, but it is most commonly associated with Down syndrome. The risk of bearing a child with Down syndrome does increase with age. The chance of having a baby with this syndrome is 1 in 1,205 for a twenty-five-year-old woman and increases to 1 in 365 for a thirty-five year old. One important note: It's a good idea to discuss with your mate and your doctor any feelings you have regarding continuing or aborting the pregnancy depending on what news you receive. While nothing will make the pain of bad news go away, beginning the discussion beforehand will help you emotionally and physically.

The present recommendation is that pregnant women who are thirty-five and older should have amniocentesis or some other form of genetic testing. Amniocentesis is the most thorough prenatal test available. There are approximately eighty metabolic diseases that can be detected with amniocentesis. However, if you and your partner have no history of genetic diseases in your families, neither of you has any known chromosomal or metabolic abnormality, and there is no history of a previous birth with genetic disease present, then the only tests done on the amniotic fluid will be chromosomal analysis and alpha-fetoprotein measurement. The other tests are usually not performed unless there is a specific risk factor because they are costly, time-consuming, and generally unnecessary. Ninety-seven percent of women who undergo amniocentesis find that their babies are free of genetic abnormalities.

The procedure is simple, and most women find it straightforward. But not all. Some find the procedure invasive, upsetting, and somewhat frightening, and say that they would like to have been prepared beforehand. Some women are glad they knew very little about the procedure. Using ultrasound as a guide, your doctor inserts a very long, thin needle through the abdomen into the uterus to obtain a small amount of the amniotic fluid, which is drawn off into a syringe. The amniotic fluid contains cells shed by the fetus that contain the "life story" of the fetus. Results are usually available within approximately three weeks.

The risks are usually minimal—especially when done by someone who performs this procedure routinely. Infection and possible miscarriage are the most frequently mentioned complications.

Chorionic Villi Sampling

Great strides have been made in improving an alternative to amniocentesis, chorionic villi sampling. CVS, as it is often referred to, can detect chromosomal abnormalities and other genetic abnormalities earlier in the pregnancy than amniocentesis. CVS is performed between the tenth and twelfth week of pregnancy. It's an attractive option becasue the results are back before most people know you are pregnant. If you should decide to, you can terminate the pregnancy quietly. An abortion at this stage is physically less arduous and the recovery is easier. Most of the time the procedure can be done in the doctor's office. And if you want to try to have a baby again, the waiting time is not quite as long.

Chorionic villi are involved in the earliest development of the placenta. This test is a biopsy of the villi, which are obtained by inserting a catheter through the cervix. (If the placenta is on the anterior wall of the uterus, a needle may be inserted through the abdomen, just like in amniocentesis.) The results are usually obtained within ten to fourteen days. CVS can give the same information as amniocentesis regarding chromosomal abnormalities, but is not as conclusive for neural tube defects. So CVS will be combined with a blood test for alpha-fetoprotein a few weeks later.

At present, the risks attendant to CVS are still being studied and have engendered some debate. Several small studies have found that there is a greater risk of limb defects with CVS. That risk may increase if the test is done before the tenth week of pregnancy. But if you talk to gynecologists who do this procedure all the time, the risks for this defect seem to be no greater than those found in the general population. The risk of miscarriage is slightly higher than with amniocentesis, but these numbers are improving as the testing procedure becomes more refined.

Screening Tests and Anxiety

The waiting period for the results of amniocentesis is from two to three weeks. At present, in many hospitals and medical centers where the test is performed, there is little if any counseling. Before you decide where to have the test performed, talk to your doctor. You should have an avenue for discussing any anxiety you may be feeling regarding the outcome of the test. Many older mothers-to-be may feel that the fate of potentially their only child hangs in the balance.

As you approach this justifiably nerve-racking time, you may want to consult your obstetrician or nurse-midwife regarding pregnancy support groups and/or counseling in your area. If you are not anxious, more power to you. And if you are, consider it normal, and don't let anyone convince you that you are being neurotic. You're not. We wait for the results of all tests with some degree of trepidation, and certainly that is a natural response regarding a test that may affect the outcome of your pregnancy and so your life. Try to relax. The odds are in your favor that everything will be fine. On the other hand, don't be too hard on yourself for the occasional case of jitters. And talk about your feelings with your partner and with friends you can trust.

Abortion After Prenatal Testing

While most expectant mothers are relieved and happy after finally obtaining their CVS or amniocentesis results, this is unfortunately not always the case. Indeed, the point of these tests is to screen for chromosomal abnormalities such as Down syndrome. So it is important to think through what decisions you feel might be appropriate for you to make if the news you get is not the news you hoped for. Some couples may consider the news of Down syndrome an aspect of fate they are not willing to tamper with or avoid and will choose to continue the pregnancy.

What is important is that you and your partner make the choice with the help of those around you, including your doctor. In the end the decision is yours. This is one subject you want to think about and talk about before you are faced with it.

Even if you have decided beforehand that you will terminate the pregnancy if you are given the news of a genetic problem, it is nonetheless a horrible blow. It's particularly painful for an older woman who may feel her chance to have a baby becoming slimmer and slimmer. If you find yourself faced with bad news, you must first of all allow yourself to feel grief—grief that you will want to share with your partner. At this point your doctor may focus on the inexorable medical procedure to come. But your tragedy is human and your emotional responses necessary and appropriate. You will probably feel angry, remorseful, and heartbroken, and you may even find yourself wondering what could be wrong with you or your family that you would produce such imperfection. There is nothing wrong with you. Such a result is no one's fault; in fact, the chromosomal damage occurred prior to and not during the pregnancy, within the substance of the egg itself or the sperm. Such a result could not have been foreseen or prevented. Biological imperfection is as much a part of nature as is the mysterious and complex process of development itself. The more you deal with the news in a factual way, the less room you'll leave for self-recrimination.

At Ten Weeks

Earlier abortions are physically easier, but an early abortion after the results of CVS cannot be compared to an early abortion chosen to end an unwanted pregnancy. Whenever pregnancy was desired, an abortion takes a greater emotional toll. The procedure is the same as that for early abortion (described on page 185), and the recovery period is relatively short, in terms of physical recovery. However, many women experience a considerable period of grief and also pangs of guilt, for they have made the decision to terminate after having made the decision to become pregnant. If you have decided to have an abortion after bad results from CVS, you should expect to have emotional repercussions for some time. If you feel unable to share your feelings of confusion, grief, or guilt with friends, you may want to seek counseling or the help of a support group. You are entitled to a period of grief. This is a normal part of the healing process after such an ordeal. What may be helpful to hear and what your doctor may not have shared with you is that most of these pregnancies would have ended in spontaneous abortions in not too many more weeks.

At Twenty Weeks

Most couples who choose to have amniocentesis have considered the possible results of the test beforehand, and it is a good idea to have a game plan in mind so that you and your partner are prepared for the possibility of unhappy news.

Since amniocentesis occurs at the beginning of the second trimester, if you plan to end the pregnancy, decisions must be made quickly. While nothing can prepare a couple for the emotional shock of such news, having a plan in place will help in terms of all the practical decisions that must be made at the same time that you are experiencing so many painful and perhaps conflicting emotions.

In most areas of the United States a woman can obtain a dilation and curettage (D&C) abortion up to 22 weeks. Otherwise, a second-trimester abortion involves inducing labor and is a great deal more complicated than the D&C. The sooner the abortion is performed, the less risk to the mother.

If a D&C cannot be performed, the abortion involves the removal of some of the amniotic fluid and then the injection of prostaglandins or a salt solution into the uterus to induce labor contractions. From the time of the injection the labor process lasts approximately twelve to fourteen hours (it usually occurs more quickly if you have given birth before). The termination mimics the birth process, except that the contractions are not intermittent as they are in labor, but occur even more rapidly and so are felt as a constant state of pain, pressure, or cramping.

141

Just as you would want someone to be with you during delivery, you should also plan to have someone with you for this.

If you decide you wish to try to conceive again, you will want to take some time, first, to heal both physically and emotionally. The enormous difficulty of what you have been through cannot be stressed enough. Although the temptation is to try again immediately to erase or cancel out this negative experience, a period of waiting will increase your chances for a positive and healthy outcome in your next pregnancy. Your body needs to rest and restore itself, and some distance between this unhappy ending and your new attempt at pregnancy can only help you emotionally. And to be asked to be a "replacement" baby is an added burden for any child. Generally, women are advised to wait six months to a year before starting another pregnancy. Talk to your doctor about the best waiting period for you.

Losing a Pregnancy in Midlife

"I just wish I hadn't heard the heartbeat. There was too much joy in that . . . . too much to get over."

Maggie Somerset (age 36)

HAVING A MISCARRIAGE is tragic, especially for a woman nearing the end of her childbearing years. As with many other situations like this, there are rarely answers for "Why me?"

I had several miscarriages in my mid-thirties before becoming pregnant with Rachel. The worst was at about four months gestation. I was really feeling pregnant and had told everyone. The spotting started on a Saturday afternoon (after a morning when nothing unusual happened). The bleeding just started out of the clear blue. Then the cramping started—like the worst menstrual cramps I ever had. I remember feeling as if I were in labor, even though at the time I didn't know how that should feel. I was afraid to take something for the pain for fear that a salvageable situation might be ruined. Of course, there was no "situation" to be salvaged. I called my obstetrician sobbing. He asked me if I felt pregnant. Funny question. But then I realized that I did not. Suddenly I became a statistic—one of the 40 to 50 percent of pregnancies that end in miscarriage.

> *"The loss of a baby is what it is, a loss, a tragedy. It is not a detour on the route to a healthy baby. It is a tragedy of its own, and its grief must be respected."*
>
> Barbara Katz Rothman, *The Tentative Pregnancy*

THAT DAY and those that followed were extraordinarily tough. The hormones that had been sustaining the fetus plummeted and I was on an emotional roller coaster. I cried at Hallmark ads. I cried if the forks weren't stacked in the drawer properly. I cried if someone looked at me cross-eyed. I realized the miscarriage was not something I would get over at once.

If you have chosen to become pregnant, a miscarriage is never easy, no matter how old you are. But there is an additional component of sorrow for many women when a future pregnancy may not be a possibility. Feelings of loss, grief, and anger are normal after such a loss; while these feelings and the experience that caused them are not pleasant, it should be stressed that they are normal and necessary.

Like all human endeavor, the birth process is not fail-safe. The fact that 40 to 50 percent of pregnancies miscarry may seem high, but many women who miscarry never know they are pregnant. Many times that "late" or "heavy" period is an early spontaneous abortion. But when you miscarry after you already know you're pregnant, the loss feels different. Even more devastating, one in eighty pregnancies ends in the birth of a dead infant. In addition, one in seventy pregnancies is ectopic—i.e., the fetus begins development outside the uterus, in a fallopian tube or the abdominal cavity. An ectopic may cause maternal death because of internal hemorrhaging.

In all three of these situations, the physician may focus on the physical problems to the exclusion of the patient's emotional state. You may find that your family is not much more helpful. At a time like this, clichés abound. It's almost as if everybody is trying to staunch your grief before you've had a chance to experience and share it. In particular, you may find that truly loving friends and family seem unable or unwilling to acknowledge that for you that miscarriage or that ectopic pregnancy was, in fact, the loss of a child. Oddly enough, these people mean to be comforting. It is as if they pretend that what was going on here wasn't really going on here to make it easier to accept that it's not going on anymore. For most women, this is not helpful.

My obstetrician has what she calls the Princess Diana rule. She notes that the British royals never seem to spontaneously abort. And there's a reason for that. They never announce they're pregnant until they are safely into the second trimester when the incidence of spontaneous abortions is much lower. She recommends not telling the world that you are pregnant until the fetal heartbeat is heard in the doctor's office at twelve weeks. After twelve weeks less than 5 percent of women will spontaneously abort. If you have to deal with the sadness of letting people know that you have miscarried, let someone close to you do the work for you. Inform those who knew about the pregnancy that well-meaning people can simply say "I'm sorry."

What you need most is to talk about how this loss makes you feel. If, for a time, this isn't easy to do with your partner or your family, you should seek professional help. As I've said, it is normal to lose a pregnancy and it is normal to experience grief afterward. There is no one way to grieve and there is no right way to grieve. After the loss of a pregnancy allow yourself to grieve in the way that is right for you for the time it takes you.

When It Happens More Than Once

Losing a pregnancy is hard enough. Going through the same loss again is more than should be asked of anyone, and yet it happens. General medical wisdom insists that two miscarriages is still within the realm of biological normality. The statistical chances of having a successful pregnancy after two miscarriages are about the same as after one miscarriage or none at all. However, if you are forty or approaching forty and have had two miscarriages, it is more than prudent to begin a full medical evaluation to give yourself the best possible chance for a successful pregnancy in the future.

When three or more miscarriages occur, the term "habitual aborter" may be used to describe this repeated loss. While it is still possible that each of the three miscarriages was caused by spontaneous and random events, your individual situation will be evaluated. You will be checked for possible difficulties such as an incompetent cervix, endometriosis, or low hormone levels. It will probably be suggested to you and your partner that you be medically evaluated before trying to become pregnant again. If adhesions from a previous surgery, fibroid tumors, or endometriosis are found to be the cause of multiple miscarriages, surgery may correct the problem.

Ectopic Pregnancy

When a fertilized egg implants itself outside the uterine cavity, an ectopic pregnancy occurs. The most common location of an ectopic pregnancy is the fallopian tube, though 5 percent of these pregnancies occur in the cervix, abdomen, or ovary. When an egg implants in the tube and begins to grow, the tube eventually ruptures because it is incapable of expanding. Although diagnosis of an ectopic pregnancy before the tube ruptures can be difficult, it can avoid a medical emergency. That's right—a ruptured ectopic pregnancy is a medical emergency.

Signs and symptoms of an ectopic pregnancy are usually caused by the stretching of the tube, rupture of the tubal wall, or hemorrhaging into the abdomen or tube. Because a ruptured ectopic pregnancy can be extremely dangerous, it is important to be aware of the warning signs and report them to your doctor immediately. These symptoms include:

- Missed menstrual period. Seventy-five percent of women who experience ectopic pregnancy have missed a menstrual period.
- Pain, either localized on one side or general pain of the abdomen, experienced as cramping, tearing, or stabbing pain. The pain may occur with bleeding. Pain may also occur during intercourse.
- Fainting and weakness.
- Bleeding or spotting.

If you experience any of these symptoms while you are trying to get pregnant, you should notify your doctor immediately. When there is a possibility of an ectopic pregnancy, it is better to be safe than sorry.

The sooner an ectopic pregnancy is diagnosed, the better the chances of saving the fallopian tube.

Today, we can diagnose tubal pregnancies through a combination of sonograms, pregnancy hormone levels, and progesterone levels. If the tubal pregnancy is diagnosed early, the drug methotrexate can be used to destroy the tubal pregnancy. Laparoscopic surgery can be done in most cases when surgery is needed. Thus it is crucial that ectopics are diagnosed early to avoid tubal rupture and more complicated abdominal surgery.

CHILDBIRTH

Labor and Delivery

"It was my third pregnancy, and I knew what I wanted.
When we got to the hospital, I said, 'Give me the drugs.'
One of the doctors said, 'Don't you want to see if you
can do it the natural way?' I said, 'I've done this before.
I know I can do it the natural way. I also know if I'm
too far along in labor I won't be able to have an epidural,
so give it to me now.' "

Jean Grayson (age 43)

F OR NINE MONTHS you've been waiting for that blessed event—the birth of your baby—sometimes more patiently, sometimes less patiently. And now, here it is—and you're still waiting! You've probably asked your doctor just how accurate your due date is at least fifty times, if not a hundred. The due date is calculated from the date your last menstrual period began, and so its accuracy is subject to the length of your menstrual cycle and your memory. But the truth is, even if you were able the recall for your doctor the very minute your last period began, when your baby actually arrives is still up for grabs, particularly if it's your first child. Here is one rule of thumb: the odds are that your baby's birth date will not be the same as your due date. Yet, when the due date is accurately calculated, 90 percent of women will deliver within one week of it. Most physicians are reluctant to let over-forty mothers go much past their due date. If your baby has still not been born and you are a week overdue, your doctor may decide to induce labor. Past this point, the placenta actually becomes too old to function properly, and the baby may begin to become malnourished. Approximately 20 percent of babies are born at least a month early. Prematurity is the number one cause of infant mortality. Multiple births, an incompetent cervix, an unusually large baby, or an infection that may cause the membranes to rupture, all may be causes for prematurity. If your baby is early, but less than a month early, it is not considered premature and the chances are that everything will be fine and your baby will be healthy.

Counting Down

If you have taken a Lamaze class or another type of natural childbirth class, you will probably be familiar with what to expect during the last weeks and days of your pregnancy. By the way, I recommend taking a childbirth class, even if you are pretty sure you will be having a cesarean. These days the emphasis in most of these classes is no longer on the natural way as the right way, but on being prepared for anything and everything that may happen. You will learn how to maintain a sense of control with the least amount of drugs necessary to get you through the pain. The goal is to get you prepared both to deliver naturally when and if it is possible and to make the decision to ask for help when you need it. Although you can never be fully prepared for such an all-consuming process as childbirth, in this case a little knowledge may do you a great deal of good.

As you approach the due date, things may change in terms of your body for better and for worse. Your feet may swell and your back may ache because the position of your baby has changed. In compensation, there will probably be that moment when the baby "drops"—that is, the head drops into your pelvis. This usually relieves the pressure in your chest and makes breathing easier.

You may also find that you are experiencing intense Braxton-Hicks contractions in the last weeks of your pregnancy. Their purpose is to help prepare the uterus for labor by softening the cervix. These contractions are evidenced by cramping or a feeling of tightening in the uterine area and are not indicative of labor—but they do cause many false alarms. It's best to prepare yourself for false alarms so that you don't end up running to the hospital at the first sign of a Braxton-Hicks contraction.

In the last few days before your labor begins you may also find that the mucous plug becomes dislodged. The mucous plug is a white or clear plug and is usually accompanied by some blood, which will appear as a pinkish discharge. This should not alarm you. It's a natural part of the preparation for labor and delivery and is not a sign of infection or in-cipient labor. (It happens less to women who've had one child already.) At your last prenatal visit, your doctor may tell you that the baby's head is engaged, which means that it is firmly fixed in the pelvis. Even though this is no assurance that labor is just around the corner, it is a good idea to have your hospital bag packed at this point.

Not all women experience their water breaking, but if your water does break, you'll know. It may happen gradually, like wetting your pants, or it may occur with a gush. If you think your water has broken, you should note the time and then notify your doctor. If you are having contractions you should begin to time them. Nowadays, if your water breaks and your labor does not progress (that is, your contractions do not become regular and closer together), your doctor may induce labor. Labor usually progresses, but if it doesn't, a cesarean section (p. 151) may be recommended to avoid any risk of infection.

Labor may be short. Labor may be long. It may be excruciating. It may just be painful. Labor is different for everybody, except for one thing: there is always some pain involved. I was lucky: both times I was in labor things went smoothly and it lasted only five to six hours. But do I remember the discomfort? You bet. Some women say, "Oh, it was nothing," but either they mean nothing in comparison to what they were expecting or they have conveniently forgotten any discomfort that might impede the decision to do this all again (or else they're fibbing). There is no such thing as a textbook labor. Each woman's experience will be different. The key is healthy mother—healthy baby. Neither an instruction book nor a report card follows the baby and the placenta out of the vagina!

The pain of labor is caused by many different things, including the size of the baby, the size of the mother's pelvis, and the position of the baby. This pain may be intensified, however, by the mother's level of anxiety. If you are anxious and afraid, you will inevitably tense your muscles automatically. This is another reason to prepare yourself as much as possible through childbirth classes, reading the literature on the subject, and discussing everything with your partner and/or labor coach. Personally, it was great to have my husband and my daughter Kate there this time around. They were both great. I didn't even need to think of having a focal point to concentrate on during the contractions—I had two: my husband's face and my daughter's face.

One other thing to take into account is who the doctors on call are at the hospital where you are planning to deliver. Since labor and delivery is not a job that responds to the regimen of a nine-to-five schedule, you'll want to know who's relieving your doctor (or midwife) on weekends and evenings and in the middle of the night. If possible, try to meet the other doctor or doctors beforehand.

Inducing Labor

As your labor reaches fruition, you should also discuss the possibility of inducing labor with your doctor. Pitocin is the trade name for oxytocin, the hormone that is administered to induce labor. Pitocin is potent and usually causes the uterus to begin contracting. Many women have heard that Pitocin causes labor to be more painful, but that's not really true. The medication makes the contractions more efficient and these stronger contractions hasten the labor. I've had Pitocin twice.

In this country, labor is generally induced only for medical reasons and not for the convenience of the patient or doctor. Reasons for inducing labor include maternal diabetes; preclampsia or general hypertension; an overly long pregnancy; and the premature rupture of the membranes (i.e., the water breaks), which happens in roughly 15 percent of pregnancies.

Vaginal Birth

It's great to be able to say that at least in the area of childbirth and medicine, times have changed, because they really have. The credit goes to the women giving birth and to their doctors. Natural childbirth is no longer a standoff between mother-to-be and physician, but an agreed-upon possibility. And an epidural or a C-section is no longer the "kiss of unnaturalness" for a woman intent on natural childbirth, but a reasonable possibility when the need is justified.

Naturally, we all want to give birth naturally. So, if you're over thirty-five and preparing for the possibility of complications during labor, you'll also want to be preparing for a natural delivery. As you probably already know, this includes enlisting your partner in your plans, and taking a Lamaze or other preparatory birthing class with your partner or whoever you've decided should be your coach.

There are three stages of labor. 1. Effacement and dilation of the cervix to ten centimeters. Effacement may take from eight to ten hours or more. 2. Birth. This includes pushing, which takes approximately an hour, but may take less time or more. 3. Expelling the placenta (afterbirth). This usually takes between 5 and 45 minutes. If your labor does not progess, you may be given Pitocin to speed up your contractions and avoid a possible C-section. If your pain becomes unbearable, you may ask for an epidural (the same local anesthetic used in many cesarean deliveries) or for a painkiller. If your labor is induced or if you choose to use painkillers or an epidural, this is not technically considered a "natural" birth, so what you will be given when should be discussed and agreed upon with your doctor during your prenatal visits. Some women instruct their doctors not to give them anything for pain, no matter how much they may plead for relief, and some insist that they begin something for pain as soon as they make this request. Once again, what matters is that you make the choice that's right for you.

These days, a woman over thirty-five has a very good chance of giving birth naturally, if that's what she wants, and she has an equally good chance of getting the help she needs when she needs it. If you choose your doctor and are comfortable with his or her hospital affiliation, you can feel comfortable with the decisions you make during the labor and delivery process, knowing that you are doing what is best for your baby and you.

If you are pregnant, there are many books on pregnancy and childbirth you've probably already read or considered reading. One of the best is, of course, *What to Expect When You're Expecting*. Two other fine books that will help you are Kathryn Schrotenboer's *Guide to Pregnancy over 35* and *Birth over Thirty* by Sheila Kitzinger. (See the Directory of Health Resources.)

Cesareans and the Over-Forty Mother

In the 1970s the rate of cesarean deliveries in the United States increased threefold. The rise in the rate of cesarean delivery was attributed to several reasons, including slow labor or labor that has failed to progress, having had a previous cesarean, breech presentations, and also fetal distress (although this last issue is controversial). Now the numbers are decreasing, in part due to more women having vaginal births after cesareans and to active management of labor. Active management of labor involves administering Pitocin aggressively so that the uterus and the mother don't fatigue while waiting for active labor to start. Currently, the chances of having a cesarean delivery are between one in four and one in five.

While there are many good reasons for the greater chance an older woman has of cesarean delivery, sometimes, unfortunately, there is no good reason. Thankfully, enough attention has been paid to the subject in recent years that the C-section rate in this country is diminishing. To avoid an unnecessary C-section, you should make sure to interview your doctor regarding the percentage of C-section deliveries she or he performs, and you should also obtain this information about the hospital where you plan to deliver. Twenty percent or less is a reasonable rate for C-section deliveries, while more than 30 percent would be considered high. However, these figures are ballpark numbers; if your doctor or hospital specializes in high-risk patients, the rates may be slightly higher.

Reasons for a Cesarean

You will want to discuss with your doctor the potential reasons for a cesarean. Here is a short list of reasonable reasons for a C-section delivery.

- **Active Herpes.** If you have had genital herpes, and if the virus is active within four weeks of your delivery date, you will be scheduled for a cesarean. There are great neurologic risks to a baby born vaginally during an inflammation of herpes—particularly, the risk of brain damage.

- **Placenta Previa.** In placenta previa the placenta covers the cervical opening. Consequently it obstructs the baby's path during delivery. If the placenta even partially covers the cervix, you will be scheduled for a cesarean section.

- **Abruption.** Abruption is the sudden, premature separation of a normal placenta from the uterine wall. This causes brisk bleeding that can interfere with the baby's respirations and circulation. It is a medical and surgical emergency and a very valid reason for a C-section.

- **Fetal Distress.** A baby is considered "in distress" if it is not getting enough oxygen. Your doctor can tell this by watching the fetal monitor and sometimes by sampling the oxygen and pH of the baby's blood with a scalp monitor. This involves placing a very small metal coil in the baby's scalp when the head is engaged in the birth canal. In this situation, an emergency cesarean is often necessary.

- **Cephalopelvic Disproportion (CPD).** Simply put, CPD means the pelvis is not large enough for the baby's head to pass through it. If you have had a cesarean delivery once because of CPD and are considering another pregnancy, you should expect to have another cesarean delivery.

- **Gestational Diabetes.** Babies born to mothers with gestational diabetes (page 134) are often very large. If you have gestational diabetes, your doctor may recommend that you have a cesarean delivery. This is called for if you do not go into labor before your due date or if your baby appears to be larger than average according to the most recent sonogram.

- **Preeclampsia and Advanced Eclampsia.** If you have been receiving consistent prenatal care, preeclampsia can be diagnosed before an emergency situation arises. Your doctor will monitor the situation prior to your due date to make sure an emergency situation does not occur and may suggest a cesarean delivery. The ultimate treatment for preeclampsia and eclampsia is delivery.

- **A Postmature Fetus.** A postmature fetus is one that is at least two weeks overdue. If your baby is overdue, your doctor will discuss with you the possibility of inducing labor or of a cesarean delivery. In many cases, the amniotic fluid begins to dry up, jeopardizing the baby's health and making a cesarean delivery necessary. After waiting so long, some women are relieved when a cesarean section is recommended.

- **Rh Negative Complications.** Rh complications are rare these days because of expert prenatal care, but if the situation does occur a cesarean delivery is necessary. In this situation a mother's blood is incompatible with the baby's and she makes antibodies against the baby's blood. The result can be severe anemia for the baby. Sometimes the baby can be treated in utero with a transfusion. Other times an early delivery is the best choice.

- **A Prolapsed Cord.** A prolapsed cord is one that has moved down into the cervix or vagina, impairing the blood flow to the baby. A cesarean delivery is not always necessary in this case, but the situation must be monitored closely. If the cord begins to cut off the baby's oxygen, an emergency cesarean may be necessary.

- **Multiple Births.** A woman expecting twins has about a 5 percent greater chance of having a cesarean delivery, depending on the maturity and position of the babies. The risk with three or more babies is three to four times greater, primarily because most of these births are premature.

Some C-section deliveries are done because of the possibility of a breech birth—when the baby's feet come through the birth canal first instead of the head. Breech presentation is a common indication for a C-section because of the risk of birth trauma. One in forty infants born vaginally in the breech position has some degree of birth trauma. Prolapse of the umbilical cord can occur in up to 10 percent of cases with double footling breech presentation. In some cases it may be possible to reposition the baby in the womb, and this technique is usually tried before a cesarean delivery is suggested.

In addition, an older mother may opt for a cesarean more readily than if she were twenty-five for the simple reason that she is planning on having only one child and doesn't want to take any chances. There is nothing wrong with this decision, as long as *you* are the one who is making it and are comfortable with your choice.

The choice to have a C-section is often made during labor—a process of extraordinary effort and physical pain—so it's important to prepare for this possibility by discussing the subject beforehand with your husband or birth partner and with your doctor. You don't want to find yourself belly to scalpel without having thought it through and accepted the possibility.

If you've been told in advance that a C-section delivery is a possibility, most books on childbirth include a section on cesareans. In addition, there are also books entirely devoted to the subject.

C-Section Delivery

If you are having a cesarean, you will be hooked up to an IV, and you will have a urinary catheter inserted before you enter the delivery room. The IV contains a lactate Ringer's solution that guards against dehydration; it is also in place in the event that further medication is necessary to counter the side effects of the anesthesia.

There are basically three choices of anesthesia for a cesarean—an epidural, spinal anesthesia, or general anesthesia. In the United States, general anesthesia is used only in emergency situations. An epidural is the preferred choice of anesthesia for cesareans. In most cases a continuous lumbar epidural will be used. A small, plastic tube is left inserted in the lower back between the vertebrae, where the original epidural was given, so that additional medication may be administered during the surgery. That the dosage may be regulated during surgery is one of the reasons that the epidural is chosen by so many doctors. Another major advantage of an epidural is that the mother is alert and awake to meet her new child.

Often referred to as a spinal block, spinal anesthesia is much like an epidural, but the effect is more far-reaching. While the effects of an epidural wear off fairly rapidly, after a spinal the numbness in your legs may last for six hours or more. The obvious advantage of a spinal block is that complete numbness is ensured during the surgery.

Once the anesthesia has taken effect, the procedure begins. The incision that is now used in almost all cesarean deliveries is called a low, transverse incision, made at the base of your abdomen, just below the "bikini line." It will take a fair amount of time for your doctor to make the incision and then cut through the skin, fat, and tissue to reach the uterus. So, don't worry, just focus on whom you are about to meet. Once the peritoneum (the membrane that lines the abdomen) is cut, the uterine incision is made and the amniotic membrane is cut, causing a gush of fluid. The baby's head is usually the first, visible part of the baby. Incision to delivery takes only about five to ten minutes. Then the placenta is removed by hand.

Stitching you up will take approximately twenty to forty minutes— stitches are required for the myometrium (the muscle of the uterus), the peritoneum, the fascia (connective tissue), and the fat layer, and usually a series of clamps or staples for the skin layer. If you have prepared for a cesarean delivery beforehand, you will probably have requested to hold and even nurse your baby immediately. Having your baby with you for even part of the time will make this phase go faster. If you plan to nurse your baby, now is the time to begin trying. If your baby doesn't latch on, you shouldn't worry. Many babies aren't very hungry right after they're born, and you will probably be exhausted enough to leave well enough alone. You'll be spending at least some time in recovery, at which point you may request to have your baby with you, at which point you may want to try nursing again . . . and again . . . and again.

While a C-section delivery is no picnic, you should not worry unduly about it before or after. This is in fact one of those times when you can thank medical science for having perfected this reasonably safe and effective procedure. If a cesarean is indicated, then this is the safest manner of delivery for you and your baby. No one embraces the notion of a surgical birth, but when it's better than the alternative (as it is in so many cases), a little perspective might help you to be more accepting of your fate. Remember, you chose the safest delivery for you and your baby, and in this case, the end does justify the means. The result—that healthy baby in your arms—speaks for itself!

Recovering from a C-Section

Some women claim that recovering from a cesarean is a piece of cake. Some women claim recovery takes a year. Wherever you fit on this recovery curve, the most important aspect of your recovery is that your own individual needs are being met. If you are so exhausted that you cannot see straight, you will have to enlist the help of family and friends so that you can get adequate rest. If the pain of your incision is so severe that it is hard for you to pick up the baby, have your husband hand the baby to you.

If there is nothing you want more than to begin to get back in shape, allot some time each day for your exercise routine. But *check with your doctor first*, and start slowly. Build up gradually and beware of any exercises that may put any undo strain on your abdominal muscles. This is a recuperative period, not a marathon training program—give yourself time.

Abdominal surgery—and a cesarean is considered to be abdominal surgery—is one of the most painful procedures to recover from. Recovery does not occur overnight. It is normal to have a considerable amount of pain the first week or so after surgery. You should take something to relieve the pain, particularly at night to help ensure restful sleep. If you are nursing, discuss this with your doctor. In most cases, you can still take acetaminophen with codeine. Only a minimal amount passes through to breast milk, and if this medication makes you more comfortable in the immediate postnatal period and makes it easier for you to care for your baby, then you should consider it. Other women consider plain acetaminophen enough. You should check your incision daily to make sure it is healing properly, and if you notice any oozing or pus, or that the scar seems to be separating, you should see your doctor.

DEPRESSION

Some women become depressed after delivering a baby and a cesarean delivery is no exception. In fact, women who undergo emergency C-sections have approximately a sixfold increase in the incidence of postpartum depression. Some therapists say that in certain cases cesarean depression may be compared to post-traumatic stress disorder. More often than not, the reason for severe cesarean depression is lack of support at a critical time: a woman who has just undergone a painful abdominal surgery is not given the help or sympathy she needs. Instead, she is forced to field such questions as "Why didn't you try harder?"—as though having a baby is some contest to prove your stamina or brawn!

If you think you may be suffering from a depression after a C-section, ask your obstetrician to recommend a therapist or counselor. There are also cesarean support groups in most areas, so your doctor may put you in contact with such a group. Not only will you gain emotional support from group members who've been through what you have, but you will be asked to help others too. This may help you in turn. Suffering alone and in silence will only add to your depression. The "baby blues" are transient, lasting only a few weeks. If you feel a depression pulling you down, talk to your doctor about postpartum depression. Therapy and antidepressants may be in order.

It's also a good idea to discuss with your doctor what happened to prompt your C-section delivery. On your six-week postpartum checkup, sit down and review the events in order to see whether steps can be taken to avoid a cesarean with any future pregnancy.

Here are the types of women who are most likely to suffer depression after a C-section.

- Women who planned for and expected natural childbirth
- Women who had emergency C-sections
- Women who felt the surgery was forced upon them by their doctor or partner
- Women who wanted to breast-feed and found that the C-section impeded their ability to do so
- Women who did not experience their C-section as a birth process
- Women who had medical complications after a C-section

And here are the kinds of women who probably won't suffer from depression after a cesarean.

- Women who know that what they wanted above all else was a healthy baby
- Women who've had other major life crises and know that things don't always go according to plan
- Women who planned their C-section with their doctor and trust their doctor's judgment
- Women who do not believe that natural childbirth is all that matters

One final note. Allow yourself to be tired, whether you have a vaginal birth or a cesarean section. Your body has just been through an arduous process and it needs rest. Try to sleep as much as possible after birth. There's a reason that mother nature delays the appearance of breast milk until the third postpartum day: she's trying to take care of you.

Breast-feeding

"When I was leaving the hospital, I asked a nurse about breast-feeding at night. I was afraid I wouldn't wake up when my baby needed me. I asked if I should set the alarm. She laughed at me, and a year and a half later, I'm still laughing at myself."

Millie Stafford (age 39)

A 1994 ARTICLE in *The New York Times* was titled "Mother's Milk Found to Be Potent Cocktail of Hormones." That breast-feeding is good for your baby cannot be overstated. In the first months of life, breast milk protects an infant with the mother's immunities while the infant's immune system has a chance to mature. Research has now shown that breast milk also helps in the final steps of the process of development of the brain itself.

If you want to breast-feed and your baby has trouble latching on, don't give up. Many babies take their time figuring out what to do next. If you are having trouble, ask the nurses or your doctor for help. Many hospitals now have nurses who specialize in providing advice about breast-feeding. Ask if there are any community programs. These steps are important because mothers can no longer stay in the hospital while they work out the nuances of breast-feeding. I think this lack of support for new and older mothers is one of the saddest casualties of medical reform. And since your mother may live across the country or have no experience herself, breast-feeding for the first time can be a frustrating and disheartening challenge to accomplish on your own.

I have three children and fed each one a different way. Kate, my oldest, is adopted and thus bottle fed. I found breast-feeding difficult with my second daughter, Rachel. Despite my background in pediatrics,

I was surprised at how bumpy such a natural process can be to get started. My daughter didn't have a great suck and my nipples were quite sore. With my third, I was determined to try again. I pumped my breasts, which toughened the nipples and kept the milk coming in regularly. I was also lucky that my son came out of the womb and just got it! He came out hungry and had a great suck, so everything went smoothly.

Of course, the most important thing is that your baby get adequate nutrition. You should feel no qualms about supplementing with formula if you feel that your baby is not thriving. The worst possible scenario is to stick doggedly to a breast-feeding regimen while your baby fails to thrive. Be careful that your baby is getting enough to eat and that your baby is not becoming dehydrated. If you don't feel that breast-feeding is right for you, try not to let anyone make you feel guilty about your decision. This is only the first of many times you'll have to trust yourself and your own instincts when it comes to your children. Many women who breast-feed worry that the baby isn't getting enough food. But if your baby is gaining weight and consistently urinating (twelve to twenty diapers a day), you're on the right track.

New Motherhood

"There's one great thing about having a second child:
you really appreciate the first few months when they can't
move."

Brenda Faunch (age 42)

WILLIAM FAULKNER is said to have remarked that work is the only thing a person can do eight hours a day. Needless to say, he was never a mother or, more correctly, a child-care giver. Child-care is a twenty-four-hour-a-day equal-opportunity employer. The needs of a newborn are endless; and for many mothers, the fascination with this new and magical life is almost as endless—clouded, perhaps, only by exhaustion.

If you have been working for twenty years and would be lost without your work, you will want to use the months you are pregnant to plan a strategy that allows the best possible way to blend the demands of your old life with those of your new life. If you feel you are ready for a change or at least a modification in terms of your work and career goals, now is the perfect time to begin to effect that change. The point is that it's up to you. There is no easy way or right way to raise children and the more you take into account your own needs in the matter, the better parent you will be.

Above all, remember that having a child does change your life and that's as it should be. As much as you can in this imperfect world, you should get the help you need in order to maintain a positive outlook and keep your options open whenever or wherever you can—whether that means working less, changing careers, or getting back in the saddle as soon as possible. It's up to you. And remember, infancy is not forever; when you're in those colicky doldrums of the first six months, just re-mind yourself how quickly these children grow up. Relish each stage. Soon they'll be in school and then begging you for the car keys! Start planning your strategy now for your work plans after childbirth.

The Second Heartbeat Phenomenon

"What having children really means is that you mortgage your peace of mind for life. Most of the time I think parenthood is really wonderful . . . and then something will happen and I think, God, this is so tough."

Joanna Seibert, M.D. (age 53)

I REMEMBER WHEN I first heard my baby's heartbeat during a prenatal exam. I lay on the table thinking, "Oh my god, I have two heartbeats now." The truth is, on some level, this feeling of attachment remains long after the umbilical cord is cut (in fact, in some form, forever). Career, marriage, turning forty, you name it . . . nothing changes a woman's life as much as having children does.

As mothers, we feed our babies with our blood before they're born, and we seem to worry about them with our blood from day one on. The upside is that this intense love can make us richer and stronger and more giving as individuals. The downside is that we really do part with whatever vestiges we might have had of that great concept, peace. We

160

worry about sleeping through the night (them and us), swallowing pennies, is she getting enough to eat? We worry about ear infections, first steps, potty training, discipline. We worry about baby-sitters, how much TV should he watch, playground accidents, preschool, playdates, learning curves. We worry when she comes into our beds when she's little and when he's not in his bed when he's big. We worry about nourishment and nurturing of all kinds all the time. And none of us gets through motherhood without some blue periods and down times when we think that not only the world, but also our spouses, parents, in-laws, nannies, baby-sitters, bosses, and even our children are against us. This is the price we pay for joy. And when your four-year-old says to you, "Mom, I can feel your heart beatin' just like mine," and you think of that time when you had two heartbeats, it's all worth it.

INFERTILITY AND THE BIOLOGICAL CLOCK

While media attention to the subject of infertility has heightened many women's fears regarding their own fertility and to some extent exaggerated the problem, it is true that as a woman ages, her fertility decreases. The eggs you are born with just age along with you.

Infertility is commonly defined as the inability to conceive after a year or more of intercourse without contraception or the inability to carry a pregnancy to a live birth. In addition to the natural decrease in fertility during the aging process, sexually transmitted diseases (STDs) and IUDs have compounded the problem of infertility for many women in recent years.

Secondary infertility is the inability to conceive after having already had one or more children. The causes of secondary infertility are the same as for infertility. The term also applies to women who have lost a pregnancy and then find it impossible to conceive again.

The Causes of Infertility

Infertility has many causes, including some forms of birth control, certain diseases, some operations and procedures, and also choices in lifestyle. However, there may also be no known cause for infertility.

- **Age.** A woman's fertility peaks about the age of thirty. One in five women between forty and forty-four is unable to conceive. As a woman ages her fertility naturally decreases. In addition, she is at a higher risk for diseases and conditions that may interfere with fertility.

- **Birth Control.** Three kinds of birth control affect fertility. The pill may cause what is known as "pill amenorrhea," which means that after you stop taking the pill you do not get your period. Pill amenorrhea may last a few months or as much as a few years. One fourth of women who have been on the pill take more than thirteen months to become pregnant. The IUD is associated with pelvic inflammatory disease (PID), which can be a cause of infertility. The diaphragm may impede fertility by causing scar tissue.

- **Ectopic Pregnancy.** One in five women who has had an ectopic pregnancy (page 145) will then be infertile. The infertility is due to pelvic scarring. If a woman becomes pregnant after an ectopic pregnancy, she has a one in three chance of carrying that pregnancy to term.

- **Endometriosis.** As endometriosis progresses and the uterine lining tissue attaches to other pelvic organs (causing pain and scarring), infertility becomes more and more common.

- **Marijuana.** Smoking marijuana regularly (four times a week or more) can interfere with ovulation.

- **Menstrual Irregularities.** There are some women who, from the beginning, never ovulate on a regular basis even if they menstruate every month. Menstrual irregularities may also be caused by anorexia, bulimia, and frequent and intense exercise.

- **Nasal Decongestants.** Some decongestants, when used habitually, dry up other mucous membranes in the body as well as the nasal passages, including cervical mucus. This may inhibit conception.

- **Nitrous Oxide.** Dental assistants who are exposed to nitrous oxide five or more hours per week are more likely to be infertile and also have a higher risk of miscarriage.

- **Pelvic Inflammatory Disease.** PID can cause scarring and also blockage of the fallopian tubes. About 25 percent of women with PID become infertile.

- **Smoking.** Women who smoke fifteen or more cigarettes a day take longer to become pregnant and are less likely to carry a pregnancy to term. Smoking also triples the risk of miscarriage.

- **Sexually Transmitted Diseases.** The STDs (page 172) that cause infertility most frequently are gonorrhea and chlamydia. The latter causes about 100,000 women per year to become infertile.

Procedures and surgeries that contribute to infertility include:

- **Cervical Conization.** This operation, which removes part of the cervix, is used to diagnose cancer. Other procedures involving the cervix may also reduce fertility.

- **Cesarean Section.** Surgical childbirth may cause scarring to internal organs and reduce fertility.

- **DES.** If your mother took DES, your fertility may be reduced. (See "DES—Past and Present," page 187.)

- **Dilation and Curettage.** A D&C, in which the interior of the uterus is scraped using a curette, may alter the lining of the uterus and decrease fertility.

- **Myomectomy.** This operation to remove fibroids may decrease fertility because of scar tissue inside the uterus or on internal organs.

- **Pelvic or Abdominal Surgery.** As with the other surgeries mentioned, any surgery causing scarring to internal organs may decrease fertility.

Coping with Infertility Problems

About one in thirteen couples in the United States is infertile. For many of these couples, this is the most difficult life crisis that they face. For some the desire to have a child begins to consume their lives. The obsession with becoming pregnant begins to affect their relationship, their jobs, and their relationships with friends and families. Temperature taking, sperm counts, the new drug, the next test, and so on . . . all begin to supplant a formerly happy life with a regimen that involves hope one week and despair the next.

For many women, the greatest indignity is the irony of having spent so many years observing the rules of birth control only to find they needn't have bothered. Others chide themselves ("Why did I wait so long?"). But all women who face this challenge experience the one moment that resonates—that moment where you say to yourself, "In some fundamental way, I must be a failure." This is the human dimension of the biological situation. Of course you're not a failure, and neither is your husband or partner. But it can take a long time to come to terms with fate. Whatever time it takes is well deserved for any woman who has spent time planning and waiting for the perfect time to have a baby, only to find it is out of her control.

We have already examined the causes of infertility in women. Infertility in men may be caused by too few or irregular sperm. In 3 to 20 percent of all couples experiencing infertility, the infertility cannot be explained. But when the reason can be pinpointed, only 50 percent of the time the problem lies with the woman.

Some couples decides not to go forward with treatment for infertility, leaving things as they are naturally (some of these couples adopt, some do not). Other couples decide to pursue treatment, but only to a point. A third group decides to accept any treatment that may help them become pregnant.

Let's look briefly at some of the options available for treatment.

If you have an ovulatory problem, you will be administered a drug such as Clomid or Pergonal to induce ovulation.

If you have endometriosis, hormone therapy, laparoscopic laser surgery, or laparotomy is possible.

In some cases of infertility, artificial insemination and in vitro fertilization (page 167) are options. Artificial insemination involves insemination with your husband's sperm or a donor sperm. In in vitro fertilization, your eggs are surgically removed from your ovaries, transferred to a petri dish, and fertilized with your husband's sperm or donor sperm. The resulting embryos are then placed in your uterus.

Infertility can take a toll on your marriage, at least temporarily, and pursuing treatment can take a greater toll.

Not to make light of a very difficult time in the life of any couple, but the sooner you share that there is something surrealistic about all that you're going through to have a baby, the sooner you'll get your sex life back and the better the chances that you'll keep your marriage healthy and well. That's what it is: a sex life—separate and apart from family life and the biological necessity of producing life. And that's what it is: a marriage—not necessarily an assembly line for offspring.

Fertility Drugs and Your Body

Recent studies have shown that women who have taken fertility drugs are approximately three times more likely to be diagnosed with ovarian cancer. These figures pertain particularly to women who never conceived. It is not clear whether fertility drugs themselves cause ovarian cancer or whether long-term infertility is the culprit. What is clear is that every time an egg breaks through the epithelial lining (and menstruation occurs), there is stress on the ovary. It follows that interruptions in ovulation—i.e., pregnancy—lower the risk of ovarian cancer.

Approximately 100,000 women take fertility drugs in the United States. Even though some of these drugs have been in use for twenty years, there have been no long-term studies yet on the women who have taken them or the children to whom they have given birth.

While so far no obvious aftereffects have emerged in those treated with fertility drugs, far more women are taking far more potent drugs for longer periods of time. With baby boomers passing forty and planning families later in life, high-tech, high-potency treatments have become more common. Although long-term effects have yet to be analyzed, there are obvious short-term side effects to fertility treatment. These include nausea, bloating, abdominal pain, hot flashes, and mood swings.

One prominent study, by Dr. Alice Whittemore at Stanford University, found that pregnancy, breast-feeding, and taking oral contraceptives all help in lowering the risk of ovarian cancer, but that fertility treatments may triple a woman's risk of getting the cancer. Because of Whittemore's results, the FDA asked drug companies to include the potential risk of ovarian cancer in their labeling. At the present time, there have been no changes in labeling to include this warning, and the approval process might take years. But the risk is still small. The lifetime risk of developing ovarian cancer is only 2 percent and the fertility treatments may raise the risk to 6 percent. For many women it is worth that chance if it results in the birth of a child.

If you are have difficulty conceiving and are thinking of taking fertility drugs, you should discuss your choices and the attendant risk factors with your doctor and decide how long a course of treatment seems advisable in your situation.

Alternative Methods of Conception

If you are forty or approaching forty, single and childless, and you wish to have a child without having a male partner, building a family can still be a real possibility—provided this is a choice you want to make. June Cleaver might blanch at all that technology has made possible in terms of family planning, but then again she might not. The reality is that the same technology an infertile couple may consider is also an option for you. Sperm banks are now easily accessible and very well monitored. By law, all sperm must be tested for the AIDS virus and genetic abnormalities and found healthy before being frozen. If you go this route, make sure that you are dealing with a licensed sperm bank and that the sperm has been frozen. Frozen sperm is the safest, healthiest choice.

Artificial insemination involves the introduction of the partner's or donor's semen into the upper vagina or cervix. Several inseminations are usually performed during a single menstrual cycle to enhance the possibility of conception. The least known, simplest, and least expensive form of artificial insemination is called *intrauterine insemination,* or IUI. IUI costs less than one third of in vitro fertilization (IVF). The technique involved in IUI is much like that for artificial insemination except that the physician uses a tiny catheter to place the semen in the uterus instead of within the upper vagina or cervix. According to a recent study, a 27 percent rate of pregnancy per couple was achieved with IUI (this rate is comparable to that of the much more costly IVF). The risk of multiple births is about the same for IUI as IVF. If you are trying to decide on a method of artificial insemination, IUI should be considered before other more costly options. There are many clinics that now perform artificial insemination at increasingly reasonable costs, making this option possible for more and more couples and single women.

In vitro fertilization involves the removal of eggs from the mother's ovary, fertilization of the eggs in a laboratory dish with the father's sperm or donor sperm, and then implantation of the resulting embryos in the mother's uterus, where the embryos develop into fetuses. IVF was first used to help women with blocked fallopian tubes, but is now used for a variety of of infertility problems, including endometriosis, male infertility, and unexplained infertility—a term used to describe infertility that lasts more than two years and has no known cause. One of the risks of IVF is the possibility of multiple births, which increases the risk of prematurity and high blood pressure in the mother. Another risk is that none of these eggs will develop into a viable fetus.

THE ADOPTION ALTERNATIVE

"Five doctors told me I would never have children because my fallopian tubes were blocked. It took me a year and half to get over the fact that I wouldn't have a baby. But then it dawned on me that what I really wanted to do was parent. I truly got over the need for a biological child. And now? . . . We have three children—two adopted and one biological. Life couldn't be better."

Connie Fails (age 46)

I CONSIDER MYSELF SO LUCKY because I have been able to experience having a child through adoption and having two the old-fashioned way, as a friend would say. Ask any adoptive parent and you'll hear the same thing: it is not necessary to give birth in order to have a family. People find and make families in a variety of ways. For all the pressures and pains of modern life, there is the advantage that the notion of the nuclear family unit has become more pliable, offering more options to childless women than there were in the past.

One reservation that I hear from people who are considering adoption is the concern that you just don't know what you're going to get. Well, the fact is that you don't know what you're going to get even when you have a biological child. Life is a crap shoot, and so is having children—whether you pop them out yourself or another woman does it for you.

In fact, there are many women who feel that, rather than undergoing extraordinary medical procedures in the hope that a pregnancy will result, they would prefer to give love and nurturing to a child who is in need of parents.

Couples decide on adoption at different times and in many different ways. Some couples have always been open to adoption, while others only begin to consider adoption as an alternative when they find their chances of having their own biological child are decreasing. Once you decide to adopt, the process of the adoption may be a lengthy one. Therefore, it is best to begin as soon as possible.

There are two basic ways to go about adopting a child: agency adoption and independent, direct, or private adoption. These two methods may be pursued simultaneously. In an agency adoption, the couple must be interviewed by the agency and meet the standards the agency has set for parents and the home environment. This process is usually called the home study. Once you've filed your application with the adoption agency, a social worker is assigned to your case. Typically this process will consist of two interviews—one at the agency and one at your home. In these interviews your social worker will explore your feelings about adoption and being adoptive parents. While it is hard to assess who will be a loving parent, emotional maturity, the present status of your family, your marital status, your relationship with others, and your feelings toward children are often areas of focus. In an agency adoption, the biological parents place their child with the agency, and the agency places the child with the adoptive parents.

For people who hate red tape or question whether they will meet agency standards, private adoption is often the preferred route to take. In a private adoption, the biological parents place their child with the adoptive parents independent of any agency. This process is handled by an attorney, so a good first step is to find a lawyer in your area who specializes in adoption. In a private adoption it is possible to meet the birth mother of the child. In fact, some adoptive parents arrange to be present for the birth. Birth-related expenses and legal fees are usually paid by the adoptive parents, and this money is nonrefundable. The cost can be anywhere in the range of $7,000 to $20,000.

In either approach, it is best to begin the process of adoption with an open mind. In fact, at some adoption agencies applications are not even considered if, for instance, a white couple wishes to adopt only a "healthy, white infant."

The recent adoption horror stories that have been played out in the press should remind anyone that it's important to be as informed about this process as possible. Adoption laws vary from state to state. Know your rights as adoptive parents and know the rights of the birth mother. Make sure you understand the grace period in which a birth mother has the right to change her mind and rescind the arrangement. This is one area where a good attorney can be worth the expense.

A third possibility for adopting a child is intercountry adoption. In an intercountry adoption, you travel to the country of the child's birth and bring the child back to the United States to live. The child is adopted either in the country of origin or in the state where you reside. The advantage of intercountry adoption is that it is usually a much faster process than agency or private adoption. Instead of waiting as much as five years to finally adopt a child, you may find that you have your child happily and legally ensconced in your home within six months. The challenging aspect of this process is that you don't often (if ever) know much at all about your child's origins. For an intercountry adoption to be successful, you will have to be prepare to accept the unknowns in your child's past and to create a transracial/transcultural family forever. Costs for intercountry adoption range from about $10,000 to $15,000, depending on the country where the child was born.

When you decide to build a family through adopting a child, you will have to prepare yourself for the unexpected, as best you can. Try to keep an open mind at all times. The process may be grueling, disheartening, and exhilarating by turns. One day you may think you have the perfect lead on the child you're sure will be right for you, only to have your hopes dashed the next day. You may enter the process prepared for it to take a year or more to find a child, only to find yourself needing to decorate a bedroom and prepare yourself for parenting in two or three weeks. Or you may hope against hope that within six months you'll have your child, only to wait for years to bring your child home. The process is nothing less than an emotional roller coaster. And this grueling and uncertain quest is often embarked upon by couples who have only recently suffered the loss of an unborn child or come to terms with the painful truth that they will never build a family by giving birth to children themselves.

SEXUALITY, GYNECOLOGICAL ISSUES, AND THE PASSAGE OF TIME

"A few days ago, I was walking down the street, and I heard men whistling, saying, 'Hey, beauty.' I didn't think they were talking about me, but they followed me and kept whistling, clearly at me. Then they came up on either side of me, and said, 'Oh, no. She's old, forget it.' I didn't know what to feel. I was offended that they were following me and whistling at me. Then I was offended that they thought I was old. Then I laughed."

Suzanne Peters (age 43)

"When I was coming into my sexual prime my husband left me. I sometimes wonder if that was the reason for his leaving."

Robin Young (age 46)

YES, LIFE ISN'T FAIR. Aging isn't fair. And sex isn't fair. Sex can disappoint us no matter how experienced we are. Sex can elude us. Sex can confuse us. Sex can even kill us. But despite these realities, midlife is the prime of life, and it's the time when sexuality really begins to blossom for some women. A woman who is forty knows her body and knows what she wants. She is also versed in the arts of diplomacy and compromise—she's had to be to survive. Suddenly, all this self-knowledge, wisdom, and gusto converge to make her more than able to take care of herself in the bedroom by asking for and getting what she wants and enjoying it more while still being a loving and generous sexual partner.

Some women continue to enjoy sex with the same partner. Some women find a new partner with whom they enjoy sex more. Some women who had always been heterosexual find they have more fun with women. For others, just when things were getting good, a partner dies or leaves. For others, a bout with serious illness may hamper enjoying sex fully. And there are also those who may simply be glad to have the whole business over with and thus are happy to use age as an excuse not to engage.

Wherever you fit into this patchwork quilt of aging and sexuality, there are two rules to observe to help ensure your mental and physical health:

1. You must find the sexual milieu and the kind of sexual activity that works for you.
2. You must remember that you are never too old to practice safe sex, because you are never too old to contract a sexually transmitted disease.

If you choose a new partner when you are eighty and you plan to have intercourse, there is just as good a reason to protect yourself as if you were twenty, thirty, or forty. The reason is AIDS and other STDs. They do not practice ageism.

Love in the Age of AIDS

There was a time, not too long ago, when the only thing we thought of when we thought of safe sex was not getting pregnant. Bad as they may have been, those were the good old days. Now it's not our hearts we worry about, but our lives.

If you find yourself dating again after all these years, the optimal way to begin a sexual relationship is for both you and your partner to be tested for sexually transmitted diseases, including HIV, and then to proceed with sexual relations using a condom, a barrier method, or both.

RATING SEX FOR SAFETY

- Petting and mutual masturbation with clean hands is safe.
- Oral sex cannot be guaranteed as safe.
- Intercourse is not safe.
- Anal intercourse is not safe.

If the person you are considering sleeping with is not interested in taking these precautions, you may want to reconsider things. Not only is he unwilling to assure you of your own physical safety during sex, he is also resisting taking the first step toward a trusting relationship. The question is: What kind of a relationship could you possibly have with such a man? The answer is, an unsatisfying and possibly dangerous one. No one, particularly someone with the wisdom of a few added years, has time for that.

Sleeping with Married Men (Who Are Married to Someone Else)

If you've told yourself married men are safe, ask yourself this: If he's sleeping with you, what makes you so sure he hasn't been sleeping with other people too? You cannot simply say to yourself, "Oh, this guy has had a monogamous relationship until now." The truth is, you just don't know. If you go ahead with a relationship, you must use a condom and you should consider a test for HIV too.

Sexually Transmitted Diseases and AIDS

"I started getting divorced when I was thirty-nine. By the time I was forty-two, I was at least living separately. I had a younger boyfriend who wanted to become my lover. I wanted him, too. We were kind of rolling around on the bed and there were no condoms. I told him I couldn't have sex if it wasn't safe. I cared about my

health, and I had small children who needed me. As safe
as a person may seem, you never know. He got out of
bed and went to the drugstore to buy condoms. I'm sure
I've felt more powerful, but I felt powerful enough at that
moment. By the way, the sex was great."

Jessica McCamce (age 44)

Chlamydia

Chlamydia trachomatis is the most common bacterial STD in the United States. Chlamydia is transmitted through vaginal or anal intercourse and by oral-genital contact. This is a sexist disease—women are more at risk for this infection, they are easily infected, and they experience most of the symptoms. At least 70 percent of females who've had sexual relations with an infected male will be infected themselves, while less than 50 percent of men who sleep with infected women will become infected. Between three and four million Americans are thought to be infected with chlamydia each year. The disease, oddly enough, is not reportable at the state or national level, so these numbers are estimates.

The disease is often asymptomatic in women and therefore hard to diagnose. If it goes undiagnosed, chlamydia can be a major cause of infertility in women. Because it can be asymptomatic, chlamydia has usually moved up the reproductive tract and caused damage before it is discovered. Fully half the women with a chlamydial infection have already experienced damage to the lining of the uterus (chlamydial endometriosis) by the time they are diagnosed. By that time 30 to 40 percent have pelvic inflammatory disease (PID) which leads, in turn, to infertility (PID often produces scarring of the fallopian tubes). It also should be noted that a single episode of PID increases a woman's chances of an ectopic pregnancy by 700 percent!

Though mild cases of chlamydia may produce no symptoms, more severe cases may be accompanied by lower abdominal pain, irregular menstrual flow, vaginal discharge, nausea or vomiting, and sometimes fever. Pain during intercourse is also common. While none of these is necessarily a sign of chlamydia, such symptoms should not be ignored. If there is any chance that you may have this or any other STD, you

173

should err on the side of caution and consult your physician as soon as you notice any such symptoms. Chlamydia can be treated with antibiotics. (Your partner must be treated, too.) If not treated, it does progress.

Genital Herpes

Genital herpes affects approximately 40 million Americans and approximately half a million new cases are diagnosed annually. Genital herpes is highly infectious. A man who has one sexual contact with a woman who is infected and symptomatic has a 50 percent chance of infection. The statistics for women are even more alarming. A woman who has a single sexual contact with an infected, symptomatic man has an 80 to 90 percent chance of infection. The herpes simplex virus enters at the mouth, the vagina, or the urethra (all mucosal surfaces), or at cracks or tiny breaks in the skin. You may also be infected if you share a sex toy such as a vibrator or even a towel that has been used by an infected and symptomatic person.

If you are infected with genital herpes, the incubation time is about three to six days. A day or two before you actually notice blisters, you may experience itching or burning in the genital area. It usually takes ten to twenty days for an outbreak of genital herpes to heal. Although once infected with genital herpes, you have it for life, at least a third of those with genital herpes never experience a second, noticeable case. In others, recurrences diminish in number and intensity as time passes.

The highly infectious nature of genital herpes is one more good reason to strictly adhere to safe sex practices, since using a condom greatly improves your chances of not being infected. If you have an attack of genital herpes, it is recommended that you abstain from sex for at least ten days after the lesions disappear. If you have a recurrence, you should abstain for at least two days after the lesions disappear. If you have a tingling or burning sensation in the genital area and know that you are infected with the herpes simplex virus, you should also abstain from sex.

When you have an outbreak of herpes, you should wear loose-fitting cotton underwear to keep the blisters from being irritated further. You should also refrain from wearing pantyhose if possible, for the sake of comfort. You should use a disinfectant spray, such as Betadine, a few times a day to cut down on the chances of a secondary infection. Avoid damp clothing, such as a bathing suit. You may also consider avoiding physical activity such as bicycle riding or horseback riding for the obvious reason of added discomfort. Wash the area several times a day and avoid feminine deodorants or harsh soaps that may cause added irritation. If you have pain or discomfort, ibuprofen or aspirin will help.

Genital Warts

Genital warts or venereal warts are also called condylomata acuminata. They are soft and dry, usually painless warts that grow on or around the genitals and around the anus. They are often pink or grayish white in color and may give the appearance of clusters of miniature cauliflower. Genital warts are caused by a virus called the human papilloma virus (HPV) that is sexually transmitted.

Until as recently as the 1950s, genital warts were not generally considered to be infectious or sexually transmitted. It actually took a study of wives of returning Korean war veterans, who found themselves quite suddenly to be afflicted with vulvar warts, for the connection to be medically verified.

The present estimate is that there are 750,000 new cases of HPV per year and 12 million cases of venereal warts in the United States today. Recent research has made clear that venereal warts are not only a cosmetic problem, but a health problem as well. HPV has been found in studies to raise the risk of cervical cancer for women. If you are infected with HPV, you should make sure that you have regular Pap smears and consider having them more frequently than once a year—once every six or nine months. Additionally, if you have been diagnosed with HPV, you should be tested for other STDs, since venereal warts are often found to coexist with them.

Venereal warts are commonly found in the labia, the opening of the vagina, the inner third of the vagina, and on the cervix. You may find small patches of gray or pink tissues in only a few locations or you may feel overwhelmed because the warts cover almost all the exposed genital area. Warts also may be found just inside the urethra. Genital warts are usually obvious to a medical examiner. Because similar lesions are found in cases of syphilis, a blood test is done routinely to screen for syphilis. Genital warts are yet another good medical reason to use condoms at all times—if you know that you have the virus, you probably also know that you may not always be able to see the lesions or warts.

At present, there is no treatment that successfully eradicates venereal warts forever. The present treatments can only help to remove a visible outbreak of warts. These include:

- Trichloroacetic acid, which is applied to the warts on a weekly basis.
- Podophyllum, which is contained in a liquid base and is applied by a doctor or health-care specialist. It is a caustic chemical that you should not apply yourself, nor should it be used if you are pregnant.
- Carbon dioxide laser surgery, which burns away the warts.
- Liquid nitrogen, which freezes and usually destroys the warts after one or two treatments.
- Interferon, which is a protein that is injected into the base of the warts.

Again, none of these treatments can eradicate HPV itself. Though venereal warts are often contracted early in the sexual life an adult, they can be passed on to anyone at anytime through sexual contact and the infection lasts a lifetime. So protect yourself and others.

Viral Hepatitis

There are many kinds of hepatitis, but hepatitis B, which has been found in semen, vaginal secretions, and saliva, is the variety that is an STD. It may be transmitted by infected blood, but it also may be transmitted by sexual activity—*any kind* of sexual activity including kissing. Recent studies show that anal intercourse or not using vaginal contraceptives during vaginal intercourse may facilitate transmission of the virus. Sex with multiple partners is also a major risk among heterosexuals.

Often, hepatitis B infections are asymptomatic—the person who has it doesn't know it. If you are considering a new partner, practicing safe sex continually is the only way to help prevent sexual transmission.

The good news about hepatitis is that there are vaccines available now for hepatitis A and B. The vaccine for hepatitis A is not licensed in the United States, but the vaccine for hepatitis B is available in this country. I believe so strongly in this vaccine that not only have I been vaccinated, but I have had all three of my children vaccinated. If you have a family member who is a hepatitis B carrier, if you are work in the health-care field, if you have taken or do take intravenous drugs or have had or do have multiple sex partners, or if you have had a bisexual partner, it is recommended that you be vaccinated for hepatitis B.

AIDS

AIDS (Acquired Immune Deficiency Syndrome) is caused by the human immunodeficiency virus (HIV), which destroys the body's immune system, thus allowing normally mundane or rare infections to eventually overcome and destroy the body. In essence, it is the lack of a functioning immune system that causes the body to fail and succumb to an otherwise manageable infection.

Normally the immune system produces white blood cells that attack foreign substances and germs. Whether it be an ear infection or a tumor, the immune system is on guard to protect us with billions of disease-fighting cells. What makes AIDS so insidious is that this virus infiltrates the immune system and individual cells. The virus uses the machinery inside the body's cells to stop fighting infections and instead start producing more virus. As this happens the immune system is literally depleted—allowing infections and tumors to set up shop.

While small groups of people who are HIV positive have been followed for more than ten years without developing full-blown AIDS, these groups are almost completely made up of men with AIDS. Very few women who are HIV positive have been followed for the same length of time. In fact, the first studies of women with AIDS were instituted only in the early 1990s and long-term data will begin to be available only in the next few years. It should also be made clear that *the signs of AIDS or HIV infection are different for women than they are for men.* It is noteworthy that research for this disease has, until recently, almost entirely ignored a major segment of the population that is at risk—namely, women.

Unfortunately, but quite clearly, AIDS is a woman's issue. In one study of women in Brazil and the United States, women with AIDS were found to live a shorter time than men with AIDS. The major reason

177

for this difference is thought to be lack of treatment, particularly early treatment prior to the development of full-blown AIDS. Often women fail to receive early treatment because they are not diagnosed early.

Recent research on women has revealed some of the symptoms of the disease that are exclusive to women. The list below gives gynecologic symptoms that may indicate HIV infection. It should be stressed that most women who have these conditions do not have AIDS, and there is no cause for alarm and no reason to worry. But if you have placed yourself at risk for AIDS and have one or more of these conditions, you should have an HIV test immediately as a precautionary measure:

- Recurrent yeast infections, when yeast infections were previously not a problem
- Other vaginal infections that are chronic
- Sexually transmitted diseases (see above)
- Pelvic inflammatory disease (PID)
- Cervical cancer

If you know you may have been exposed to the virus—even if you don't have any of these symptoms—err on the smart side and get tested anyway.

HIV is found in significant concentrations in semen, vaginal secretions, blood, and breast milk. It is through the exchange of these body fluids that the infection can be passed from one person to another. The virus is not found in high enough concentrations in other fluids or the skin to make casual contact a concern. It is not contracted from such everyday events as shaking hands, and it is not transmitted by being exposed to someone's tears. Nor is it possible to contract it through the saliva exchanged in kissing. Although one study, taken out of context and blown out of proportion in some newspaper headlines, stated a remote chance of the presence of the virus in human saliva, it would take gallons and gallons of saliva to present any risk at all of infection—certainly more saliva than the most passionate of deep kissers may exchange.

A person who is HIV positive is considered to have AIDS when one or more of the serious illnesses related to HIV (such as Kaposi's sarcoma or Pneumocystis carinii pneumonia) is diagnosed or when the functioning of the immune system has been significantly reduced. Immune-system function is measured by how many T4 cells (also referred to as CD4+ lymphocytes) are in the blood. When the count of T4 cells, which are white blood cells that normally fight infection, goes below 200 per cubic millimeter of blood, the immune system is said to be significantly impaired.

HIV is a slow-acting virus and may exist in low levels in the body for years, causing few, if any, problems. But over time, as other organisms that cause illness find their way into the bloodstream and the immune system is activated again and again, the immune system begins to wear down and the HIV spreads. This is why maintaining the best health possible, avoiding infections whenever possible, and obtaining treatment for any infection immediately are all paramount strategies in the defense against AIDS.

Sometimes a person who is HIV positive may go twelve years or more without developing serious AIDS-related illnesses. Although such longevity in HIV positive patients has been considerably rare, as AIDS-related illnesses are better managed, more and more people are living nearly illness-free for greater periods of time. Researchers are now studying those HIV positive patients who are living for long periods of time without full-blown AIDS to try to find out what self-protective mechanisms the body develops to keep the virus at bay.

"Safe sex, sure. Condoms, sure. But who teaches Condoms 101 for grown-ups? When I was married, I used a diaphragm. When I was divorced, I was forty-two, and my doctor said, 'Always use a condom when you have sex.' This seemed like such a remote possibility at the time that I didn't ask him the particulars regarding how to use one. Well, eventually I did have sex again. I did use a condom. We were both a bit awkward about the whole thing and lo and behold, the condom ended up being left

*behind inside me. So there I was, in the ER getting
a condom removed. Well . . . we got the hang of
it, and I'm still seeing him. Maybe we'll give a
course."*

Hilda Carlson (age 46)

W E LIVE in a world where anyone can get AIDS, but we also
live in a world where we can avoid this disease. Information
is readily available to us regarding how to minimize our risk
for AIDS. Here are some steps that are absolutely necessary to take to
help avoid contracting AIDS:

- Always practice safe sex. This means that your partner must use a
  condom whenever you have vaginal or anal intercourse.
- Do not have sex with a stranger. This is a tough one, because even
  the love of your life was a stranger once. But when I say "stranger,"
  I mean the following: Don't sleep with a man you don't know. Don't
  sleep with a man you can't trust or can't talk to about issues such as
  AIDS. Don't sleep with someone who isn't willing to have an HIV
  test with you.
- If you use IV drugs, do not share needles.
- Do not have sex with someone who uses IV drugs.
- Do not have sex with a man you know sleeps around.
- Do not have sex with a hemophiliac. Hemophiliacs are almost always
  male, and almost all the hemophiliacs in the United States born
  before 1985 have been infected with HIV.
- Be monogamous with a monogamous person after ascertaining that
  neither of you is HIV positive. If this seems easier said than done,
  remember that life—by which I mean healthy life—is more important than sex.
- Store your own blood if you are planning to have surgery and may
  need a transfusion.
- If you are planning to be artificially inseminated, use frozen sperm
  that has been tested several times, over more than a period of a year,
  for the AIDS virus.
- Do not have sex with a homosexual or bisexual man.

Birth Control After Forty

"I knew I wasn't going to have any other babies. And this was in the days before everyone worried about sexually transmitted diseases, or husbands getting vasectomies. So I had my tubes tied and discovered a new sexual freedom."

Joy Marion (age 63)

A S A WOMAN AGES, her needs for birth control change, as does her perception of which control methods are comfortable. In particular, in an older woman, the traditional barrier methods, such as the diaphragm and the cervical cap, may become increasingly uncomfortable to use. Only you can be the judge of what's comfortable and what isn't. However, if you find that you're avoiding sex because the method of birth control you're using just doesn't make you feel good, explore other options.

The preferred method of birth control for older women is sterilization. For married couples over thirty, sterilization is the most common choice for birth control. Sterilization is a permanent and irreversible method of surgical birth control. Women and men often choose sterilization in midlife because they are very sure they will not want any more children. The failure rate is 0.4 percent for men and women, making sterilization the most reliable form of birth control available.

It must be stressed, however, that sterilization has been abused flagrantly in the United States when treating women who are middle-aged, of lower socioeconomic standing, or African American, or women who speak a language other than English. Because of pressure from minority and women's groups, regulations were enacted in March 1979 protecting women seeking federally funded sterilization. These regulations prohibit any threat, overt or implicit, of the loss of welfare or Medicaid benefits if a woman does not consent to sterilization; they also prohibit the use of hysterectomy for the purpose of sterilization.

Tubal ligation, the process by which sterilization is achieved for women, involves dividing or tying off a woman's fallopian tubes so that

181

eggs cannot pass through the tubes to the uterus. Vasectomy, the sterilization process for men, is a simpler and less expensive procedure that involves fewer possible complications than tubal ligation. It also has a lower failure rate. A vasectomy is not immediately effective, and you should continue to use another method of birth control for approximately fifteen days or ten ejaculations after the process and after follow-up tests have been done. Your partner is considered to be sterile only after two negative sperm counts.

If you have relied upon the pill until now, you should reevaluate your choice of birth control as you approach forty. Some physicians recommend that women over thirty-five avoid the pill because of the increased risk of heart attack and stroke. Much of this depends on your family history and lifestyle—i.e., your overall health, exercise patterns, use of cigarettes, and obesity. If you are over thirty-five and smoke, you will be strongly advised to avoid taking the pill.

The IUD is the most widely used method of birth control in the world. Many physicians love the IUD for women over forty because of its ease and reliability. Nonetheless, this method can have complications. One of the major risks associated with the IUD is infection—a risk at any age. The three most dangerous IUDs—the Dalkon Shield, the Majzlin Spring, and the Birnberg Bow—have been taken off the market, but some women may still have them. If you think that you may still be using one of these three IUDs, you should have your IUD removed immediately. A common symptom associated with the IUD use is midcycle bleeding, which may also be a sign of one of the reproductive cancers—another reason to check with your doctor to see if there is another method of birth control that might be better for you. The obvious concern is that if you use an IUD, such a symptom might be dangerously disregarded. One other problem for women using an IUD over forty is that the uterus becomes smaller, causing the IUD to be deeply imbedded and difficult to remove.

The diaphragm and the other barrier methods are commonly recommended forms of birth control for women over forty who do not wish to pursue sterilization. You should have your diaphragm refitted regularly and be conscientious about removing it as soon as it is safe to after intercourse, since diaphragms have been associated with urinary tract infections. You should also clean your diaphragm thoroughly and get a new one regularly to avoid infections and tears in the diaphragm wall.

The diaphragm is 98 percent effective when used with a spermicidal cream or jelly.

The most important thing for a woman undergoing menopause to remember is that she should use birth control for a full year after she ceases to get her period. Once you stop getting your period regularly, the inclination may be to throw your hands up in the air and go, "Hurray, no more birth control!" Don't: missing your period may or may not mean that you haven't ovulated. Many women become irregular before their periods cease altogether and thus may ovulate, though infrequently. (See "Birth Control and Menopause," page 217, for further information.)

Abortion

"Abortion is the most divisive social issue to face this country since slavery."

C. Everett Koop, M.D.

THE CLINICAL DEFINITION of abortion is the deliberate removal of fetal tissue from the uterus in order to terminate a pregnancy. There are many methods for aborting fetal tissue and many reasons women choose to have an abortion. Abortion is not considered to be of greater risk to a woman over forty who is in good health.

It is inevitable that there are widespread misunderstandings regarding such a controversial procedure. Some of these misconceptions include the notion that a woman has been irresponsible about birth control. This tendency to blame a woman for negligence exists among both the general population and doctors. The truth is there is no form of birth control that is 100 percent effective. And while vasectomy is the simplest, safest, cheapest, and most effective form of birth control, there are many men, even those who have already become fathers, who refuse to even consider a vasectomy. Thus women often remain responsible for birth control, relying on those methods that are 98 percent effective. Yet they are blamed for being irresponsible when they wind up in the 2 percent for whom birth control did not prevent contraception. And women who have had more than one abortion are often seen as having some deep-rooted psychological problem. Would a sexually active man who had been responsible for more than one abortion be stigmatized in the same way?

Any woman, no matter how conscientious she may be, may face an unwanted pregnancy during her reproductive years. On average, women are fertile for approximately thirty-five years. A lot can happen in thirty-five years (two world wars were fought within a thirty-five-year period). And yet women are consistently blamed for unwanted pregnancies, as if this were a situation they created all by themselves.

The decision to have an abortion is often hard to make for a woman, and the process itself is not pleasant. No sensible woman makes this decision lightly. To insist otherwise—to claim that women breeze through it—is, as Betty Friedan once said, like saying women are gung ho about having mastectomies. When a woman makes this difficult decision, we need to remember that a man was involved in the decision as well, because he wanted to sleep with this particular woman, but not to share a child with her, felt that it was the right decision for both of them, or was completely absent—and irresponsibly so—after having, at least sexually, committed himself to a woman.

Abortion was legalized by the Supreme Court in 1973, but the debate about abortion only grows more intense over time. As outlined by the landmark decision *Roe* v. *Wade*, during the first trimester (the first 12 weeks) of pregnancy, the decision to abort is stated to be a private matter between a woman and her doctor. In the second trimester, individual states may require that abortions be done only at licensed hospitals for the sake of the woman's health. As individual states pass legislation restricting abortion rights, what a woman can or cannot do legally becomes more difficult to ascertain, so each individual needs to be aware of the rules in her state. In more and more states, if a woman requests an abortion, the spouse's consent is required, which for some women becomes restrictive. And there are many groups and many elected officials now fighting to overturn *Roe* v. *Wade*.

Choice Means Choice

"I was shocked to find myself pregnant at forty-nine.
Our daughter was a sophomore in college and I didn't

*hesitate in my decision to terminate this pregnancy. If I
had been ten years younger, it might not have been such
an easy decision."*

Diana Williams (age 50)

W HAT YOU CHOOSE to do if you find yourself pregnant at
forty-two, and what you chose to do at twenty-one may be
a world apart. That is what choice is all about. Take the
time to thoroughly consider all your options, and if you find the choice
you are facing to be a particularly difficult one, seek help, from both a
professional counselor and friends. Do everything you can to ensure that
the choice you make is truly your own.

A standard pregnancy test is not accurate until the pregnancy has
reached six weeks, though newer special tests may be accurate at
twenty-four days. Nevertheless, most women do not know that they are
pregnant until they've missed one period and are at least four to six
weeks pregnant. An early abortion must be performed before a woman
is twelve weeks pregnant. Thus, you usually have only about a month
to make this decision. At least 5 percent of women who initially choose
to have an abortion do not go through with this decision. Thus, counseling and the procedure are usually not scheduled for the same day.
Before going any further, you will want to have your blood pressure
taken and have your blood tested to see if you are anemic. You will also
want to find out if you have Rh positive or Rh negative blood—if you
are Rh positive and pregnant with an Rh negative fetus, the opposing
cells could enter your blood during an abortion procedure and cause an
antibody reaction.

If you do choose to terminate the pregnancy, you'll want to be aware
of what procedures are available to you.

- *Early Vacuum Abortion.* This is the most common method of early
  abortion and is usually performed within four to twelve weeks. A
  tube is attached to a suction device and inserted through the cervix
  into the uterus. Then the uterus is gently vacuumed. This procedure,
  which is usually done under local or general anesthetic, has the few-

est side effects. In some instances it can be performed in the doctor's office or clinic without anesthesia.

- *Dilation and Evacuation Abortion.* D&E is usually performed within thirteen to twenty weeks. The procedure is a combination of the suction curettage done in early abortions and a surgical procedure in which a sharp curette (a scoop-shaped surgical instrument used to remove tissue from body cavities such as the uterus) is inserted to remove any remaining fetal tissue.

- *Prostaglandin Vaginal Suppositories.* In this process, vaginal suppositories are inserted every three to four hours to induce uterine contractions. This method is new and may cause nausea, intense contractions, and other side effects. It is also associated with fairly high rates of incomplete abortion and a D&C (dilation and curettage) may be necessary immediately afterward to remove remaining tissue.

For abortion procedure used in the middle trimester, see page 141.

RU-486

In 1980 an abortifacient drug called RU-486 was synthesized and eight years later it was marketed in France. Three years after that, the drug became available in England. It has yet to be made available in the United States, but is currently undergoing clinical trials. RU-486 is the first in a new category of drugs called antiprogestins. Among other effects, RU-486 interferes with the production of progesterone, which is the hormone that nurtures a developing pregnancy. When deprived of progesterone, the placenta will wither and then decompose, and if an embryo has recently implanted, it separates from the uterine wall and is discharged from the vagina.

RU-486 must be taken approximately seven to nine weeks after your last period, when you are five to seven weeks pregnant, for it to be effective. Taken alone, RU-486 is about 80 percent effective, but it is about 95 percent effective when taken along with a booster dose of prostaglandin. Prostaglandin is the hormone that causes the uterus to contract. In France, a woman is given three 200 mg tablets of RU-486 and sent home; taking these is sometimes enough to cause a woman to miscarry (at this point in a pregnancy, a miscarriage is similar to a heavy period with noticeable cramping). Two days after taking RU-486, a woman is then given a vaginal suppository of prostaglandin or a dose of Cytotec—an ulcer medication in the prostaglandin family. Ninety-five percent of women miscarry within four hours after taking prostaglandin.

Almost all of the physical effects associated with the combination of RU-486 and prostaglandin combination are attributable to the latter. These effects include:

- Moderate to severe cramping for the hours before the abortion occurs
- Bleeding for anywhere from four to forty days
- Dizziness, nausea, vomiting, and/or diarrhea

As an abortion method RU-486 has one primary advantage—since no instruments enter the body, there is little or no risk of infection. One of the disadvantages is that, at least at present, when RU-486 is administered in France, the procedure takes four visits. Doctors stress that the prostaglandin must be given and women must keep their appointments.

Other Gynecological Issues

DES—Past and Present

"When I found out that my mother took DES I was paralyzed with fear. My first impulse was to rent space in my doctor's office! But now I just get checked regularly and spend time telling my mother that it's okay—it's not her fault."

Kate Summers (age 41)

I N THE 1940s and 1950s diethylstilbestrol, or DES, was given to women to prevent miscarriages. A generation later, clear cell carcinoma, a very rare vaginal cancer, was diagnosed in seven young women—all of whose mothers had taken DES to avoid miscarriage. While there is a relationship between in utero exposure to DES and this rare cancer, the incidence of clear cell carcinoma among DES

187

daughters is much lower than was initially expected—the range is somewhere between 1 and 2 per 1,000 and 1 and 2 per 10,000. About 300 DES daughters in total have been diagnosed with vaginal cancer. There may also be an increased risk of cancer of the cervix or precancerous cervical changes (dysplasia), but the increased risk is small and whether there is a connection at all is still being debated.

Approximately 80 percent of DES daughters, however, do have benign changes of the cervix or vagina due to in utero exposure to DES. Most of these changes would be impossible to detect without a pelvic exam. Sometimes a fold of vaginal tissue called a vaginal collar surrounds the cervix. Also, glands that are usually found only in the cervix may be found in small numbers in the vagina as well. This condition is called adenosis and may lead to increased vaginal discharge. Of those DES daughters diagnosed with vaginal cancer, 90 percent also have adenosis, leading to the theory that vaginal cancer may develop in areas of adenosis. However, this is as yet only a theory.

STRATEGIES FOR A DES DAUGHTER

DES daughters should have an annual pelvic exam, including a regular Pap smear, a Pap smear of the upper vagina where vaginal cancer occurs, and iodine staining of the vagina, beginning at the age of fourteen. If there are any abnormalities in your Pap smear, you should have a colposcopic examination and begin to have regular exams every six months. Any abnormal or irregular bleeding should be reported to your doctor immediately. You should avoid the use of estrogen, either in birth control pills, after-intercourse contraception, or hormonal replacement therapy after menopause. If you become pregnant, pay special attention to signs of premature labor and ask your doctor to check your cervix for signs of early dilation frequently.

IF YOU HAVE TAKEN DES

There is much debate about whether or not having taken DES increases your chances of breast cancer. Since there is not enough evidence to conclude that there is a cause-and-effect relationship between taking DES and increased risk, the best advice is to take the same precautions you should take anyway—practice self-examination, have a breast and pelvic exam annually, and have periodic mammograms after the age of forty.

PMS—What It Is and What It Isn't

"Now that I'm in my thirties PMS doesn't take the toll
on me that it used to. I understand it more now. I know
what to expect. I'm not saying I like it—but at least there
aren't as many surprises."

Angela Bates (age 34)

THE TERM "RAGING HORMONES" has dogged the path of women's emancipation for decades, and it is probably time to lay this phrase to rest once and for all. Hormones do not rage. Hormone levels in the body change, as they are designed to. This is natural, this is biology. And the power of hormones is not a female issue—it's a human issue. Women and men have hormones, need hormones, and have more or less of certain hormones at certain times. The systems are different, the cycles are different, but both sexes have systems and cycles. However, we know only too well that estrogen seems all too often to take the rap for that truant family member, testosterone. We never hear about the "raging testosterone" present in the street brawl between two "reasonable" men over a car alarm that whined all night. At the very least, it is clear that the spectrum of acceptable female behavior is much more narrow than the spectrum of acceptable behavior that men enjoy.

The sooner we deal straightforwardly with hormonal changes as an aspect of human biology and not a value judgment upon one sex, the better. And the less we imbue hormones with magic powers, the closer we will be to an unbiased and biologically sound assessment of what hormonal changes do and what we can expect from these changes.

Although progress in this area seemed to be at least visible as a blip on the radar screen, that blip now seems to be moving off the screen. Take, for example, PMS. At first, we were delighted that we were finally being taken seriously when we said, "This thing called the menstrual cycle . . . you know, believe it or not, when there are changes in hormonal levels at different times of the month, there are sometimes changes in the way that I feel." We thought we were being freed from that old, catchall, sexist dismissal, "It's all in your head." Perhaps we were, but we were being incarcerated in a much more confining, if

189

insidious, methodology of dismissal. To use an analogy befitting the consequences women sometimes face in this society, once again the punishment does not fit the crime. Suddenly, PMS is listed as a new psychiatric disorder. Now PMS appears in the American Psychiatric Association reference manual as Late Luteal Phase Dysphoric Disorder or LLPDD. Supposedly this legitimization, via serious title and initials, refers to symptoms so severe that they may interfere with or curtail work or social activities or relationships. Well, yes and no. I by no means want to dismiss the existence of PMS, but I do want to stress that such severe cases are few and far between; and even then, this condition (part of the natural, biological cycle) is being branded—and thus stigmatized—by the medical dogma that insists that to be female is to be other and therefore dismissable.

Estimates tell us that between 20 and 80 percent of menstruating women suffer some form of PMS. This disparity in numbers is reflective of the confusion and vehement disagreement that plagues the debate regarding what PMS is, what PMS does to the women who suffer from it, and how to treat PMS.

Believe it or not, two hundred different symptoms have been reported in association with PMS. The most common physical symptoms include: breast tenderness, a craving for salt or for sweets, abdominal bloating, headaches, and leg swelling. The most common psychological symptoms include: irritability, a sense of things not quite working right or going right or being right, depression, a loss of self-confidence, and hostility.

PMS is most common after the age of thirty or thirty-five. It often begins or becomes more pronounced after childbirth or some other significant interruption in the hormonal and menstrual cycle, such as when a woman stops taking birth control pills. It also increases in severity with age. In fact many women confuse menopause with an exacerbation of PMS.

This is another area in which you will do better to trust yourself before you trust anybody else. You are the best judge of your PMS. If you think you have symptoms of PMS, keep a chart for a month or two. Record your patterns of menstruation—the number of days and the amount of bleeding. Record your thoughts, moods, headaches, and food cravings or intolerances. Then share this chart with your doctor. If you feel you have a serious condition and your doctor agrees, she or he will prescribe medication. Diuretics are used to alleviate bloating. Progesterone may be used in the treatment of PMS and is taken orally or vaginally, though results of this therapy are mixed. Antidepressants, such as Xanax or Prozac, may also be prescribed. PMS is due in part to a deficiency of the chemical serotonin. So it makes sense that certain medications (like Prozac) that inhibit the uptake of serotonin work in alleviating PMS symptoms. In a recent study published in the *New England Journal of Medicine*, women who took Prozac because of severe PMS symptoms showed four to six times more improvement than those who took a placebo. Women treated with a low dose of 20 mg had reduced symptoms with few side effects.

However, do not underestimate the effect of diet and exercise on your symptoms. You yourself and your attitude are the best weapons you have in protecting yourself from serious effects of PMS. You know how your body changes before you get your period, and you know how to help yourself through these times. Many women find that adding a morning exercise routine helps relieve some of the tension and symptoms that they experience. Others find that taking Tylenol at night for a few nights before their period is due helps relieve discomfort. Some women add a vitamin B supplement to their daily routine the week before their period.

If you find that as the years pass you can "tell" you're getting your period in more insistent ways, you may want to talk to your gynecologist about how to help yourself through these times. Behavior changes, such as additional exercise, drinking plenty of fluids, and eliminating wine or other alcoholic beverages from the diet, can help you counteract your symptoms before you consider other courses of treatment.

The Effects of Aging on Your Sexuality

"I've been with the same man for fifty-two years. That may sound odd by today's standards but this relationship has been the cornerstone of my life. And sex has always been important to both of us. We may not go as fast or as often as we used to. But we still take the time to touch each other."

Lida Samuals (age 72)

S EX IS PLEASURABLE, and great sex is even more pleasurable. Sex is a way of sharing intimacy. It's also a way of communicating without words. Safe sex is good for you and good for your health. Above all, sex is and should be fun, and the good news is, sex can be even more fun for women in the prime of life.

Women approaching forty or in their forties may find themselves at a sexual peak of sorts, lusty, arousable, and knowledgeable about what they like and how and when they like it. Remember to consider yourself in your prime and enjoy it. Of course, once we've been around the romantic block a time or two, there is one thing we all know: as much as we might like sex to be a constant in our lives, no one has the sex she wants to have with the person she wants to have it with the right number of times a week she wants to have it all of the time. That sex comes and goes is a fact of life. Put another way, sex lives—like life itself—are changeable, and if we're experiencing a sexual drought of sorts, there is no reason to think of it as permanent or to allow the absence of sex in our lives to make us feel less sensual, sexy, or womanly. As we grow into ourselves, becoming comfortable with our mature bodies and confident that we have the wisdom and knowledge to take good care of ourselves, we can also feel good about being sensual and expressing our sexual and sensual selves—no matter what sort of sex life we might be experiencing. The truth is, we are sexual beings all the time—not just some of the time—and this is something to enjoy.

Sex and Society

As a society, we Americans don't deal very comfortably with the topic of sexuality in general. We consider it to be roughly equivalent to violence and place many of the same prohibitions upon filming and viewing it. We tell one another that it's the last thing we want our teenage children to be exposed to, and then we neglect to talk to them about the very thing we don't wish them to be discovering and exploring on their own without our guidance.

Our media declare again and again that sex is the province of the very young—and basically very heterosexual young—with a few enlightening, but always acerbically drawn film portraits of the exceptions. Of course, in fact, sex is for the living; as long as it is safe, sex is healthy and restorative for any adult at any age with a disease-free, consenting adult who is not a blood relation.

In addition, we certainly don't deal well or openly with sexuality in the second half of life. We act as if, after a certain age, sex doesn't exist or ought to be practiced extremely discreetly, without fanfare (as if it were the taking of tea). Nothing could be further from the truth.

It's not sex that vanishes—sometimes, sadly, it's the loving partner who does, and sometimes, just as sadly, it's the willingness to make the effort to enjoy it. When it comes to sex after forty and fifty and sixty and seventy, the most important thing to remember is that your sex life can and will last a lifetime—if you want it to.

Changes for a Male Partner

What changes most noticeably when it comes to sex in the middle and later years involves timing. To put it another way, it's not how you have sex, but how long it takes you to have sex. This may actually be a very thinly disguised gift for most women and men. Arousal time becomes time for foreplay—and after all those times you've said, "Don't rush," now you have your wish. If you play your foreplay cards right, taking a little longer at it can hardly be considered a negative. Indeed, it can become a truly life-enhancing positive. We could all benefit from taking more time for pleasure and intimacy.

In general, when men age, the following occurs:

- Getting an erection takes longer.
- Erections are not as hard.
- Unless there is an existing problem with premature ejaculation, the time it takes to reach orgasm and ejaculate is longer, and ejaculation may not be as powerful.
- After ejaculation, the time before a second erection is possible is longer.
- More direct physical stimulation is necessary to obtain an erection and orgasm.

Men often report feeling a great deal of pressure regarding performance. Therefore, the best favor that you can do your partner is to take the pressure off. This can include actually verbalizing your assurance or showing how you feel in physical ways, or both.

Foreplay can be verbal as well as physical. In fact, it can be anything you and your partner want it to be. Remember, freedom of choice extends to the bedroom. Even though foreplay may not be everything, remember that great preludes can be wonderful introductions to even greater music. You never know: once you begin to say "what's the rush?" and since you know from experience what works for you, you might find that sex is actually better now that you have the wisdom and maturity to appreciate it. Try it often, so you can make it a habit if it isn't already.

Changes for a Female Partner

"I had breast cancer, and I thought I was really cool about it. I was sure my husband would be fine about my body, as I was sure I would be. Well, the first time we were in bed for reasons of desire and not exhaustion, I started crying and couldn't stop. The best thing my husband did was to appreciate my tears. That did more for my libido than any false compliment."

Mary Bockman (age 54)

IN TERMS OF ATTITUDE, some women report being more self-conscious about their aging bodies. In other words, society's attitudes do take their toll. Often women are brainwashed into confusing what the culture deems "looking sexy" with actually feeling sexy. Feeling sexy is your own personal, inalienable right at any age; and as long as you take good, physical care of yourself and devote attention to your mental well-being as well, feeling sexy is possible—whatever your age. If you do feel insecure about your aging body, you can ask your partner to remember to make compliments part of the play of foreplay.

Here are some physical changes you may experience as part of your sexual response:

194

- Lubrication takes longer than it did.
- If you were used to your skin flushing readily, it may not any longer.
- Your breasts may not swell as much.
- Your nipples may not harden.
- Your labia may not become as engorged.

As the sexual organs of the female are less visible than those of the male, so the physiological effects of aging on the sexual responses of women are also less visible, as well as less predictable, than those of the male. The most common complaint among older women is that vaginal lubrication takes longer and is often inadequate at best. This is not an insurmountable problem. A vaginal estrogen cream may combat vaginal dryness, or K-Y Jelly or another lubricant like Astroglide may be used during foreplay. The problem for some women, however, is that they are used to judging their level of sexual arousal by how moist their vagina feels. Thus, they may tend to interpret vaginal dryness to mean that they don't feel aroused, and this may dampen their actual level of arousal. Try new things and rely on external lubrication. Practice and a reassessment of your mental cuing can help solve this.

Vaginal dryness can make intercourse very painful and therefore unpleasant. While you don't want to avoid intercourse, you do want to avoid painful intercourse, as you may begin to associate your sex life with not only lack of pleasure but also pain. To avoid adding negative reinforcement to the pain of the experience, discuss your problem with your partner and take measures to solve it as soon as possible, so that you may keep sex pleasurable and continue to look forward to sex with positive anticipation.

In addition to a decrease in vaginal lubrication, the lining of the vagina begins to thin with age. This can sometimes lead to the shrinking of the vagina or vaginal atrophy, which may cause painful intercourse. If you find that intercourse is painful for you even when using an estrogen cream and taking other precautions to ensure vaginal lubrication, you may want to see your gynecologist for a pelvic exam to see if vaginal atrophy is causing the problem. Many women report that hormone therapy helps immensely in maintaining vaginal lubrication; ERT may also help to preserve vaginal tissues, thereby preventing vaginal atrophy.

All of this may not sound so heartening if you're planning on great sex in the prime of life, but the following will. The clitoris, which is so wonderfully sensitive to stimulation, does not seem to be affected by aging at all. It remains sensitive and continues to increase in size when sexual arousal occurs and it becomes engorged with blood, just as it did when you were first exploring the pleasures of sex.

In addition, a woman's capacity for orgasm is not hampered at all by age, as long as she is in good health. In fact, many woman report that they are more orgasmic after menopause. Some studies suggest this may be related to the peace of mind women feel when they know they cannot become pregnant. In one study, the frequency of orgasm for women tended to increase during each decade of life, through the eighties. Although the ability to have an orgasm does not decline for women as they age, many women do report that, much like men, the intensity of the orgasm lessens.

Nonetheless, if you like sex, the news is good. Finally, the pleasure may really be yours.

Inhibited Sexual Desire

"For two years my husband and I were not at all sexually involved . . . maybe we had sex once every six months. Then we had a crisis. He lost his job and started to confide in me again. He was great about working to find another job . . . and somehow, during all this sharing, we got back together in bed again. It can happen."

Carole Salmon (age 42)

JUST WHEN YOU THOUGHT it was safe to jump into bed with your long-term, significant other, now there is inhibited sexual desire (ISD), the shark in the love bed of the nineties. The bad news is, it's true. You or your partner (male or female) may suffer from a lessening or extinguishing of sexual desire for a number of reasons, both physical and psychological. The good news is ISD is very responsive to treatment, both physical and psychological.

I'd like to make it very clear that having sex less often than you used to does not mean you necessarily suffer from ISD. Let's face it, with the job and family obligations that come with the territory of the late thirties and forties, most of us have sex less often than we used to and less than we want to. Whether it's the kids, the job, the parents, the in-laws, or that recent fight about squeezing the toothpaste tube in the middle, there are a host of ordinary reasons that sex gets postponed or even deleted from the roster now and then.

ISD develops because for a variety of reasons sexual feelings and thoughts are considered dangerous in and of themselves. Even though ISD is a real problem, most of those who suffer from it believe that they do not feel desire (or rarely do) and are not conscious of inhibiting their sexual desire. ISD commonly occurs in couples where desire differences exist—that is, one partner desires sex consistently more than the other partner. Often the lack of desire on the part of one partner actually begins to suppress desire in the other partner.

There are also different types of ISD. *Primary ISD* is less common than the other types and refers to a lifelong absence of sexual desire. *Secondary ISD* is far more common and refers to a loss of interest in sex. In *global ISD*, lack of desire occurs across the board, that is, in all sexual situations. As the name would suggest, *situational ISD* affects sexual appetite in certain cases but not all situations.

A person suffering from ISD shuts off sexual feelings and responses, either by evoking negative images and thoughts, focusing on the most unattractive aspects of the partner or their own flaws, or thinking obsessively about stressful topics (such as money worries or problems at work).

Here are the types of women and men in the middle years more likely to suffer from ISD:

- Type A career-oriented people, who suffer from job-related stress and are often too exhausted from or preoccupied with professional obligations
- Those recently divorced or widowed
- One or both members of a couple who have recently experienced catastrophic illness
- Those who feel pressured to perform sexually or may have failed to perform sexually in the past
- Those suffering from depression
- Those suffering from alcohol or drug addiction

In most, if not all, of these circumstances, the situation can be reversed with proper medical attention and appropriate therapy. (It should be noted that psychological issues regarding sex are the issues treated most successfully by psychotherapy.) If you think you or your partner might be suffering from ISD, you should see your medical doctor first. If all things are go physically, you will want to ask for a referral to a general therapist or a sex therapist.

Partner, Partner

"Men talk to have sex. Women have sex to talk."

Anonymous

I WAS DOING some research on this chapter—reading some of the literature recently published—and I came across an amazing statement in an otherwise fairly wisely written, informative study regarding heterosexuality. To paraphrase: as men age, changes in the pattern of ejaculation, including a longer arousal time and a softer erection, cause distress in "female sex partners" and that "female sex partners" misunderstand what is happening. Misunderstand? I doubt it. Time is time. An erection is an erection. Misinterpret? Maybe. But probably not before that "female sex partner" (what a nickname, huh?) has tried to understand by asking questions about how her "male sex partner" likes to be touched and is feeling, and to reassure him by sharing the well-understood fact that we get a little older—we go a little slower.

Then there's another scenario. Maybe, as always, he's just not talking. I mean, talking, sure, but about *Monday Night Football*, not "stuff." Let me put it this way. Just like he forgot to tell you about the Visa bill that didn't get paid last month or the fact that things at work haven't been going so well, he's probably not lying there saying, "Honey, I want you to know I really, really want you and I really want to have sex right now, even though I'm not hard . . . at least not yet. These are just the physiological changes that occur as a man gets older. Trust me, it's got nothing to do with lack of desire. If you'll be a little patient and rub me a little here, pull me a little there and a little harder, while I massage you just the way you like me to, this will all be fine."

If he is lying there saying and doing all of this, then do what he asks. You've got yourself a rare one. But since he's probably not, here are a few things he's not telling you.

As men grow older, they may want sex just as much, but the physical signs of desire are manifested more slowly. Used to counting on a strong and immediate erection, an older man may become tentative about initiating sex. If you begin to worry that he is not in the mood or not attracted to you and you become tentative, you'll end up missing out on what you both want. Instead, you may want to spend some time massaging his penis and scrotum gently, in an exploratory fashion. Even if you've known this man for decades, your partner has probably brought some issues of prowess and ego to bed with him as well. Vanity, you might say, thy name is man in contemplation of his phallic self. He's probably as worried as you are, but for different reasons. While you're wondering if he's lost interest, he may be saying to himself, "Holy———, what can I count on, if I can't count on that?" You may be able to help reassure him by sharing that you understand this is all part of the aging process, and that while you may not have all the time in the world, you certainly can spend a little extra making sure your time together in bed is a pleasure.

Remember, sex is not a race. There's no one in your bedroom clocking your performance or waiting to award a medal for speed, hardness of erection, or endurance during intercourse. You may want to remind your partner of this too. And above all, don't take a lack of immediate erection or a somewhat softer erection personally. These changes are part of the physiology of aging and have nothing to do with anything you have or have not done. For that matter, try to think of developing creative techniques for his arousal and yours as part of the challenge of aging gracefully and pleasurably.

Sexual Fantasies

"Women tie sex to love. . . ."

Lonnie Barbach, Ph.D.

IT WILL COME as no surprise that the sexual fantasies of women differ substantially from those of men. And it will shock no one that only recently have researchers discovered just how different the female fantasy life is from the male fantasy life and begun to take this difference seriously and to conduct studies that deal specifically with the fantasy lives of women.

Whereas past sexual research seemed to indicate that men had more sexual fantasies per day than women, recent studies make clear that when the differences between male and female sexual fantasies are factored into sexual research, women have as active a fantasy life as men. It's just different. We could have told them that, right?

We could have told them what the differences were too. Women tend to connect the emotional to the physical more than men do—to imbue sex with feelings, if you will. For women, romance (and the feelings it brings) opens the door to satisfying sex. While a man's fantasy may focus on the successful completion of the sexual act (by the way, the woman in the fantasy is always ready, as well as willing), a woman's fantasy will proceed from romance through intimacy and the foreplay that enhances such feelings on to sexual satisfaction. What researchers are only beginning to discover is that you can't judge a woman's fantasy life simply by immediate genital arousal. Remember, any fantasy you want to have is yours to have. And if any of your fantasies sometimes surprise you, it might help to remind yourself that chances are a million other women have had the same fantasy, too.

Sex is not just an act, but an activity that is enhanced by atmosphere and the sharing of emotional feelings as well as physical sensation. Whatever turns you on—whether it's flowers and perfumes, a sweaty workout at the gym in tandem, massage oil, bubble baths, dinner and dancing, a picnic in bed, candlelight or daylight—is as important to the sensual quality of the experience as the physical aspects of sex. Sometimes it's even more important!

Other Issues

"After my husband had his heart attack, I treated him as if he were a tiny bit fragile. Finally, he said to me, 'Oh, come on. If I'm going to die, I'm going to die.' Now, we're right back at it."

Helene Shatan (age 60)

THE TWO MOST COMMON obstacles to a fulfilling sex life as we age are health and the lack of a partner. Many health problems that were once thought to be insurmountable when considering a satisfying sex life can be controlled or corrected, so that sex may be enjoyed. These include diabetes, heart disease, and many forms of can-cer and vascular problems. If you are afraid to have sex because of your physical condition, you should discuss the problem with your doctor. She or he may be able to help with medication and in reassuring you that you are not going to jeopardize your health by resuming a sex life. If your partner has had prostate surgery, you will want to discuss with him and his doctor how this might affect your sex life. Some men are not at all affected by the surgery, while others are.

Lack of a partner may be a more difficult problem to overcome. Sometimes a woman who has been without a sexual partner for some time becomes uninterested in sex altogether. This is usually psycholog-ically protective. It's like Aesop's "The Fox and the Grapes." We think, This is something that I can't have. Therefore, I will make it something that I don't want. One common form of male sexual dysfunction stems from the loss of a loving spouse and is referred to as widower's syndrome. After losing a wife of many years, a man may find that when confronted with a new sexual relationship he finds he has sexual difficulties he's never had before, such as becoming erect or maintaining an erection. While women who are widowed may undergo all of the same emotional trauma when becoming involved with a new partner, the "evidence" of such feelings of conflict is not as obvious. In addition, many women who are widowed choose to remain celibate, rather than face all of the complications of a new relationship. In fact, widowers tend to remarry much more frequently than widows do. If you find yourself becoming involved with a widower, remember to give him plenty of time and understanding when it comes to the bedroom. Waiting a little longer than you might actually want to wait to begin the sexual aspect of your relationship may be one way to ensure that once you do commence your sexual relationship, it is satisfying for both of you.

Practical Tips

- Have sex in the morning instead of the evening. The end of the day is when you are the most tired, and while this may not have been an issue when you were an indefatigable twenty-nine, you may notice that by eleven at night you are now more interested in sleeping than sex. Try having sex when you've just awakened, refreshed and filled with energy after a good night's sleep.

- Get plenty of exercise and stay physically active. When you're in shape, you have more energy—and that includes more energy for sex.
- Don't measure or judge your sex life by impossible standards. If you're fretting about the time it takes to achieve an erection or vaginal lubrication, you'll be obsessing yourself right out of the mood.
- When you can have sex, do have sex. Sure, you don't forget how to ride a bicycle, but you do get rusty at it without practice. The same goes for sex. The more you do it, the more in practice you will be.
- Skip toasting your sex life with alcohol. Alcohol is a depressant and as such will simply put a damper on your sexual appetite.
- Talk about it. One of the simplest ways to relieve the tension or the pressure associated with sexual performance is to get your fears and anxieties off your chest. If you feel you've been keeping up your end of the conversations and he's not talking, ask him a question he'll have to answer, like "Should I stop?" He'll probably say no, and leave it at that. But you can keep trying.
- Get help for any physical or emotional problems that may be adversely affecting your sex life.

PART 4

THE REAL M WORD— MENOPAUSE

"What changed her was what changes all women at fifty. . . . A weight fell away from her; she flew up to a higher perch and cackled a little."

Isak Dinesen

ALTHOUGH WOMEN LIVE longer than men, society frowns on women aging. After menopause, a woman is considered to be somehow less than a woman, or at least older than society would want her to be. Our terrific longevity is often not appreciated because of such attitudes. Though still firmly in place in society's collective consciousness, this mind-set would seem to be a throwback to a time in history when childbearing was considered to be not just a woman's role, but her only job. If she ceased to menstruate, then she was jobless. The world has changed, and so have the job descriptions of men and women; nevertheless, attitudes, sluggish as they are, seem to have a long way to go to catch up.

Add to this the terrible demands of a youth-oriented culture—tuck this, nip that, and most of all, never divulge your age—and many women come to dread their menopause. While not synonymous with dying, for many it is still synonymous with deterioration and the beginning of "the end."

Menopause, of course, is none of these things. What's most important to remember is that life goes on much as it always did after this so-called change of life. If you like where you are in life and what you're doing and you have good friends, life is fundamentally just as good as it ever was. And if you're in reasonably good health, it's nowhere near over. Finally, don't forget—sometimes it even gets better!

MAMA NEVER TOLD ME THERE'D BE NIGHTS LIKE THIS

"I'm out of estrogen and I have a gun."

Anonymous

A SEA CHANGE in our approach to menopause might involve the following: whereas the mothers of baby boomers rarely shared the story of their own menopausal experiences with their daughters, those daughters are already planning to mark and remember this time in their own lives to share with their daughters when the right time comes.

The first time my mother and I really spoke about her menopausal symptoms was when she told me she was getting the blues. This admission was alarming since my mother has always been known for her sunny outlook on life and her high energy level. Now she was dragging and felt very fragile. She expected the hot flashes, but a change in her psyche took her by surprise. Fortunately she wasn't afraid to talk about these changes and ask questions. If this was menopause, fine—she could accept that, as long as this part of it was temporary. But she wasn't about to live the rest of her life in some kind of gloomy, depressive state. So she asked questions, sought help from her doctor, and embraced this new stage of her life.

One of the historically significant factors in the mystery of this inevitable passage in a woman's lifetime is the dead silence with which the subject has been treated until very recently. The medical jargon was cursory, cryptic, or indicting. Women too were silent on the subject, perhaps because of the pressure of society's silence, or perhaps because of their personal shame or regret at the end of fecundity and beginning of what they'd been taught to believe was the "end of life." Through their silence—unintentionally, of course—the mothers of our mothers and now our own mothers have contributed to the negative mystique surrounding this passage.

The very presence of silence indicates that there is a secret, and everyone knows that by definition secrets are considered to be powerful. Secrets are often thought of as dirty and a big deal. Inadvertently, this notion of a "secret" passage has imbued an ordinary biological process with more power and significance that it really needs to, or ought to, have in women's lives. It's a change, but it's not nearly as significant as moving around the world, losing a spouse, changing careers, or any number of changes that people successfully navigate in midlife or at other times. Menopause is inevitable. It's the right thing to have happen to you—not the wrong thing—and it is biology doing its job. You don't die from menopause. You are still you when it's over. These are blessings. One other thing: the end of fertility can be more of a boom than a bust. You're free.

This notion of a silent secret is changing now. Talk to your mother if she is alive. Talk to your friends and your friends' mothers. This is something all women go through, and sharing our thoughts and feelings about the experience is a way in which we can help one another. Many women still suffer the discomfort of night sweats and the fear of extreme bleeding in silence. This self-imposed silence is one form of suffering that we can avoid. It's time for us all to accept menopause for what it is—not a dirty secret, not even a silent passage, and certainly not an indication of old age or a nail in your coffin, but a part of the biology of being female. To do this, we need to begin to separate fact from fiction.

TWICE CURSED

"I just kept thinking . . . god, menopause? Does that mean death is just around the corner?"

Anna Nicholson (age 45)

WHEN YOU WERE very young you discovered that getting your period was getting "the curse." Now as menopause approaches, you'll discover that there are as many whispers and rumors about the change of life in these enlightened times as there were about "the curse" all those years ago—and your mother still isn't talking. Only recently have books like *The Silent Passage* by Gail Sheehy, *The Change* by Germaine Greer, and other thoughtful reconsiderations of menopause been published.

Whether it be the biblical notion that women were "unclean" when they were menstruating, the ancient Roman belief that menstrual blood was not only unclean, but deadly, the early-twentieth-century notion that women experiencing the climacteric (menopause) were considered "insane," or the modern debate regarding classifying certain types of PMS as a mental illness, the menstrual cycle, from beginning to end, has seemed to confound those who would define and explain it. Perhaps this might have something to do with the fact that until recently most, if not all, of the people doing the defining and explaining were men.

A woman goes through physical and hormonal changes that have always been subject to value judgment and interpretation, while a man's physical and hormonal changes seem to be exempt. This may be an example of reigning party politics, and it may also reflect upon the mystery associated with birth and all the connected processes, or it may occur because the changes in women are so dramatic. Whatever the reasons, it's unfair.

In the early twentieth century, women were sometimes institution-alized during menopause. Of course, what was often termed a nervous breakdown was not a breakdown at all, but a temporary imbalance in hormones while hormone levels shifted and realigned into a new post-menopausal balance. Some women, however, paid a price for simple biology and lived through menopause as patients on a mental ward.

CHANGING HOW WE VIEW "THE CHANGE"

"I kept asking my mother about her menopause. I wanted
to know for myself. She said, 'Oh, it was nothing.' I
pressed her. She said, 'My period just stopped. I can't
remember when.' I kept wanting this to be true for me,
but of course, childbirth for me was a lot different than
it was for my mother. She had said that was nothing, too.
And for me, menopause was something . . . not bad,
but something . . . and it happened early."

Carol Mathers (age 45)

UNTIL RECENTLY, one of the common myths associated with menopause was that it was a "deficiency disease." Not only did women have to suffer through their physical changes, they were also told there was something wrong with them. Even today jokes about menopause enjoy a wider circulation than equivalent sarcasm regarding testosterone rampages.

There were compelling reasons why our mothers' mothers were afraid to tell our mothers about menopause. Years ago, it just wasn't done. The topic was taboo: women were not supposed to be sexual, and anything that was connected to a woman's physicality was not discussed. Ironically, what was once taboo for reasons of prudishness is now taboo because women want to be perceived as sexual, and the loss of fertility is still erroneously confused with the loss of sexuality. It's easy to say that you should share the process of menopause with your family and peers, but it can be hard to do. Often women don't discuss their menopause because they fear that their friends aren't there yet. It will take a while before we all feel as comfortable discussing menopause as we do pregnancy.

Fifteen percent of women who experience menopause say they experience no discomfort at all. But many women looking back on their menopause say that they did indeed have signs and experience discomfort, even though they were unaware that these signs were related to menopause until they had ceased to menstruate. The discomfort usually ceases when a new hormonal equilibrium is reached. By the time a woman realizes that, indeed, she has been in such physical flux because she is experiencing menopause, it may be closer to the end of the process than the beginning. It's a little hard to ask people to talk about what they're not sure they're going through.

That brings up one very interesting point. A woman may not yet be going through menopause—even though she thinks she is. Here's why: as we get older (into our forties) the hormonal swings and symptoms from PMS may become more severe (see page 189). At the same time, a woman's periods may get longer and be associated with heavier bleeding. A physician may start hormone replacement therapy (erroneously, I believe—because it's too early to start giving replacement estrogen if the body is still making some of its own) and everything comes crashing together. The result may be that you are on a hormonal and emotional roller coaster, but it's not really due to menopause.

Nonetheless, while there is still a great deal of research to be done on the topic, menopause is now out of the closet, and that is perhaps the most important step.

THE FACTS

"For one whole winter, I kept saying to myself, 'Gosh, you're getting a lot of colds . . . and what about these aches and pains?' Oh, and there were other things. I just kept thinking, 'Gee, I'm really aging before my time. . . . Gosh, maybe I've got some dreadful, terminal disease' . . . and then one morning I woke up and said to myself, 'Oh, I get it . . . this is menopause.' "

Barbara Milston (age 47)

ALTHOUGH WE MAY NOT live in the age of enlightenment, we do live in the age of information, and information can only serve the menopausal woman well.

Even the word "menopause" is not particularly accurate or reflective of the complex process of hormonal change. A commonly used definition of menopause is the final cessation of menstruation, but the end of menstruation is merely the most obvious result. Menopause is a process that occurs over time. The amount of time varies from woman to woman, but the menopause always takes more than one month or one menstrual cycle and is almost never, as some old clichés would have it, like the shutting off of a faucet. The process of menopause takes from one to ten years to complete for most women. The symptoms of menopause may last ten years, but the process to reach low estrogen levels is shorter. Menopause usually begins in the forties. The average age for completion is 51.4 years.

The Terms

The term "menopause" is used in a variety of ways. Menopause describes that period of time in which a woman's body is undergoing adaptive hormonal changes that will signify the end of fertility. But menopause is also used to refer specifically to the date of the final period. In the medical literature, three stages regarding menopause are distinguished:

210

1. *Premenopausal* signifies the menstrual years.
2. *Perimenopausal* refers to those years in which we may notice changes related to the beginning of menopause.
3. *Postmenopausal* refers to the time after the last period.

The Hormones

Hormones are complex chemicals produced and secreted by glands that regulate or control the activity of other organs in the body. A hormone is released by one specific gland, travels through the bloodstream, is absorbed by the target organ, and sets off the desired chain reaction. The hormones that are involved in the reproductive cycle are estrogens, progestogens, and androgens. These are secreted by the ovaries in women, the testes in men, and the adrenal glands in both men and women.

Estrogen

Estrogen—specifically, the diminishing of estrogen levels—is the hormone most commonly associated with menopause. Estrogens help to regulate the menstrual cycle. They also affect a woman's body in many other ways, including promoting cell growth and repair in the genitals, regulating vaginal mucus, and keeping the vaginal walls healthy. Estrogens also protect the bones, aid in the absorption of calcium, trigger and control the development of the breast, help lower the cholesterol level, and protect against heart disease.

Progesterone

Progesterone is actually one of a group of hormones called progestogens. At the time of ovulation, when the egg is released from the egg sac, this empty sac transforms itself into a mass of tissue called the corpus luteum, where progesterone is then produced. The chief function of progesterone is to make a home for the fertilized egg by thickening the lining of the womb (the endometrium) with increased blood supply. What is most important about progesterone when it comes to menopause is that it counteracts some of the deleterious effects of pure estrogen replacement therapy in postmenopausal women.

Androgens

Testosterone, the principal androgen, is responsible for the development of male sexual characteristics. It is produced primarily in the testes in men. In women, it is produced in the adrenal gland or converted from androstenedione, a substance secreted by the ovaries and the adrenal gland. After a woman experiences menopause, her testosterone level is comparatively higher because her estrogen level has decreased substantially.

An Honest Confusion

Even in these enlightened times, the treatment of the often experienced side effects of menopause is inexact and unsatisfactory because the entire process so dramatically defies exact analysis. The confusion often occurs because there are many signs that may be associated with the process of menopause that are hardly common knowledge, not just for patients, but for doctors as well. (Then again, these signs may not be associated with menopause.) From fatigue to frequent urination, neck pain to a tingling in the fingers, signs of menopause are open to interpretation and are often indications of unrelated infections or diseases.

Signs of Menopause

"The first time I had a hot flash, I would say the worst part was just how anxious I was. When I got used to them and learned to talk myself through them, they were just mildly uncomfortable. It was like I had to come to terms with them before I could manage them."

Martha Sullivan (age 41)

THE FIRST TIME I ever really knew anyone going through menopause was when I was a staff surgeon at the University of Arkansas. One of the operating-room nurses would roll up the legs of her scrub pants and wear the largest scrub shirt she could find. At first I thought this was just a hilarious way to dress and quite unusual since operating rooms are often quite cold and most people complain that they're freezing. But then I saw the reason for her attire. One day I looked across the table at her and she was red-faced and perspiring. In a matter of seconds she was drenched in perspiration.

Expect the best when you are approaching menopause, but be prepared for anything. Here are some signs that are classic menopausal indications, some of which often go unrecognized.

Hot Flashes

Perhaps the most famous sign of menopause is a hot flash. This most common symptom of menopause is experienced by 75 to 85 percent of all women. A hot flash is a vasomotor response to changes in the hormonal levels: the vascular system, driven by hormones that trigger responses in the brain, misfires. The brain perceives that the body is overheating and relays to the nervous system that it is time to try to cool the body down. Blood vessels near the skin dilate and the blood supply to the skin surface increases, bringing with it heat.

Flashes often begin in the face and sweep across the body. You will feel flushed, perhaps sweat profusely, and feel a vague sense of unease and in certain situations (say, a formal dinner party), an unavoidable sense of embarrassment. During the night, hot flashes take the form of night sweats. Many women wake up bathed in sweat. The most important thing to remember is that there is no reason to panic. This is a natural, if uncomfortable, process, and it will pass. Many women are familiar with the sensation, having experienced it in pregnancy, so the experience does not seem so strange. However, the intensity of the experience may be much more extreme during menopause than during a pregnancy. The frequency of hot flashes and night sweats varies greatly from woman to woman.

If you find that you are experiencing hot flashes or night sweats, just bear with your body and try not to worry. Try to make yourself as comfortable as possible—for example, by removing layers of clothing or bedclothes. Talking about the situation with your partner or friends can also help. Most important, remember that hot flashes are a physical response to a normal process. They will cease when a new hormonal balance is achieved by the body. (See "Preparing for Menopause," page 233.)

Exaggerated PMS

"I always had trouble with PMS and could tell my cycles by clockwork. But this was a little overwhelming. Suddenly I seemed to be on edge all the time. I was snappy and jumpy and not at all comfortable with myself. The hot flashes were nothing compared to this!"

Tamara Davis (age 59)

FOR MANY WOMEN, extreme discomfort surrounding their periods is a sign that the perimenopausal stage has begun. PMS definitely worsens for many women in their forties; some physicians confuse this with menopause and then prescribe estrogen, often with disastrous results. If you experience what you consider to be an intensification of your personal version of PMS, you may want to look for other physical clues that might indicate the approach of menopause. Talk to your doctor. This can be a difficult aspect of aging to handle alone.

Other Signs

Heavy Menstrual Bleeding. Long periods with very heavy flow frequently indicate menopause. This situation often requires medical attention, such as a dilation and curettage (D&C) or the addition of or an adjustment in hormone therapy. If the situation is severe enough, a hysterectomy may be indicated. (For more on heavy menstrual bleeding, see page 216.)

Irregular Menses. Some women begin menopause by missing a period, returning to their normal cycle, then missing a period again.

Frequent Urination. Frequent urination is chronic for some women, or it may indicate the onset of adult diabetes in others. It may also be a sign that you are entering menopause. If you begin to urinate more often than usual or more at night, consult your physician.

Vaginal Dryness. With the drop in estrogen levels and the lowering of mucus levels, the vaginal walls become thinner and drier, which may lead to discomfort during intercourse. Usually women who are experiencing vaginal dryness have already begun to miss periods or have finished menstruating, but this is not always the case.

Decreased Metabolism. You may find it difficult now to drop that five pounds, which was so easy in the past. Cutting calories may not get the same fast results that you expect.

Bladder Infections. Because of the proximity of the bladder to the vagina, the thinning of the vaginal wall affects the bladder as well. Frequent bladder infections are common among women experiencing menopause.

Flatulence and Gastric Upset. Gastric distress may be a sign of anything from cancer to irritable bowel syndrome, but the same symptoms can also be a symptom of menopause.

Joint and Muscle Pain. The pain you might be considering to be the commencement of arthritis may actually indicate the beginning of menopause.

Mental Fuzziness. Some women liken this to a fog, with diminished concentration and short-term memory. If you are feeling uncommonly distracted or forgetful, check for other signs that you might be entering menopause and talk to your doctor.

Skin Sensitivities and Acne. Your skin does change with age. However, if you notice an outbreak of pimples or unusual facial redness or rashes, discuss the possibility of menopause with your doctor.

Headaches. Some women experience severe, migrainelike headaches during menopause, while other women who have been prone to headaches find that their number of headaches decreases with menopause.

Mild Depression and Mood Swings. Deciding what constitutes a mood swing or signs of depression isn't easy, but if you notice that you're "not yourself," you will want to pay attention to other signs that you might be entering menopause and see your doctor.

Pain During Intercourse. Because of vaginal dryness or even the infrequency of intercourse, due to lack of desire, intercourse may become painful.

While all of the above may be signs of menopause, they may also be symptoms of disease, such as gallbladder disease. The wide range of these signs reflects the fact that as menopause begins, the hormonal balance of estrogen and progesterone (and even testosterone) in the body is entering a period of great flux and eventually permanent change. This hormonal balance directly affects our entire body, especially the digestive and nervous systems. It might help if you keep in mind that Heracleitus established thousands of years ago the law of stability and flux by pointing out that "structures" that fluctuate are the most stable. And, most important of all, remember it's only temporary.

Changes in Your Period

"It seemed like I was bleeding all the time. At first I thought, Oh, God—I must have cancer. Then I talked to my mother and she said the same thing happened to her."

Cynthia Rappaport (age 54)

FOR SOME WOMEN the cessation of menstrual flow may take years, while for others it is literally over within months. But during their forties, the vast majority of women notice some changes in the length of time between periods and the amount and duration of the flow of their periods; sometimes this happens in a woman's thirties.

Heavy bleeding (menorrhagia) is the most disconcerting of the menstrual changes. In many cases, pads or tampons cannot contain the flow and a woman may be embarrassed or even terrified by so much blood. Sometimes periods become so extended that it seems that one period blends into the next in a continuous flow.

Many women say they find relief through a healthy diet and getting lots of rest. Some women find that acupuncture helps. Others turn to medication. One way medication is used to control menstrual flow is to administer a progestogen at the very beginning of a period. The progestogen causes the uterus lining to slough off more completely, which will, in most cases, make the next period lighter.

Some women miss a period now and then and this is their introduction to menopausal changes. Others experience bleeding long after their periods have ceased (usually at times of stress). Any of these changes should be reported to your physician so that a proper diagnosis may be made.

BIRTH CONTROL AND MENOPAUSE

"My periods were so infrequent and the bleeding so scant that I never gave a second thought to the possibility of being able to conceive. And then one day my husband and I faced the fact that I was pregnant at the age of fifty-one. I wish we had never had to face that dilemma."

Diana Chipworth (age 57)

THE MOST IMPORTANT THING to remember regarding birth control later in life is that you should continue to use some form of birth control until one full year after the cessation of your period. Even if you are one of those women who never got pregnant easily, or even if you have never been pregnant, you should not dismiss the possibility of pregnancy. Pregnancy can occur during the menopausal years, and using birth control will give you peace of mind during those perimenopausal months, where you might miss a period and wonder at the significance of this absence.

As you grow older, you will also want to reconsider your choice of birth control. What worked for you comfortably at twenty-one may not work at forty-one or forty-five. As your body begins undergoing menopausal changes, what was comfortable for you may become uncomfortable. For example, if you are experiencing very heavy flow, you will not want to use an IUD, which can be associated with heavy bleeding.

The Pill

Over and over again in recent studies, the pill has been found to be safe for women. The Nurses' Health Study data associates using the pill early in life with a decreased risk of breast cancer—even though in later life usage is associated with a slightly increased risk for breast cancer (this added risk disappears as soon as a woman stops taking the pill). The estrogen in the pill may mask some menopausal signs, such as hot flashes. So if you are still on the pill in your late forties or early fifties, you may not even know that you've entered menopause until you go off the pill. If you are uncertain, your doctor can check a blood FSH (follicle-stimulating hormone) level at the end of the week after you finish a cycle of birth control pills to rule out menopause.

IUD

In the past decade, the IUD has been marketed toward older women, since in association with PID it can cause infertility. The most common problem associated with the IUD is heavy bleeding. Obviously, if you are having heavy periods related to menopause, this will not be the method for you. In fact, about 20 percent of women fitted for the IUD discontinue use because of increased bleeding. If you are still using an IUD in your forties, you will want to report any changes in your menstrual bleeding to your physician immediately. The changes in bleeding may be related to menopause or an underlying medical condition and not the result of the IUD. The IUD is recommended only for women in monogamous relationships who are less likely to be exposed to sexually transmitted diseases, and it is not recommended for women with a history of PID.

Barrier Methods

Barrier methods, which include the diaphragm, cervical cap, and condom, are the most commonly recommended form of birth control for older women. Probably because women become less fertile with age, the barrier methods become more effective. The diaphragm is 98 percent effective—as effective as the IUD or pill—when used as directed. With women in their forties, the condom is 97 percent effective when used alone and almost 100 percent effective when used with a contraceptive cream or jelly. Contraceptive creams and jellies can also be helpful to women who are experiencing vaginal dryness related to menopausal changes.

Women in their forties, however, often experience increased discomfort with barrier methods. If you experience discomfort with your diaphragm, you may want to ask your gynecologist to fit you for a new one. (If you have a prolapsed uterus, you will probably not be able to use a diaphragm.) Also, be aware that the diaphragm is associated with an increased risk of bladder infections, so make sure to urinate before and after intercourse if you are using a diaphragm.

Sterilization

Interestingly enough, sterilization is rapidly becoming the leading contraceptive method for couples in the United States. Male sterilization, or vasectomy, is particularly easy. It can be performed in a doctor's office under local anesthetic and takes about half an hour. Female sterilization is a much more involved surgical procedure requiring general anesthesia. In any surgery there can be complications and this should be taken into account. Some women arrange for sterilization during another necessary surgical procedure, such as gallbladder surgery or delivery by cesarean section. Sterilization should be considered permanent. For a women who's already had her family, this information is usually greeted with relief.

Natural Birth Control

Natural family planning methods, such as the rhythm method, are not recommended for women in midlife. Because duration of the menstrual cycle and vaginal mucus secretions are subject to continual variation, it is much more difficult for a woman at this stage of life to tell when she is ovulating. Therefore, miscalculations are likely. The average cycle for a woman at age thirty is 28 days. At age forty the cycle shortens to 24 days.

SURGICAL MENOPAUSE

"I had a hysterectomy when I was thirty-five. They were worried about something. I can't even remember what. All I remember is that suddenly I was having hot flashes and every lining of my body seemed dry."

Josephine Rotenberg (age 80)

WHEN A WOMEN undergoes a hysterectomy with an oophorectomy (removal of the ovaries) before menopause, she experiences a surgical menopause. Her period ceases suddenly. Her hormones shift suddenly. Hormone replacement therapy, which keeps estrogen in the system, is almost always advisable to make the menopausal transition more gradual.

Hysterectomies

Each year 600,000 hysterectomies are performed. While many hysterectomies are necessary and well advised, it has been increasingly recognized that the hysterectomy was, for years, the operation of choice for the doctor and not for the patient. The stereotype in the fifties and sixties was that a hysterectomy could be performed in the morning and the doctor could be free by noon with plenty of time for a round of golf. The financial payback for the doctor was high—high enough to pay the dues at the country club, hence the nickname "the golfer's surgery." Economics certainly played a role in the high rate of hysterectomies. In the past a doctor could make money performing a hysterectomy, rather than "watching and waiting." The revenue from hysterectomies also helped hospitals compensate for the declining birth rate as the baby boom ended. Hysterectomies have even been used as a form of surgical birth control among poor, less informed minority women. In general, the more surgeons and hospital beds in a given area, the more unnecessary surgeries were recommended and performed.

That was yesterday. Not only do doctors not have that much disposable time anymore, but the entry of women gynecologists and obstetricians into the field has helped to change the image of the procedure and to question its necessity when appropriate.

> *"I was diagnosed with fibroids and medications hadn't helped. One physician told me that because of the size of the fibroids I wouldn't be able to get pregnant anyway, so I should proceed with a hysterectomy. I was only thirty-two. I got a second opinion. I needed surgery—but not a hysterectomy. Today I have two children who wouldn't be here if I had rushed into things."*
>
> Rachel Simpson (age 39)

TODAY WOMEN ARE AWARE of alternatives to surgery, and surgeons are learning new ways to treat benign diseases of the uterus. While the number of hysterectomies performed is declining, this operation is still presented as a treatment option for women with extreme menopausal symptoms, such as excessive bleeding due to fibroids or menopausal changes. Only a very small portion of hysterectomies are performed because of life-threatening diseases such as cancer—about 8 to 12 percent. If a hysterectomy is recommended to you, *seek a second opinion.* A hysterectomy may be the right choice, but many times it is not necessary. The bottom line is not to rush into this decision. Talk with your doctor and make sure you understand your options.

Some Negative Reactions

The medical profession used to report that a woman's reaction to hysterectomy was purely psychological, and that, for example, hysterectomy had no effect on sexual response. But medical perceptions are changing.

Women report, variously, a loss of sexual feeling, memory loss, and fatigue following a hysterectomy. Many also report *that their doctors did not warn them beforehand* regarding how they might react to the surgery. One study reported that 46 percent of women experienced diminished libido and sexual responsiveness following hysterectomy. Today physicians often leave the cervix in place with this operation. However, if it is removed with the uterus, a woman may not be able to experience orgasm due to the loss of cervical stimulation.

Many women report depression as a common response to hysterectomy. Studies have found that approximately 70 percent of women experience some depression. This may be due to the postoperative recovery period and the inability to exercise. It may also be a reaction to the actual and figurative loss of fertility.

Other women experience no such adverse reactions. What is most important is that you become aware of the possible reactions to hysterectomy prior to undergoing surgery. As with all aspects of the experience of menopause, the best advice is to follow the Boy Scout motto: be prepared.

Reasons for a Hysterectomy

In this day and age, there are still several extremely valid reasons to undergo a hysterectomy:

Cancer. In the case of invasive endometrial cancer, a hysterectomy is usually necessary.

Hemorrhage. Hysterectomy may also be necessary when severe hemorrhaging (uncontrollable bleeding) is present, if the situation has not been improved by D&C or hormonal therapy (like Lupron).

Fibroid Tumors. Fibroid tumors are growths in or around the uterus. Nearly 40 percent of white women over the age of 35 have fibroids, and even more black women do. More than 99 percent of fibroids are not cancerous, and fibroids usually can be removed by myomectomy, removal of the tumor alone. If bowel or urinary function is obstructed and the tumors are too large for removal by myomectomy, a hysterectomy may be necessary.

Advanced Pelvic Inflammatory Disease (PID). Each year approximately 1 million American women develop pelvic inflammatory disease. Also called salpingitis, PID was originally defined as an infection of the fallopian tubes. The diagnosis is now applied to infections of the ovaries, uterus, and cervix. The bacteria responsible for the infection are almost always sexually transmitted. Fifteen percent of women with gonorrhea develop PID, but it may also be traced to childbirth or sometimes endometrial biopsy or a D&C. If the infection has spread to the peritoneal cavity, the membrane that lines the abdomen, a hysterectomy may be necessary.

Extreme Uterine Prolapse. The pelvic floor supports the organs contained within the lower abdomen, including the bladder and uterus. When the pelvic floor is weakened, as in childbirth, or if there is a hereditary weakness, these organs may sink farther down, or prolapse. If the uterus has descended through the vagina, a hysterectomy is necessary.

Advanced Endometriosis. Endometriosis develops when fragments of the endometrium, the tissue that lines the uterus, find their way from the uterus and become implanted on other organs. These cells imitate the menstrual cycle and the blood they produce has nowhere to go. Blood blisters or cysts may form, eventually causing scarring and adhesion (tissue binding organs together). When endometriosis cannot be treated with hormones or other drugs and causes severe pain and bleeding, a hysterectomy may be advised.

When Hysterectomy May Not Be Necessary

*"I was diagnosed with fibroids when I was thirty-one.
My main symptom was pressure. I tried medication, but
I just got hot flashes and the fibroids didn't get any
smaller. So I had a myomectomy and the fibroids were
removed. I was never pressured to have a hysterectomy.
My only concern was whether the tissue would be benign."*

Martha Snyderman (age 37)

223

The Case of Fibroids

Fibroid tumors are the most common reason for hysterectomy between the ages of thirty-five and fifty. As stated before, fibroids, which are almost always benign, are very common in aging women. Fibroid growth may be stimulated by estrogen, so women with fibroids should avoid taking high-dose birth control pills or high levels of hormone replacement therapy during menopause. Low-dose oral contraceptives may conversly cause a decrease in the size of fibroids for some women. Fibroids usually recede after menopause. Surgical removal of fibroids (myomectomy) is recommended if the fibroid has grown beyond the size of a twelve-week pregnancy, or is about the size of a grapefruit. Sometimes surgeons recommend surgery for much smaller fibroids if they are in the submucosal area. In this situation, they may not protrude into the center of the uterus but can wreak havoc with bleeding. If you are bothered by fibroids and are approaching menopause, you may want to wait until menopause to see if your fibroids recede.

There are four indications for operating on a woman with fibroids: pain, pressure, bleeding, and growth of the fibroid of 25 percent or more over one year. With the first three symptoms it is really up to the woman to decide how these factors influence the quality of her life. With a sudden growth in size of a fibroid, your doctor will likely urge you to consider surgery because of the concern that there may be an underlying malignancy. Once again, unless your fibroids are obstructing your bowels or urinary tract, a hysterectomy is probably not necessary, though the decision of whether or not to have surgery is always up to you. You should get a second opinion if hysterectomy has been suggested for removal of fibroid tumors that are not causing undue discomfort.

TWENTY TIMES THE TESTOSTERONE, OR POSTMENOPAUSAL ZEST

"Our lives are always changing. Menopause is just another change. If you let yourself change, you're a lot better off. Like everything, attitude really does help a lot."

Lisa Jamieson (age 43)

MENOPAUSE IS A time of transition, and transitions involve a certain amount of complication and travail. But change can also be positive. Menopause is the process by which the hormones in the female system seek new levels and achieve a new balance, and once the job is completed, a woman produces less estrogen. Thus, the ratio between estrogen and testosterone in the system changes as well, with the balance tipping in favor of testosterone for the first time in a woman's life.

Many women report a surge of strength and independence and a feeling of power once the menopause has been achieved. Some find that they can make positive changes in their lives in a variety of ways—changes in the ways they make their living or express their anger or perceive their place in the world.

THE POLITICS OF ESTROGEN THERAPY

Several years ago I interviewed a a gynecologist from a very prestigious East Coast medical school about the pros and cons of estrogen replacement. Something she said caused me to laugh, and I've never forgotten it. She said that if testicles failed the way ovaries do, we would know everything there is to know about hormone replacement. Obviously, she was slamming the fact that in our male-dominated medical culture, learning about estrogen has been on the bottom of the need-to-know list for a long time. Now we are playing catch-up.

Estrogen or hormone replacement therapy is here to stay. Every woman with the means and at a certain age and stage of life will probably at least briefly consider if it is right for her; she will also probably feel a bit daunted by the prospect of making this decision. Simply put, when it comes to estrogen, you may have begun to think you're damned if you do and damned if you don't. So much has been written recently about the pros and cons that it may seem hard to assess your own situation before the swirling data regarding benefits and risk factors. But great progress has been made in the field—both in calculating a patient's risk factors, and in minimizing these factors by manipulating the therapy itself. Until recently, estrogen was used alone to restore the premenopausal levels of that hormone; little attention was given to mimicking the premenopausal pattern of the secretion and interaction of hormones. With the addition of progesterone to most therapies, all this has changed. Although the new combination therapy is more accurately referred to as hormone replacement therapy, or HRT, both terms are still used.

Estrogen has been used in the treatment of menopausal complaints for the last half century. In fact, by 1947 the hormone was available orally and as a vaginal cream. By 1975, the sale of estrogen had reached the phenomenal amount of $83 million per year. There was a great deal of hype associated with ERT, from preventing wrinkles to keeping breasts firm and even the promise of that quixotic carrot, eternal youth. All of this is just that—hype. When the therapy was new and estrogen was used alone, many women suffered side effects in the popular quest for the unattainable. But things have changed. Estrogen therapy today is more sophisticated than ever. The dosages are generally lower and estrogen is combined with progestins (synthetic forms of progesterone). Taking estrogen and progesterone daily (with no breaks and no periods) is very popular. The progestin protects against developing uterine cancer. This combination of drugs restores the hormones but does not imitate the "natural" cycle (hence, no bleeding). Also, it should be noted that a woman without a uterus can take estrogen alone.

What Estrogen Can Do

Estrogen therapy can:

- Relieve vaginal dryness
- Lower low density lipoproteins (LDL), the "bad" cholesterol

- Protect against heart disease
- Reduce bone loss, thereby helping to prevent osteoporosis
- Delay the onset of diabetes
- Limit the risk of stroke
- Improve cognition
- Relieve hot flashes
- Improve your sense of well-being

What Estrogen Can't Do

Estrogen therapy will not:

- Cure depression, unless the depression is secondary to hot flashes or sleep loss
- Prevent weight gain
- Impede the progress of aging
- Help you lose weight

Types of Regimens

Oral Estrogen

Oral estrogen was the most common form of estrogen replacement therapy until recently. It has been used in this form for over fifty-five years. Oral estrogen must pass through the digestive system and the liver. The liver, which is the organ that detoxifies what goes through the body, can be damaged by potent doses of hormones, prescription drugs, other chemicals, and, of course, alcohol. The use of pure oral estrogen is on the wane because of improved techniques that lower the risk of liver damage and other side effects.

The Patch

The development of a patch was a major breakthrough in the delivery of estrogen. Because the estrogen can be absorbed through the skin slowly, it avoids the peaks and valleys that take place with oral administration and the medication is in more of a steady state. It also avoids the effect of oral estrogen on the liver. However, some women have trouble with skin rashes where the patch is placed.

Other Methods

Vaginal pessaries, rings, or gels for topical application are also available. These methods also bypass the digestive system and the attendant risk to the liver.

Combined Estrogen and Progestogen Preparations

As stated earlier, progesterone is the female hormone responsible for preparing the lining of the uterus to accept a fertilized ovum. Progestogen usually refers to a synthesized form of progesterone. Estrogen with progestogen is often the ERT treatment of choice for women who have not undergone a hysterectomy because of the increased chance of endometrial cancer when estrogen is used alone. In fact, women taking estrogen and progesterone have a lower incidence of endometrial cancer than women taking no hormones at all. The addition of progestogen to ERT, however, has been associated with a 40 percent rate of breakthrough bleeding—that is, bleeding between periods, or bleeding in general if the period has already ceased. This is particularly common in the first six months of therapy. But the incidence of bleeding depends on how the hormones are taken. With cyclical progesterone, periods are appropriate. However, if taken daily, breakthrough bleeding is less common and light.

Is ERT for Me?

"I wasn't sure I wanted to take estrogen. I had been on it years ago when I was just beginning menopause and I had terrible mood swings. Then I found out the mood swings were from my PMS instead of the menopause. So I gave it another try and I feel so much better on it. Quit? Not on your life."

Roselynn Goldberg (age 72)

N O ONE CAN DECIDE if estrogen therapy is right for you except you and your doctor, but the more information you have, the more informed your choice will be and the more confident you'll be about making that choice. If you have a family history of heart disease or osteoporosis, you may decide to take the hormones. With a family history of breast cancer, you may decide to defer. If you fall in the middle, with no risk factors, you will have to weigh the pros and cons very carefully.

The Duration of Treatment

One of the first questions many women ask is: How long will I be on this? The answer is complicated and varies for each individual.

If you are on ERT primarily because of discomfort associated with menopause, you may be on it no longer than a year or two. But if you feel that you like being on ERT and are happy with the attendant lowered risk of heart disease and osteoporosis, you may choose to continue on ERT for much longer—even indefinitely.

If you are taking ERT for menopausal discomfort and have a familial risk of breast cancer, you will probably choose to come off therapy as soon as your discomfort dissipates.

If you have osteoporosis (or are at risk for it), you may be on ERT for the rest of your life. This is because estrogen enhances the absorption of calcium from your intestines, and as soon as you cease to take it, calcium absorption decreases and your bones may return to their original state of deterioration.

The choice is yours to make in consultation with your physician. If you do remain on ERT for a longer period of time, you will want to continue to consult with your physician regarding any physical changes you may experience. Then you can be sure that ERT continues to be right for you.

Estrogen and Relief of the Discomforts of Menopause

It is the deficiency of estrogen in the system that causes most of the noticeable symptoms of menopause. There are two predominant types of symptoms for which lack of estrogen is responsible:

1. Vasomotor disturbances (disturbances in function of the vascular system—e.g., hot flashes as discussed on page 213) and their attendant side effects, such as insomnia. Although between 75 and 85 percent of menopausal women are affected by vasomotor symptoms or hot flashes, only about 30 percent seek medical help for their symptoms. About 25 percent experience hot flashes for longer than five years and a very small number of women experience hot flashes for the rest of their lives. Hot flashes and their secondary symptoms are usually relieved in the first cycle of ERT treatment, sometimes in a matter of days.

2. Discomfort resultant from genital atrophy. The decline in estrogen in the system causes atrophy of the vagina and urethra. As discussed earlier, during menopause the vaginal wall becomes thinner and the glands in the vagina atrophy, which may cause a lack of lubrication. These changes are at least partly reversed by ERT. Since vaginal secretions contain estrogen receptors, if vaginal dryness is your only symptom, the local application of an estrogen cream may be the only treatment you need. If you find that vaginal dryness is impeding your enjoyment of sex, there are estrogen creams that will help with lubrication, as will a contraceptive jelly or cream. A water-based lubricant like Astroglide may also help. If you find that what used to work in terms of stimulation doesn't work so well now because of changing sensitivity, experiment. Don't give up; just change your approach and help your partner in changing his or hers, too.

Estrogen and Heart Disease

Atherosclerosis in women increases after the menopause (especially if you've undergone an oophorectomy). So far the evidence is good that ERT helps protect against heart disease in postmenopausal women. It lowers the risk of coronary heart disease in postmenopausal women by 40 to 50 percent, and it may also protect against stroke.

In addition, oral estrogen has been shown to raise the level of HDL or "good" cholesterol and lower the LDL or "bad" cholesterol level. The addition of progestogen does tend to lessen the positive effect on the HDL level a tiny bit, however. There may also be a positive effect on blood pressure levels and circulation, but this area is less well studied, and generalizations cannot be made. Nevertheless, so far the odds are overwhelming that ERT will help in preventing heart disease in postmenopausal women.

Estrogen and Osteoporosis

Although many factors are associated with the development of osteoporosis, estrogen deficiency towers above them all. The evidence that ERT protects against osteoporosis is abundant. In numerous studies, ERT has been shown to help keep bones strong by minimizing bone loss and increasing bone density. As mentioned above, estrogen also improves calcium absorption. When therapy is discontinued, however, there is an immediate resumption in bone loss at the same rate as in an untreated woman. Therefore, if you suffer from osteoporosis or are at risk for it, you will probably want to remain on ERT indefinitely, as long as there are no uncomfortable side effects or other symptoms. ERT also helps to prevent spinal column and hip fractures. The best results for minimizing the chances of osteoporosis and fractures in postmenopausal women occur when ERT is begun right at the time of menopause. (See "Osteoporosis," page 274.)

Estrogen and Uterine (Endometrial) Cancer

Evidence shows that unopposed estrogen therapy (oral estrogen alone) significantly increases the risk of endometrial cancer. The addition of progestogen to the therapy decreases the risk. In a woman who has not undergone a hysterectomy, the combination therapy is always the therapy of choice. The Postmenopausal Estrogen/Progestin Institute confirms that the risk of uterine cancer is 1 percent for women taking estrogen plus progestin, as opposed to 34 percent for women taking estrogen alone.

Estrogen and Breast Cancer

The bulk of the controversy regarding ERT centers around the risk of developing breast cancer. Depending on what you read, ERT increases, decreases, or has no effect on the risk of breast cancer in postmenopausal women.

The most up-to-date data comes from the Nurses' Health Study from Brigham and Women's Hospital and Harvard Medical School and was published in *The New England Journal of Medicine*. This study reported that women who use postmenopausal hormones for five years or more are at increased risk of developing breast cancer compared with women the same age who never used the hormones. The protective effect that progestin exerts over the development of uterine cancer appeared to offer no protection in the development of breast cancer. In this study, a sixty-year-old woman who used hormones for five years had a 3 percent risk of developing breast cancer over the following five years if she continued to use ERT. If she never used hormones after menopause, the breast cancer risk over the five-year period was 1.8 percent. The evidence does suggest that ERT increases the risk of venous thrombosis (blood clots) in postmenopausal women.

PREPARING FOR MENOPAUSE

"When I hit my forties, I found it easier to eat nutritious foods. I didn't crave the junk as much. Somehow I finally realized that the machine ran better on good fuel. In many ways, facing menopause made things clearer and the choices easier."

Barbara Hanson (age 49)

An "Accurate" Diet

As a culture, what we eat is very much affected by fads. We'll eliminate this and add that to the diet after one news update. From fat content to vitamins, we're driven by the desire for the quick fix. However, the fact is there are no quick fixes when it comes to the body.

What you require from your diet changes with age. You may need less protein now, but you still need some protein. You may want to add more roughage to your diet to aid digestion. On the other hand, you don't want to overdo it and thereby strip nutrients from your system.

If you are at risk for heart disease, you will want to be particularly careful about fat content. However, if you are also at risk for adult diabetes, you will want to keep some monosaturated fats and a certain amount of pure protein in your diet, because these foods are metabolized at the slowest rate, minimizing the risk of high blood sugar.

I realize this can all get complicated. You may want to consult a nutritionist to help you in coming up with a food plan that is tailored to your needs.

In terms of menopause, you will want to be aware of what foods are high in calcium and iron. Add these to your diet, if you don't already eat them on a daily basis. Bone loss (exacerbated by calcium deficiency) and anemia (often caused by lack of iron) are common problems for postmenopausal women. Here, cut down on empty calories from sugar, junk food, and alcohol; make sure you don't overindulge in fat, but do get enough protein; and eat more vegetables, fruits, and whole grains and other complex carbohydrates.

233

ERT and Diet

If you are taking hormone therapy, pay particular attention to your dietary needs. ERT tends to deplete the body's store of certain B vitamins, including folic acid and pyridoxine. Folic acid is responsible for the production of healthy red blood cells; when it's not in good supply, anemia becomes a possibility. Pyridoxine is a natural diuretic, protecting against water retention. Thus, some nutritionists recommend B vitamin supplements to women taking estrogen.

Water: The Most Needed Nutrient

Water is the most underestimated, unappreciated, important ingredient in our diets. Without it we die. With it in abundance, every organ in our bodies—from our skin to our heart—flourishes. Although it is important at every stage in life, it's particularly crucial to maintain a state of good hydration during the menopausal years.

With the dramatic changes in hormone levels during menopause, every lining in the body will change. Skin becomes drier, tears decrease, nasal mucus thickens, and vaginal lubrication becomes scarce. Water can help minimize the effects in every case. I'm not talking about tea, coffee, or fruit juices—I'm talking about water. (Coffee and tea are diuretics that will cause you to lose more water. Sugary soft drinks and fruit juices will pull water into your stomach and intestines, making it unavailable to your body's tissues.) If you can't remember to drink eight glasses a day, buy a large plastic bottle of water (around 64 ounces) and make a pact with yourself that you will finish it by day's end. You won't believe the difference.

Nothing you do can help your system more. Water transports nutrients, hormones, and oxygen to your cells and takes waste products away via the bloodstream and the lymphatic system. Water also lubricates the joints and literally makes you feel better. It makes sense that when your body is in a time of remarkable change you would want to give it all the additional help you can. This is a great place to start.

Easing Menopause with Exercise

Exercise is the body's other food. No matter how hard it is for you to exercise and no matter how little exercise you are capable of doing, you should do what you can. *Any amount of exercise is better than none at all.* Many women who begin exercising only during menopause say it changes their lives. Even though there is no fountain of youth, exercise may be the next best thing. Recent studies have shown that many of the changes—both physical and mental—that we associate with aging and menopause are really at least partially the result of inactivity.

Here are some of the irrefutable benefits of exercise:

- Your heart will be healthier.
- Your bones will be stronger.
- Your stamina and energy will be greater.
- You will help your system detoxify itself.
- You will get an exercise "high."
- You will lessen the frequency and intensity of your hot flashes.
- You will fight encroaching fat cells.

If you do not already exercise regularly, you should include an exercise program in your life.

Va Va Va Vitamins

You will want to discuss your vitamin regimen during menopause with your physician. Although we don't need a lot of each vitamin, what we need we absolutely do need.

The most important supplement for a menopausal woman to take is calcium. The usual daily dosage is 1500 mg of elemental calcium. Calcium carbonate and calcium citrate are the most easily absorbed combinations. Most of the generic supplements are fine. If you have questions, check with your pharmacist. While there is debate regarding how worthwhile vitamins may be, there is no debate about the importance of a calcium supplement. We all need calcium, and it is never too late to start taking calcium supplements and minimize your bone loss.

You may also want to consider a folic acid and vitamin B supplement and/or an adequate general vitamin supplement.

Alcohol and Hot Flashes

Alcohol is a known trigger of hot flashes. Alcohol is also an antinutrient. In large quantities, it depletes the body of vitamin C, calcium, and important B vitamins, including folic acid, niacin, and thiamine. If you drink alcohol and are on hormone therapy, you will be at an increased risk for anemia, since your supply of folic acid will be doubly taxed. Alcohol is also a depressant and the calories from alcohol are empty ones, providing few nutrients and having almost as many calories per gram as fat (7 per gram as opposed to 9 per gram). There is little to recommend alcohol for a woman who is experiencing an uncomfortable menopause, and the best advice is probably to avoid it altogether, except on special occasions.

Caffeine and Hot Flashes

Caffeine is also thought to trigger hot flashes. By causing the blood vessels to constrict in the skin and thus raising body temperature, caffeine may set off a hot flash. Because caffeine also acts as a diuretic, it may strip the body of needed nutrients, including the B vitamins and calcium.

Caffeine intake should be kept to a minimum during menopause. If you drink a lot of coffee and sodas containing caffeine or if you eat quantities of chocolate, you should cut down on your caffeine intake gradually. Giving caffeine up cold turkey may have as many side effects as having too much. It's best to try to cut down by one cup of coffee every other day and lower your caffeine intake over a week's time.

Sex in the Third Season

"The symptoms of the climacteric should not be misinterpreted as signs of mental imbalance or emotional disturbance caused by sexual deprivation."

Germaine Greer, *The Change*

A S WITH MANY ASPECTS of menopause, your sex life is really up to you. And whether or not you have a sex life is not indicative of your mental health. If you enjoyed sex before menopause and considered your sex life an important part of your life, then you probably will want to keep it that way afterward. If this is not the case, then that's fine, too. The important thing is to have it the way you want it whenever you can.

The indispensable component to the enjoyment of sex is arousal. Arousal is an internal process, specific to the individual and harder to measure in women than in men for obvious reasons. One of the great inhibitors of arousal is anxiety, and in a menopausal woman who's suffering from vaginal dryness, anxiety because of physical discomfort is common. As stated in the section on hormone therapy, a lubricant like Astroglide or an estrogen cream may be even more effective than a jelly such as K-Y Jelly in relieving vaginal dryness (and, therefore, anxiety). If there are other physical aspects to your anxiety, such as hot flashes, the best remedy is probably sharing your worries with your partner. Remember, everything that you are going through is natural, including issues regarding your sex life.

This may also be a good time to stop comparing yourself to others. Your sexual frequency is no one's business but your own. If you have sex one to two times a month, then fine. So much talk about sexual frequency is hype and the hype causes women to feel like outcasts and alone if they don't crave sex. Remember, there is no norm except what is right and best for you.

Attitude

As you head into menopause, try to remember the bright side of the picture—no more tampons, no more pads, no more accidents, no more fear of pregnancy, and eventually no more PMS. You now know that this perfect state of nonfertility takes time to achieve, but it is best to set your sights on a cycle-free horizon and look forward to this new way of living—a unique experience after all those cycle-bound years.

If a Sense of Well-being Continues to Elude You

While statistics show that women tend to experience severe depression less frequently during menopause than at other stages in life, nonetheless, there are women who do sink into severe depression. For some this is transitory. But if you sense it is not, get help for your depression. If you are experiencing extreme and chronic mood swings, or if you suffer from a continual lack of energy or feel a sense of foreboding or despair, consult your physician. If you are not on hormone therapy and your doctor determines that the risks associated with the therapy are not prohibitive in your situation, he or she will probably advise the therapy; it will relieve the symptoms that may be adding to your depression, such as hot flashes and the associated insomnia. You will probably also be advised to see a therapist and explore other avenues of treatment. The most important thing to remember is that you needn't suffer in silence.

While menopause is a natural change in life, it's possible of course to have problems at any time in life. If you feel that your personal issues about menopause are extreme, or that you are having trouble coping with daily life or dealing with the physical changes you are going through, you should seek help.

ALLOWING FOR REBIRTH

"The menopause is nature's original contraceptive that freed women for leadership in the extended family and in the broad community. In many traditional cultures a woman's status increases with age, as one might expect, on this sociobiologic basis."

Germaine Greer, *The Change*

"You are no longer young,
Nor are you very old . . ."

Elizabeth Jennings

EACH WOMAN'S LIFE is her own, and she deals with the process, the stages, the conflicts, and crises in her own way. A woman approaching menopause will do herself a great service by allowing herself to be influenced by what women who went before her have to say on the subject of menopause and the positive possibilities for life after menopause. Reading the literature beforehand and choosing role models for yourself can help.

In our present world, menopause may come to a number of women at the same age, and yet at any number of different stages of life. One woman might have toddlers in the house, another might have kids leaving home for the first time for college, and another may be single again after many years.

Menopause is reflective of biology and not personal worth. Taking note of how varied women's lives are now as they go through menopause is yet another affirmation of this fact. The more you know about menopause and the more postmenopausal women you talk to, the greater your sense of control and perspective will be as you move on to this new stage in life.

239

A Final Note

While it is important to take menopause seriously and examine it scrupulously in terms of what medicine can do to make this passage as positive and healthy as possible, it is also important to demystify the process and stress that it is natural. It happens to every woman. The details may vary, but we are connected by this rite of passage; and it's time that we accept this commonality, by sharing our information when it's comfortable for us to and also by learning that it's okay to simply take it in stride. Menopause is not the end of life, it is simply the beginning of a new and promising stage of life. Most important, the choice regarding how you proceed with your life is yours.

PART 5

CHRONIC AND PROGRESSIVE CONDITIONS AND DISEASES

"When I turned forty I suddenly noticed that I bruised more easily and cuts didn't seem to heal as quickly. But, other than that, I wasn't about to settle for any chronic ailments."

Millie Stone (age 51)

W ITH AGE COME WISDOM, a few more headaches, and a less vital immune system. Rather than despair over the march of the small, physical annoyances that aging may bring, you can counteract time's markers with knowledge and self-treatment. This part explores the most common serious diseases and conditions that we are at risk for as time passes. You will learn what you are at risk for medically and how much you may be able to do to counteract the degenerative effects of conditions ranging from diabetes mellitus to multiple sclerosis.

While learning to live with a chronic condition or a progressive disease is not exactly what we might choose as our next challenge, it is nevertheless heartening to know that you can make a difference in your quality of life as you do so. What's more, by taking an active role in your medical care, you'll be able to face your situation with a sense of purpose that will contribute to your emotional equilibrium.

Adult-Onset Asthma

"One day while playing racquetball I began to wheeze—
loudly enough for my friends to hear me. It never dawned
on me that it could be asthma. I thought that was a disease
that only happened to children."

Jane Young (age 41)

O NLY 3 TO 5 PERCENT of the adult population have asthma. Yet, when asthma occurs in later life, it can become progressively more serious and have lasting complications. Symptoms include a painless tightening in the chest, wheezing, difficulty breathing, and sometimes a cough that brings up excess mucus. The breathing becomes difficult because the airways swell and become inflamed. Asthma, which is often inherited, may be exacerbated by exercise, change in temperature, certain foods, and other environmental triggers. Cigarette smoke and air pollution aggravate asthma.

Asthma attacks are usually more irritating than dangerous, although in some cases they can be life threatening. The attacks usually last minutes or hours. Other times they can linger for days. The more the airways swell, the greater the difficulty in breathing and the more serious the attack. Asthma attacks may worsen as you age. Emergency symptoms may include severe anxiety, extreme difficulty breathing, a bluish tinge to the skin, high pulse rate, and sweating. In such a situation, emergency care should be sought immediately.

If you have asthma, you should be under a physician's care. The most important thing during an asthma attack is to keep calm. If you become more nervous or agitated, the attack may worsen. This is easier said than done. Many people report, however, that simply keeping their metered-dose inhaler (MDI) with them at all times lowers their anxiety when an attack occurs.

An MDI administers such asthma medicines as bronchodilators, cortisone, and cromolyn into the lungs in exact amounts. The MDI helps to mix the medication with incoming air and move it into the lungs slowly and efficiently.

If you have asthma, cigarette smoke should be avoided. Poor air quality due to smog or lack of ventilation in a home or workplace can also contribute to asthma attacks. If you find you have a sensitivity to any analgesics, such as aspirin, you will want to avoid them. Keep away from dust, animals, and foods you may be allergic to. Sulfites, in particular, may cause asthma attacks; added to wines and beers as preservatives, they are also used to keep lettuce and fruits looking fresh.

Adult-Onset Diabetes

"My grandmother was a diabetic and so is my mother. I don't know if this is in the cards for me or not. But at least I know that if I take care of myself now, I'll be in good shape to handle diabetes if that day comes."

Kate Gallagher (age 45)

ADULT-ONSET DIABETES is the colloquial term for Type II or non-insulin-dependent diabetes mellitus (NIDDM). Type I or insulin-dependent diabetes mellitus (IDDM) usually develops in childhood or early adulthood. Type II diabetes mellitus often develops in middle age and can be controlled with diet and exercise. Type II diabetes mellitus is far more common than you might think—shockingly so. The truth is ten million Americans have been diagnosed with diabetes, and it is estimated that another five million are not aware that they have the disease. Nine out of ten of these cases are Type II diabetes (NIDDM).

Adult diabetes is more common in women than in men. Women who develop gestational diabetes (also known as temporary or maternal diabetes) during pregnancy are particularly at risk for developing the disease later in life. In fact, those women who develop gestational diabetes and are overweight throughout their pregnancies have a 65 percent chance of developing diabetes. Although women constitute less than 40 percent of diagnosed diabetics, it's estimated that 70 percent of those undiagnosed are female.

While there is no exact known cause of diabetes, certainly heredity adds risk, as does having had gestational diabetes. One other major factor in the onset of adult diabetes is obesity. Between 80 and 85 percent of those diagnosed with adult diabetes are overweight. If you are overweight and a member of your family has diabetes, you should make every effort to lose weight. In general, if you are over forty and overweight, you have a higher risk of diabetes, heart disease, and other health complications. If you are unable to lose weight, you should seek help from your doctor in choosing a healthy weight loss program that best fits your dietary and emotional needs.

Diabetes mellitus is a condition that causes you to have too much sugar in your blood. The reason there is too much sugar in your blood is that your pancreas is not producing enough insulin—the hormone that helps your blood assimilate sugar and turns the sugar into energy (Type I diabetics produce no insulin). High blood sugar, the indicator of diabetes, means that your body is not getting enough fuel. When this occurs, the body begins to convert its own fat and muscle into fuel. To add to this process of deterioration, when the body begins to burn itself for fuel, excess ketones are produced. Ketones are substances that form when fat is digested. Excess ketones can poison the body.

The tough news is that diabetes is a serious disease. But the good news is really good news. These days, if you are willing to participate in treating your own diabetes, it can be controlled. Type II diabetes is perhaps the disease that best exemplifies the benefits of self-care and self-maintenance. If not treated, the disease may lead to blindness, amputations, kidney disease, and a shortened life span. With proper self-care, diet, and insulin therapy when necessary (usually in pill form), a normal life is not only possible, but probable.

My father-in-law was recently diagnosed with this disease. Sure, it was a shock—he'd never been sick a day in his life. Suddenly his zero-handicap golf game was suffering and as he listened to the doctor about the dietary and lifestyle changes that would have to be made, he saw his business trips, cocktail parties, and social life taking a nosedive. But then he saw the silver lining. He refused to accept this as a disease and saw it as a way of improving the quality of his life. He dropped forty-two pounds, began a regular exercise program (which he confesses to love!), and made a game out of knowing which food elements could be substituted for others. The bottom line? He's trim, healthy, and feels great. This is the way it can be for many people.

If you are diagnosed with adult diabetes, an important first step is to realize that you have quite a bit of control over this condition. You can make a difference in your own treatment. Become an expert on your dietary requirements, in order to keep your blood sugar stable throughout the day. While this may sound like an almost insurmountable task, these days it is almost as easily done as said. There are many competent guides to living with adult diabetes.

A healthy diet will not only keep your diabetes under control, but also keep you healthy. In fact, the diet now recommended by the American Diabetes Association is much the same diet recommended for all Americans as a way to good health. It consists of 55 to 60 percent carbohydrates (you should choose complex carbohydrates such as beans, sweet potatoes, and brown rice, since simple carbohydrates are metabolized directly into glucose), 12 to 20 percent protein, and less than 30 percent fat. Instead of bemoaning your fate as a diabetic, you might want to think of this as an opportunity to become as healthy as you want to be.

After making when and what you eat an artful discipline, you can make exercise your ally. Exercise itself has been found to lower blood sugar. In addition, exercise improves your circulation and keeps your weight down—important components in controlling diabetes.

Alcoholism and Drug Abuse

"One night a girlfriend and I had a long dinner and drank
a bottle of wine. When I realized that I drank half a bottle
of wine on my own I was horrified. I was panicked for
days wondering if I would turn out to be an alcoholic like
my mother."

Jeanne Willand (age 39)

ALCOHOLISM IS A chronic and degenerative condition. Not only may the disease begin to impair your mental functioning and ability, but it will also endanger your overall health. Chronic abuse of alcohol will affect your digestive system, leading to a decrease in nutrients your body is able to utilize from the food you eat. Malabsorption may also lead to folic acid anemia (page 255), as your body is unable to absorb folic acid into the system. Abuse of alcohol may also put you at higher risk for high blood pressure. Although a certain amount of alcohol may help prevent heart disease, more than one or two drinks a day will actually increase your risk of heart disease. If you have a problem with weight, it will be exacerbated by the extreme use of alcohol. If you are a diabetic, drinking too much and drinking without eating will progressively worsen your condition. The situation is equally grim if you suffer from osteoporosis or almost any other preexisting condition.

"Never drink before five in the afternoon. Never
drink by yourself and never drink when there is
work to be done."

H. L. Mencken

I HAVE ALWAYS THOUGHT that Mencken's words are sound—providing a framework of social responsibility when it comes to alcohol. While alcohol tastes good to many and provides an outlet for others, its use comes with great responsibility.

If you do drink, here are some guidelines that will help you protect yourself from having an alcohol problem.

- Never use an alcoholic beverage to quench your thirst. Drink a glass of water if you're thirsty—then think about what else you may want to drink.
- If you have a drink, drink it slowly.
- If you find that you are using alcohol to relax, try other methods, such as exercise, relaxation techniques, a quiet walk, or a hot bath.

If you think you may have an alcohol problem, but are not sure, consider the following:

- Do you think about having a drink and consider this important?
- Do you drink every day?
- Has anyone in your family expressed concern about your drinking?
- Do you find that you have physical or psychological symptoms when you do not drink?
- Do you drink alone?

If you answer yes to any one of these questions, you could have a drinking problem.

If you have a problem with alcohol, you may also have a problem with prescription drugs. The two problems can feed on each other when used in tandem and generally worsen your overall health more quickly.

> *"I took my grandmother to see the doctor because*
> *she was feeling dizzy and nauseated. I rounded up*
> *the medicines she was taking and was shocked to*
> *find out she had stuff from four different doctors.*
> *It turned out she wasn't feeling well because the*
> *medications were interacting with one another.*

Now she's on two medicines and she carries a list
with the proper dosages in her purse."

Allison Gibson (age 41)

MISUSING OR ABUSING DRUGS, both legal and illegal, is becoming an increasing problem in this country. If you take any drug for purposes other than those for which it was intended in a quantity or manner other than as directed, this is considered drug abuse. In this country, for example, more than 1.5 million people take tranquilizers for more than four months, which is considered the time period that may begin to reflect addiction.

The Federal Controlled Substances Act has classified the potential drugs of abuse in five categories, from Schedule I, the most addictive and most easily abused, to Schedule V, drugs with the least potential for abuse and addiction. Schedule I drugs include heroin. Schedule II includes cocaine, opium derivatives such as codeine and morphine, and PCP. Schedule II drugs cannot be prescribed over the telephone. Schedule III and IV drugs can be prescribed over the telephone, but no more than five refills are permitted. Schedule III drugs include those that combine a narcotic such as codeine and nonnarcotic drugs. Schedule IV drugs include tranquilizers, such as the benzodiazepines (including Xanax and Valium) and some sleeping pills, such as pentobarbihypnotics (often sold under the trade name Nembutal).

Sometimes drugs are not abused, but they are misused out of ignorance or carelessness. Among the elderly, drugs may be underused in order to save money. Many elderly women see more than one doctor, each of whom may be prescribing medicines without another's knowledge. These medications can interact or have a cumulative effect. Once more than one drug is being taken at the same time, confusion regarding the dosage of each may add to the problem.

A standard adult dose may prove to be too strong for an older person, because drugs are cleared less effectively from the body as we age. Another problem for seniors is the mail-order medicine business: it's easy for an older person to get the wrong medication or the wrong dose, and in many instances, the generic substitution may not be as good as the trade-name drug.

The most common illegal drug in the United States is marijuana. It is estimated that there is a $10 billion a year marijuana harvest in the United States, which would make marijuana the third largest agricultural crop in the country. While marijuana has been both misrepresented and misunderstood by many in this country, it is clear that this drug can create dependence. In addition, the inhalation of marijuana smoke, which many smokers hold deep in their lungs for a period of time, can damage the lungs. Chronic marijuana smokers show decreased lung capacity and also chronic bronchial irritation. If you have used marijuana for a prolonged period of time, you may be dependent upon it. If you try to stop using marijuana, you may find that you have symptoms such as irritability, sleep disturbances, tremors, and sweats—as well as other symptoms associated with drug withdrawal. As with all drugs, prolonged use indicates some degree of dependence.

Women receive prescription drugs from their doctors at approximately a ten-to-one ratio to men, including painkillers and tranquilizers, both of which may become addictive. Women tend to keep secret a dependency on prescription drugs (as they also often do with alcohol), rather than seek help immediately. This is partly because of fear of what family members and others may think, but also because they tend to put the needs of others before their own. If you have been taking any prescription drug for more than six months, you should discuss the situation with your doctor.

Shame and secrecy, which are not helpful attitudes when it comes to chemical dependency, will only prolong your problem and your battle with it. When you simply tell someone you are worried, whether it be a friend or a doctor, you will have already taken the first step in helping yourself take control of *a chronic problem that can be controlled.* You will need to replace your negative habit with some positive habits, and you will likely need help in doing this—many people do. Seeking help for your problem does not mean you are weak. On the contrary, seeking help is a sign of strength.

The most important thing to realize is that if you feel you may have such a problem you are not alone, and there are many places and ways to seek help. Begin by telling your doctor. He or she may not have all the answers, but should be able to point you in the right direction. If you feel that you cannot tell your doctor, you should find another doctor. You will need information regarding drug and therapy programs in your area.

Alcoholics Anonymous (AA) has chapters all over the country and there are meeting times to accommodate almost any schedule. AA is also helpful for those who are dealing with a dependency on prescription drugs or with other forms of addiction. AA collects no dues and asks only that you be committed to staying sober. The twelve steps of the program are suggestions that may help you lead a sober life, but following them is not a requirement of the organization. Al-Anon is an organization sponsored by AA that is designed for those dealing with a loved one's alcoholism. Consult your telephone directory for a local listing of Alcoholics Anonymous or Al-Anon.

Allergies

*"I moved to Arizona twenty years ago to get away from
my allergies to trees and grass. But now it seems that half
of the people in New Jersey have moved here too! Everyone has planted grass and trees to make things greener
and I'm sneezing now more than ever."*

Trudy Kominski (age 54)

THERE ARE DIFFERENT kinds of allergies, including skin allergies, respiratory allergies, and allergies to foods, drugs, and insect bites.

An allergy is the result of the immune system's response to a foreign material. It may be pollen, animal dander, food, or a chemical. When the immune system recognizes this material as foreign and a threat to the body, it goes into gear to do battle with what it thinks is the enemy. Mast cells release histamine, which causes the nose to get stuffy or run, the eyes to redden and itch, the skin to itch, and the throat to feel like it's going to close up.

Food allergies, and allergies in general, often worsen with age. The best treatment for allergies is to avoid the cause of the allergic reaction.

251

Since this is not always possible, drugs are often prescribed for severe allergies.

Among the myths associated with allergies are:

- Allergies are psychosomatic. While emotional stress may affect the severity of an allergic reaction, emotions do not cause allergies.
- Short-haired pets are less of a problem for an allergic person. It's not the animal's fur, but the dander—or the shedding scales of the skin—that causes an allergic reaction. The saliva and urine may also cause a reaction. If you are allergic to animals, the safest pets are fish and reptiles.
- Allergies are not dangerous. Most allergies are not dangerous, but some are. Anaphylaxis is the most severe allergic response (and thankfully the rarest). About 10 to 15 percent of the population may have an anaphylactic reaction to almost any allergen, including insect bites, pollens, some vaccines, and even some foods. It occurs most commonly after an insect sting or bite or an intravenous injection of a drug. The reaction is almost instantaneous and it is systemic (in other words, your whole system is affected). Symptoms include difficulty breathing because of the constriction of the throat and airways, rapid pulse, hives or swelling, and in some cases shock and cardiovascular collapse. Anaphylaxis must be treated immediately with an injection of adrenaline to open the airways.

Alzheimer's Disease

*"I just wish I didn't have to put Nancy through the ordeal
that I know is inevitable with this disease."*

Ronald Reagan

ALZHEIMER'S DISEASE IS CAUSED by a disintegration of brain cells and is considered a form of dementia. In fact, Alzheimer's accounts for more than 50 percent of all cases of dementia. Behavioral characteristics of the disease depend on what part of the brain is affected. More than 2.5 million people in the United States have Alzheimer's disease. It usually affects people over sixty.

Symptoms include gradual memory loss (particularly of recent events), an inability to learn new facts, an increasing tendency to repeat oneself, increasing confusion and disorientation, irritability, anxiety, and a slow disintegration of personality, judgment, and social skills. The diagnosis is usually made by the presence of the constellation of symptoms, since there is no foolproof test (other than a brain biopsy) to clinch the diagnosis. One of the many difficulties in Alzheimer's disease is that those who suffer from the disease lack an understanding of their condition—they simply don't notice. So, if you have a loved one who appears to have symptoms that may indicate Alzheimer's disease, you will probably have to encourage her or him to see a doctor for an evaluation.

Alzheimer's disease is a degenerative condition. Living with Alzheimer's—whether you suffer from it or are caring for someone who does—is not easy. Despite President Reagan's concerns in the statement above, it is *not* inevitable that the experience of Alzheimer's constitute an unbearable ordeal. You will want to maintain a daily routine that does not vary too much and maintain good general physical health through proper diet and a moderate exercise program. Notes will help remind yourself, or the person you are caring for, of daily activities, calls to make, pills to take. As much as possible, you will want to avoid disruptions to the routine, such as moving to a new home.

The only bright spot in the past few years with regard to treatment is a medication called Tacrin. In many patients it improves the ability to perform certain tasks and may help with memory. Talk to your doctor about whether this medication should be considered in your situation.

Anemia

There are many different types of anemia, the most common blood disorder. All anemias involve diminished levels of hemoglobin and in most cases a decrease in the number of red blood cells, or erythrocytes. Hemoglobin is a complex protein in red blood cells that carries oxygen from the lungs to all the tissues of the body. Thus, when levels of hemoglobin are low, your body is slowly but surely being deprived of oxygen.

The signs and symptoms of anemia are initially so mild that you may not notice them. As the condition progresses, however, you will notice that you are paler and more tired than usual. To check for pallor, look at your nail beds, or the underside of your eyelids or lips. Also examine your palms: if you are anemic, the creases in them will appear to be almost white or as pale as the surrounding skin. You may also notice a shortness of breath when you exercise or walk up stairs or that your heartbeat seems faster than normal.

There are many different kinds of anemia with different causes, but the symptoms in all cases are almost always the same. If you are experiencing any of the above symptoms, if you are suffering from reduced endurance, low appetite, numbness in the hands and feet, or diarrhea, or if you are just "not feeling yourself," you should consult your physician. Women who are experiencing menopause may be especially prone to anemia. Anemia is not a condition to take lightly and in almost all cases is not related to an inherited disorder. It is correctable. So don't worry. Just make an appointment with your doctor or at your clinic if you notice any signs that might indicate anemia.

Kinds of Anemia

IRON-DEFICIENCY ANEMIA

The most common form of anemia is iron-deficiency anemia, which can be corrected by diet and supplemental iron pills. Your physician will want to make sure that you are not receiving too much iron, because iron itself can be dangerous in large quantities.

PERNICIOUS ANEMIA

Pernicious anemia is rare; it usually occurs in older people and is hereditary in nature. It involves the lack of absorption of vitamin B_{12}. If you have a relative who has pernicious anemia, you should inform your physician so that he or she can help you prevent the development of symptoms. The condition was labeled "pernicious" before there was an effective treatment for it. Today, however, it need not be as harmful if caught in time and treated.

Folic Acid Anemia

Folic acid anemia involves a deficiency of folic acid and can result if you do not get enough folic acid or if your system cannot absorb it. Folic acid is a B vitamin also known as folate. This anemia sometimes occurs in pregnant women, when the demand for folic acid is greater than the body's supply. It may also occur in alcoholics, who can become malnourished if drinking becomes their major source of calories and their digestive tract ceases to absorb nutrients as well as it used to. The condition is treated through diet and folic acid supplements, and in the case of alcoholism, immediate abstinence. Foods rich in folic acid are raw fruits and vegetables, beans, liver, and kidneys. Remember that excessive cooking can deplete the folic acid in a food. Many cereals are now fortified with folic acid.

Sickle-Cell Disease

Also called sickle-cell anemia, sickle-cell disease gets its name from the sickling that occurs in the red blood cells, which become rigid and crescent- or sickle-shaped. The red blood cells then break up and he-moglobin is released into the blood plasma, causing anemia. Sickle-cell disease is inherited and is relatively common among African Americans. Interestingly, when red blood cells sickle they may have, accidentally, a protective effect against malaria. And while the sickling plays an important role in preventing malaria among Africans, the same protec-tive effect can be a liability in the Western world, where malaria is not a health threat. In addition to the usual symptoms of anemia, other symptoms include vision problems, skin ulcers on the lower legs, delayed growth and development in children, and increased susceptibility to infections.

The disease is chronic and over time affects other organs, including the kidneys, lungs, liver, and central nervous system. As of now, there is no effective treatment, though new treatments are being tested. The most important thing you can do if you have sickle-cell disease is to limit infections and make sure that all infections you do get are treated immediately. You should also take a daily supplement of folic acid, since sickle-cell disease increases your body's need for this vitamin.

HEMOLYTIC ANEMIAS AND OTHER ANEMIAS

Hemolytic is a Greek word that means the destruction of blood. Hemolytic anemias involve the destruction of red blood cells and the subsequent liberation of hemoglobin into the bloodstream. These anemias are inherited or acquired. Certain medications and infections may cause hemolytic anemia. If your anemia was caused by a drug, your doctor will take you off that drug. Medications such as prednisone, a corticosteroid, are often prescribed to prevent the destruction of red blood cells. While some types of hemolytic anemia are hard to cure, they are seldom fatal. Other rare anemias include thalassemia and glucose-6-phosphate dehydrogenase deficiency, both of which are inherited disorders.

Anorexia

Even though anorexia is often seen as disease of the young, many women continue to suffer from varying degrees of this disorder in their middle years. As you grow older, chronic anorexia can cause anemia and can make you more susceptible to osteoporosis. (See "Anorexia Nervosa and Bulimia Nervosa," page 347.)

Arthritis

One day in my mid-thirties, I became acutely aware that my ankles hurt when I walked down the steps in the morning to make coffee. I was not pleased. I knew the pain could only be one thing: I had arthritis. Fortunately, after fifteen minutes of walking, the flexibility improved and the pain went away. Then I was able to forget about the whole thing—until I was reminded again the following morning.

Every morning I know to expect the same thing. The pain hasn't really changed over the years. But it does remind me that there is a price to be paid for the wear and tear on the joints.

It is hard to live a long life without having some form or degree of arthritis. The word "arthritis" refers to an inflammation of the joints. The most common form of arthritis is osteoarthritis. A certain amount of osteoarthritis is almost inevitable when the joints get a great deal of use over a great deal of time—in fact, it is also known as wear-and-tear arthritis. (Because osteoarthritis is as much a fact of the aging process as it is a chronic condition, it's discussed in Part 6, "Aging and the Body"—see page 285. This section focuses on rheumatoid arthritis.)

Rheumatoid Arthritis

Rheumatoid arthritis, the most debilitating form of arthritis, is not the natural result of use over time, but an autoimmune disease. In rheumatoid arthritis, the immune system attacks itself. Although this is still not well understood, the theory is that when stimulated by an unidentified agent the disease-fighting cells of the immune system turn on the joints and attack them; the joints then become inflamed. Rheumatoid arthritis is also systemic in nature (affecting the entire body) and may affect not only the musculoskeletal system, but also organs such as the heart, lungs, and eyes. It usually affects more than one joint, but in a symmetrical fashion—i.e., both feet, both knees, both hands. The disease strikes most frequently between the ages of twenty and fifty. Among the 7 million Americans suffering from the disease, there are approximately three times more women than men.

Rheumatoid arthritis first attacks the synovium—the membrane lining the joints, which secretes a lubricating fluid called synovia. First, this tissue becomes inflamed. Then the cartilage begins to proliferate, which in turn causes the erosion of the surrounding ligaments, muscles, and bones. The result over a long period can be bent and disfigured hands and feet. The fingers and toes can become so bent and gnarled that they lose their ability to function.

Initial symptoms include pain and swelling in the small joints of the hands and feet and an overall stiffness or aching that may be particularly noticeable upon awakening or after having been seated for a long time. In addition to the swelling and pain, the affected joints may be warm to the touch. Some people experience sweats and fever as well. Rheumatoid arthritis may come and go, or it may become chronic. If you have had continual symptoms for four or five years, you will probably have to cope with the condition for the rest of your life.

Self-treatment for rheumatoid arthritis depends upon maintaining an optimum balance between rest and exercise—a balance only you can discover for yourself through a certain amount of trial and error. During flare-ups, you will want to minimize motion in the affected area—concentrate on rest and not exertion. During periods of remission, you will want to exercise the area to encourage muscle building and the restoration of mobility. Embrace moderate activity, but don't stress the affected joints unduly. In the case of rheumatoid arthritis, overdoing may be just as damaging as not doing at all—it's a balancing act, like so many things in life. Often working in conjunction with a physical therapist can help you develop the strategy that works for you.

One thing to beware of when dealing with arthritis is the notion of a miracle cure. *There is no miracle cure for arthritis.* All so-called miracle remedies rely on the nature of the disease, which almost always includes periods of remission. For example, you buy a copper bracelet. You wear it. You have no flare-ups. You may attribute this to the bracelet, as the purveyor of this miracle cure would want you to do, but in fact this period of remission is due to the nature of the disease. It's better to spend your money on a lightweight, removable splint that you can use to immobilize the joint when you do have a flare-up, and to spend your time engaging in physical activities you enjoy when you don't.

Anti-inflammatory drugs, particularly aspirin, are almost always used to treat the pain and inflammation associated with this condition. Sometimes corticosteroid drugs, including prednisone, are also used. Experimental medications that may suppress the overactive immune system are now being tested.

Chronic Fatigue Syndrome

Chronic fatigue syndrome (CFS) used to be known as Epstein-Barr virus or chronic mononucleosis. People who suffer from CFS feel a bone-weary flulike fatigue that lasts for six months or more, is not the result of another disease or condition, and does not go away when you get adequate rest.

CFS is diagnosed more frequently in women than in men and occurs most often in white people who are between the ages of twenty-five and fifty. CFS has been referred to as the "Yuppie flu," but this is probably because your standard Yuppie will pursue a second and third opinion and not spare expense to find out what is wrong: she feels she has a right to know and she also has the means to find out. Many other people who suffer with CFS are never adequately diagnosed. The symptoms can be nondescript, so it can be difficult to put together a diagnosis.

If you have eight or more of the following symptoms for more than six months, you should explore with your doctor the possibility of your having CFS and keep asking questions until they are adequately answered.

- Mild, but continuous sore throat
- Recurrent fever and chills
- Muscle weakness or discomfort
- Inability to concentrate
- Forgetfulness
- Sleep disturbances
- Headaches
- Irritability
- Depression
- Joint pain
- Excessive fatigue after exercise

It is not clear what causes CFS, though some doctors believe it is an immune system disorder and may be caused by exposure to the Epstein-Barr virus or the live rubella virus used in the vaccine for German measles. There is no cure for CFS at present, though your doctor may offer treatment to relieve your symptoms. If you think you may have CFS, the following can help:

- Get plenty of rest.
- Exercise moderately every day.
- Contact a local CFS organization or your local medical school for more information.
- Look into alternative treatments, such as acupuncture and vitamin therapy (see pages 402–410).

See also "Fibromyalgia," page 262.

Chronic Pain

*"I never understood why my aunt was such a crab all
the time until I developed chronic hip pain like she had.
Then I found myself morose and short-tempered. Pain
erodes you, like a bad relationship."*

Suzette Riga (age 47)

P AIN IS THE BODY'S most accurate warning signal, but pain is an
individual experience. Just ask any woman who's gone through
labor and you'll realize that everyone has a different gauge when
it comes to pain. A debilitating headache to one woman may be
something that can be treated with one aspirin by another. To quantify
pain, a doctor must rely on the patient's perception of that pain, at least
to some degree.

Chronic back pain is the most common chronic pain complaint. It
is estimated that 100 million Americans suffer from some form of back
pain (see page 309). Until recently, doctors have had a laissez-faire
attitude toward pain—undermedicating in order not to overmedicate,
in keeping with the credo "First, do no harm." Women's complaints
about pain, in particular, have been ignored, dismissed as "female,"
"feminine," or simply not real.

But all of this is finally changing. Chronic pain is a very real condition that has only recently begun to get the recognition it deserves.
If you suffer from pain, you know your pain is real. Keep reminding your
doctor of this, because only you can. Remember, even if your doctor
cannot find the direct cause of your pain, your pain is real and must be
addressed.

Some doctors subspecialize in the management of pain. Usually anesthesiologists are best trained to do this work because of their background in using medications in the operating room. Many hospitals now
have pain clinics that are committed to treating patients with chronic
pain that has been resistant to normal medications.

Painkillers and Analgesics

Painkillers or analgesics can give you temporary relief if you suffer from chronic pain. There are two basic kinds of painkillers, nonnarcotic and narcotic. The most common nonnarcotic painkillers (which are the most widely used of all medications) are aspirin, acetaminophen, and ibuprofen. The most common side effect of aspirin and anti-inflammatory painkillers such as ibuprofen is gastrointestinal irritation.

Narcotic painkillers include natural or artificial forms of opium, called opiates or opioids. Codeine, propoxyphene (such as Darvon or Wygesic), meperidine (Demerol), and morphine are examples.

Combinations of narcotics and nonnarcotics are popular. One of the best known is acetaminophen with codeine, such as Tylenol with Codeine No. 3. These drugs are used on a short-term basis for pain relief when dealing with surgery, broken bones, or cancer.

In most cases, narcotic painkillers should *not* be used for the relief of chronic pain. However, if you feel you need such relief, it is a clear sign that you should be discussing the issue of chronic pain with your doctor. If your doctor does not understand your problem or continues to prescribe a narcotic painkiller without discussing your situation further, you should find another doctor or at least seek another opinion.

Alternatives

There are other options beside painkillers if you suffer from chronic pain. These include physical therapy, chiropractic medicine (for back and some joint pains), myofacial pain relief therapy (a form of deep muscle stimulation and massage), acupuncture, and electrostimulation (a technique that includes implanting electrodes at the site of the pain and stimulating them to prevent pain messages from reaching the brain). Hypnotherapy and relaxation techniques play very important roles in helping a person with chronic pain and can complement any other treatment you opt for. You should consider surgery as a last resort.

Chronic pain is a very serious condition that millions of Americans suffer from. It is finally getting the attention it deserves from the medical community—more and more research is being done regarding the treatment of chronic pain and the results are promising. It is heartening to note that while there is no way around suffering pain at certain times in life, the relief of pain is now a major goal of medicine—not only are patients being encouraged not to suffer in silence, the goal is to help them not suffer at all.

Cigarette Use

There is no other single habit responsible for more degenerative conditions and eventual deaths than cigarette smoking. Whereas there is evidence that one glass of wine may be a good thing in life, there is no good cigarette. From the first cigarette you smoke, you begin to put yourself at risk for a number of conditions, from emphysema to heart disease and lung cancer. In addition, smoking weakens the immune system, plays havoc with your sense of taste, ages your skin prematurely, and adds to the toxins your liver and bladder must process. Because of the female anatomy, the toxins in the urine may increase the risk of vaginal cancers, cystitis, and bladder cancer. Cigarette smoking is also a major culprit in heart disease, including high blood pressure and atherosclerosis.

If you smoke and want to quit and are having trouble, get help. Expressing a need for help is a sign of strength, not weakness. There are many programs and methods that can work to help you quit smoking. If you ask for help and take control of your situation by researching what may be the best method of quitting for you, you will be giving yourself the best gift you could imagine—health and every chance for longevity. (See "Lung Cancer," page 107.)

Fibromyalgia

Although it may seem as if the last thing you want to hear about these days is a new disease, the truth is, the more adept we doctors become at differentiating one ailment from another, the better your chances are of getting the right treatment for the right disease. So often, people suffer needlessly because they have been misdiagnosed—or, even worse, been told that there is nothing wrong with them when something is indeed terribly wrong. Enter fibromyalgia.

Until recently, fibromyalgia was called simply fibrositis—an inflammation of the connective tissue, considered to be a rheumatic in origin and related to arthritis. What confused doctors was that they were never able to pinpoint an inflammation in the joints of patients who suffered from fibrositis. Thus, they renamed the condition fibromyalgia, which means, basically, pain related to soft tissue.

Women are affected by this disorder far more than men; roughly 80 percent of those diagnosed are women, generally between the ages of twenty and fifty. One of the reasons fibromyalgia is so difficult to diagnose is that the symptoms are wide-ranging. In addition, many symptoms overlap with other disorders, making misdiagnosis common. Some of the most common symptoms include fatigue to the point of exhaustion, general muscle pain, sleep disturbances, cold hands and feet, numbness in the hands and feet, headaches, stomachaches, and depression. Sometimes Raynaud's disease (page 277) may be suspected when coldness and numbness are present in the hands and feet. It is also important to note that many women who seem to be suffering from chronic fatigue syndrome (page 258) actually have fibromyalgia. And there is some debate over whether or not the two diseases are, in fact, the same condition.

Recently, a simple diagnostic test has made diagnosing fibromyalgia much easier. The test involves checking eighteen specific points on the body for tenderness. These include points on the front and back of the neck, the chest and shoulders, the elbows, the hips and the knees. Women with fibromyalgia are highly sensitive in these areas. If such sensitivity occurs consistently, a diagnosis can readily be made.

Even though the disease is surprisingly common, there is no known cause. Sometimes, trauma appears to be the cause, such as a severe accident, extended periods of extreme stress, or even something as seemingly minor as the flu. What is clear is that interrupted sleep and lack of sleep, as well as lack of exercise, can exacerbate the condition.

When treating fibromyalgia, Flexeril and Elavil and low doses of tricyclic drugs are usually recommended to counteract sleep disturbances. A program of regular exercise is also recommended; generally the program includes aerobic exercise that begins gradually and increases in intensity. Also, simple painkillers may be prescribed, such as acetaminophen; however the stronger, anti-inflammatory drugs have been shown to have little effect. As with so many conditions of aging, the most important thing to remember is, once again, to get your rest and get your exercise. Nothing works as a better prevention and both are invaluable as remedies, particularly in the case of fibromyalgia.

Interstitial Cystitis

"I never even heard of this problem. I thought I just had
a urinary tract infection but it wouldn't get better. The
pain was excruciating and I felt the need to urinate all
the time. Now I find out that I will have to live with this.
And I'm just twenty-nine."

Samantha Reinhold (age 29)

INTERSTITIAL CYSTITIS (IC) is a chronic condition that is extremely hard to diagnose. It involves an inflammation of the bladder wall that, when chronic, lessens the elasticity of the bladder and often reduces the capacity of the bladder by more than two thirds. IC may cause you to feel the need to urinate fifty to one hundred times a day. IC is often confused with a urinary tract infection, which can increase the time it takes to get an accurate diagnosis. If there are no bacteria present in your urine culture and antibiotics have given you no relief, IC should be considered as a possibility. If nobody brings up the topic of IC, you should introduce it.

Nine out of ten people diagnosed with IC are women. Interstitial cystitis is most commonly diagnosed in middle-aged women, perhaps because by this time in life the symptoms of IC have progressed far enough that the condition is now noticeable. If you are seeing an unenlightened doctor, you may be told that it is psychological in origin.

There is no clear cause of IC, though some researchers do think that the condition might be the result of an earlier bladder injury. IC may also be linked to chronic urinary tract infections earlier in life. Some environmental factors have also been considered, including chemicals; chronic fatigue syndrome (page 258) has also been indicated as a possible cause.

Although there are treatment options, there is no cure for interstitial cystitis. There are treatment options that work to decrease the frequency of urination and to relieve pain. Pyridium is one medication that may help. Another treatment includes filling the bladder with water, while the patient is under general anesthesia, in order to stretch the bladder. A drug called Rimso 50 is also used in some cases to encourage the regeneration of the bladder wall. To relieve pain, a type of electrical nerve stimulation called transcutaneous nerve stimulation (TCNS) is sometimes used.

If you suffer from IC, here are some helpful hints:

- Avoid acidic foods and beverages as much as possible, including citrus fruits, apples, tomatoes, cantaloupes, cranberries, pineapples, strawberries, vinegar, fruit juices, carbonated drinks, and alcohol.
- Avoid artificial sweeteners.
- Drink plenty of water and clear liquids.
- Mix a teaspoon of baking soda with 8 ounces of water and drink this concoction once a day.

Lung Diseases

Bronchitis

Acute bronchitis occurs when the mucous membranes lining the bronchi become inflamed. Breathing is difficult, and coughing spells are unavoidable. Almost everyone has had acute bronchitis at one time or another. Symptoms include a cough, chills, soreness or tightness in the chest, and sometimes fever.

The best thing to do? Drink extra liquids, take aspirin, and rest. Usually bronchitis disappears in a matter of days with no lasting effects. If your doctor suspects that you have a bacterial infection, you will be started on antibiotics. If a cough keeps you up at night, talk to your doctor about getting a cough suppressant. Unfortunately, most over-the-counter preparations won't do the trick. The best cough suppressant is codeine and you will need a prescription for that. If you suffer from emphysema, asthma, or congestive heart failure, or if you are coughing up blood, check with your doctor to see if bronchitis is complicating the problem.

Chronic bronchitis involves the ongoing inflammation of your bronchial tubes. These air passageways may be narrowed enough to interfere with your ability to breathe and to cause fits of coughing. Chronic bronchitis is often present in chronic obstructive pulmonary disease (COPD) and usually, but not always, in conjunction with emphysema. Smoking is usually the cause of chronic bronchitis, although air pollution, dust, or toxic chemical gases in the workplace may also be responsible. While the disease was once more common in men, this is changing now because more women are smoking.

The major symptom of chronic bronchitis is a chronic cough. The diagnosis is based on the presence of a cough for at least three months of the year for two consecutive years. Treatment involves throwing those cigarettes away and avoiding smoke altogether. You should also avoid inhaling fumes, such as exhaust fumes, paint odors, and even perfume. You will also want to avoid exposure to anyone with a cold, since even a minor respiratory infection can severely aggravate your bronchitis. Your doctor may also prescribe an antibiotic, such as erythromycin or tetracycline, if there is a change in the color, thickness, or volume of your sputum—an indication of an infection.

Chronic bronchitis is a serious disease and in severe cases may decrease a person's life expectancy. If you are a smoker and you quit smoking, the outlook is, of course, far more optimistic.

Emphysema

"I remember how difficult it was for my grandmother to take a breath. I found myself laboring to breathe just hanging around her. But did she ever think about quitting—even as she was suffocating to death? No. She is a constant reminder of why I never picked up the habit."

Beth Famon (age 35)

EMPHYSEMA IS ALMOST always caused by smoking, though heredity and asthma are sometimes responsible. Deaths caused by emphysema are far more frequent in those who smoke. Emphysema used to be more common in men, but now that more women are smoking, emphysema is affecting us too. Emphysema occurs when the alveoli (the cells in the lungs that exchange oxygen and carbon dioxide with your blood) lose their elasticity. Air gets trapped in the alveoli and can't escape. As air gets trapped, the lungs become hyperinflated and breathing can become quite difficult. Emphysema is also characterized by the narrowing of the smaller breathing passages. This

A NOTE ON TOBACCO SMOKE

According to the Environmental Protection Agency, cigarettes kill 434,000 people every year. The agency has now listed secondhand smoke as a group A carcinogen—putting it in the same category as asbestos and benzene, which are known to cause cancer in humans. Cigarette smoke contains almost four thousand chemicals, fifty of which are known cancer-causing agents. These chemicals include lead, arsenic, ammonia, nicotine, benzene, vinyl chloride (used to produce plastics), and cadmium (used in the production of batteries). Between 2 and 6 percent of cigarette smoke is carbon monoxide, a toxic gas that binds with hemoglobin, making it impossible for the hemoglobin molecule to transport oxygen to the tissues of the body.

causes shortness of breath because air takes much longer to flow in and out of your lungs.

By the time you have symptoms of emphysema or COPD, such as difficulty exercising, a chronic cough, or shortness of breath, damage has already been done to your lungs. Unfortunately, there is no specific treatment to reverse the changes in the lungs due to emphysema. But if your disease is diagnosed early, before symptoms are present, you may prevent further progression of the disease *if you stop smoking.*

Lupus

Systemic lupus erythematosus, or lupus, is a disease of the connective tissues. It is a chronic inflammatory condition in which the body's own autoimmune system attacks the network of fibers that binds the tissues and organs of the body together.

Nine out of ten people who are diagnosed with lupus are women; it often strikes minority women, especially African Americans. What triggers lupus is not particularly clear, but it is known that both heredity and hormones are partly responsible for triggering the disease. Environmental causes, such as excessive exposure to the sun, may also play a part. Lupus, which is most likely to appear in women during the childbearing years, is not contagious.

A woman who is suffering from lupus may find that getting an accurate diagnosis is so difficult it takes its time and toll along with the disease. Because lupus may flare up and then seem to disappear, a woman may be told it is all in her head. As in any medical discussion, never take this explanation as an answer. If it is the explanation that you are given, keep asking questions and getting other opinions.

Here are some symptoms that may be indicative of lupus, particularly when they appear in conjunction with one another:

- A butterfly rash—a rash that appears over the bridge of the nose and across the cheeks, much like the shape of a butterfly
- Joint pain that mimics arthritis
- Redness or swelling at a joint that then moves to another joint in the body
- Extreme sensitivity of the skin to the sun
- Skin rashes, which may be mild or severe enough to develop into skin ulcers or scabs
- Loss of hair
- Anemia
- Fatigue
- Purple fingers and toes after exposure to cold or to stress
- Bladder and kidney problems
- Nausea, sometimes accompanied by vomiting
- Enlarged lymph nodes
- Depression

If you do have at least some of these symptoms and have been told not to worry, it's all in your head, you should get another opinion and research the situation further.

Treatment options for lupus include aspirin to reduce pain and swelling and antimalarial drugs to alleviate skin problems. Cortisone may also be used to reduce all symptoms. There is no cure for lupus.

If you have lupus, here are some things you can do for yourself.

- Avoid exposing your skin to the sun.
- Do not take the pill, which has been found to trigger lupus.
- Avoid all other drugs, except those you are taking for your disease.

- Exercise to strengthen your muscles, improve your overall condition, and reduce the risk of osteoporosis, a risk that the drugs you are probably taking may increase.
- Eat a low-fat diet, including a great deal of fresh fruits and vegetables and complex carbohydrates such as lentils, brown rice, and beans.
- Get plenty of rest to avoid infections that may trigger attacks.

Multiple Sclerosis

"One day my sister complained that her right foot seemed
to drag. In front of our very eyes it got worse and worse.
It took months before the doctors were able to diagnose
her with MS."

Julia McComb (age 33)

ULTIPLE SCLEROSIS, commonly known as MS, is a disease of the central nervous system. The disease proceeds in episodes that may last for days, weeks, or months; between these episodes there may be long periods of time in which symptoms abate or even disappear. Thus, periods of remission are possible, but attacks usually do recur. Attacks are generally most frequent three to five years after the disease has been diagnosed. The first attack usually occurs between twenty and forty years of age; often it's so mild that it may be attributed to something else and not even explored with a doctor. If you have a relative with MS, you are at greater risk for the disease. The risk for MS is slightly higher for women than for men. Your risk also varies geographically—the risk of MS is greater in northern states than in southern states. More than 200,000 Americans have MS.

MS attacks and permanently damages the myelin sheath that coats your nerves and aids in transmission of nerve impulses. There appears to be some connection between the misfiring of the immune system and the presence of MS. Although the cause of MS is not clear, it is known that when MS is present, the concentration of immune cells in the central nervous system is high. The presence of a virus in the immune cells or in the cells that produce the myelin sheath is one possible cause of MS.

Symptoms include numbness or paralysis in one limb or more, impaired vision, tremor, and involuntary eye movements. Because these symptoms may be indicative of many different neurological disorders, accurate diagnosis is extremely important. One of the first real signs of MS is that these attacks vanish and then recur. If you have had two or more attacks, this is considered a reliable first step toward a diagnosis when combined with altered reflexes, lack of sensation, and other observable alterations of the functioning of the central nervous system. The symptoms of MS vary widely because lesions of the myelin sheath appear randomly throughout the brain and spinal cord. An MRI, a spinal tap, and other neurologic tests may be obtained in order to make the diagnosis.

The course of this disease varies widely. After diagnosis, the life expectancy is now thirty-five years or more; this is increasing because of better medical care, particularly in dealing with complications of the disease. Most people with MS are ambulatory, although MS is the number one cause of major disability in adults of working age.

While there is as yet no cure for MS, physical therapy, exercise, occupational therapy, and psychotherapy are extremely valuable in slowing its progress. At the present time, research is under way on drugs that suppress the immune system and may be beneficial in the treatment of MS.

Most women who have just been diagnosed with MS are scared and depressed. All they've been exposed to are the worst-case scenarios, and those images are indeed frightening. But the truth about MS is that the progress of the disease is very individual. Life does not end or even change dramatically when you've been diagnosed. And, as with so many other conditions, *how you live your life can have a positive impact on how your disease progresses.*

Yes, there is no cure, but if you are lucky and if you have a healthy lifestyle, long on a nutritious diet and appropriate exercise and short on bad habits that may help impair your immune system, you can play an active part in keeping the disease at bay and your situation stable.

Obesity

"If you eat it, and you don't burn it . . . then you sit on it."

Dr. Ben Saltman, professor of biology, UCLA

FAT IS A FEMINIST ISSUE, but it's also a health issue. Obesity means an excess of body fat, and obesity is one of those conditions that only worsens with age. Physically, obesity is caused by consuming more calories than your body can use. If you weigh 20 percent more than what is considered normal weight for your height and age, you are considered to be obese. If you are 100 pounds over your normal weight, this is considered morbid obesity. At least one out of five middle-aged women is overweight or obese.

Interestingly, there are some advantages to obesity. An overweight women produces more estrogen. Therefore, she may have fewer hot flashes during menopause and less risk of osteoporosis over the long term. She is also less likely to give birth to a premature baby or a baby whose birth weight is low. However, the disadvantages of obesity far outweigh the advantages. As you age, obesity is considered to be a risk factor in high blood pressure and diabetes. In general, obesity increases your risk of heart disease. While a woman's body has more fat in proportion to a man's, you don't want to use this biological truth to rationalize being extremely overweight. There is little to recommend obesity; that includes the fact that once you do gain weight it is usually extremely hard to lose that weight— a lot harder than it was to put it on. It also causes backache.

Recent studies have also shown that frank obesity (weighing at least 30 percent more than the desirable weight for your height and frame) may shorten a woman's life span. In particular, the sixteen-year study of over 100,000 female nurses has found that approximately 300,000 American deaths per year can be attributed to obesity. While this may seem alarming, it's important to note that other factors in addition to weight, such as a family history of heart disease or diabetes (two conditions in which obesity may be a cause), may also have been part of the profile of risk factors of any one of the participants in the study.

It's true that throughout this century women have battled the fashion prototype of the day. Even as many of us may long for the days of

271

Rubens's women, the reality is that we battle the image of the rail-thin woman. Just as diet and exercise should be approached with common sense, so should weight. Moderation is the key. You don't want to be too fat or too thin. If you are obese there are many reasons that make you eat too much, and no one should judge you for being overweight. You are who you are; you are not what you weigh. But by the same token, you should examine your reasons for being overweight and try to find a healthy and acceptable way to get help in changing your eating and exercise habits and losing weight—not because of anyone else's values but for your health's sake. Never let anyone dismiss you or treat you unfairly because you are obese. But, if good health is your goal, do not dismiss your problem either.

Heredity determines, at least partially, how many fat cells your body has and how large these fat cells are. Your genes may also contribute to what is called your body's set point—that weight at which your body feels most comfortable and needs a great deal of prodding to go below.

Several studies have shown that identical twins, separated at birth, have similar body types, including obesity, when reunited years later. It makes sense that the genes that determine everything else about us also play a role in obesity.

Obese people may also have slower metabolisms. That means they burn food for fuel at a slower rate than thin people, no matter what kind of food they are eating.

Repetitive dieting or yo-yo dieting, in which women lose weight only to gain it back and then lose it again, appears to slow down the metabolic rate altogether and eventually makes losing weight even more difficult.

In addition, it should be noted that as a culture we are overweight, and at lower socioeconomic levels we are even more overweight. In this country we drive everywhere instead of walk. We eat processed foods that are higher in fat at the expense of grains and roughage. It makes sense that a sedentary lifestyle and a high-fat diet are a dangerous combination . . . and yet these factors are totally within our power to change.

A diet low in fat that concentrates on more helpings of fruits and vegetables and whole grains, combined with a diligent exercise campaign, is the only safe and stable way to lose weight. If you need help with this endeavor (and most of us do), consult your physician. There are many reputable meal plans that may help you with the challenge of losing weight.

However, there are also a lot of fads that will be looking for your business as well. Here are some things to avoid:

- Do not go on a liquid diet without consulting your physician.
- Do not decide on a surgical procedure, such as gastric bypass surgery, also called stomach stapling (in which part of the stomach is stapled shut so that you feel full when you've eaten less), unless you have truly tried everything else—including moderate exercise with a low-fat diet and counseling over at least a year-long period. This surgery is usually reserved for morbidly obese people whose weight is causing other medical problems.
- Do not take diet drugs without consulting your physician.
- Do not think that liposuction is a treatment for weight loss. At the most, liposuction removes six to eight pounds and only works for women who want to rearrange their proportions.

Remember, a fad diet may help you shed some pounds, but it will not help you keep the weight off. So in a sense it can make your situation worse. The only weight you can keep off is weight that's been lost slowly on a healthy diet. You must develop the habit of a healthy diet and a healthy exercise plan if you want to keep weight off. Just as weight is put on our bodies over time, so goes weight loss.

The truth is that obesity is rarely treated successfully, and the only dependable factors in keeping weight off are a consistent exercise regime and a low-fat diet. If you do not exercise, you will not be successful in losing weight and keeping weight off over the long term. Sadly, there's another cultural stereotype at work here, and that is woman as dieter. We've all watched, read, or listened to countless ads appealing to our desire to be thin or thinner, and no matter how little we pay attention to such an inundation of propaganda, we have all considered or tried various diets at one time or another. However, we have probably never seen a diet ad that stressed the exercise part of the diet. We are being sold a bill of goods—that if you just cut this out, consume some tiny amount of calories, cut that out, stop chewing, and swallow this shake here and there, you will lose weight—as if a diet were a magic bullet. The truth is the only magic bullet is daily routine, making exercise and a low-fat diet a lifelong habit.

All this involves a lifestyle change—one that works for you. For me, it means lots of water, moderate exercise, and constant attempts to eat more fruits and vegetables. Yes, I still have pizza every now and then, and I love a cold beer. Modifying your eating habits isn't meant to be an austerity program, but a healthy change that you can live with.

Osteoporosis

"Life is a struggle . . . against hydrogen ions."

H. L. Mencken

As WE AGE, our bones thin. A woman's bones reach their peak density at the age of thirty-five and lose density from then on. Osteoporosis is one of the most common and most preventable problems for the elderly, especially women. It affects an estimated 20 to 25 million Americans. Often it is called the "silent disease" because there are no early warning signs or symptoms.

The bones of the body are made of hard, rigid tissue with a liquid marrow center. Our muscles attach to our bones, and our organs are located within the skeletal structure the bones make up. Bones are built mainly of proteins, sugars, and minerals. And bones are alive. The marrow produces blood cells and stores those all-important minerals calcium and phosphate.

Like most of the tissues of the body, the bones are constantly regenerating themselves. This never-ending process is called remodeling. It is remodeling that keeps the bones strong and enables the body to keep the level of calcium in the blood constant—a necessity for blood clotting and the continuous beating of the heart.

As we grow older, new bone is formed more slowly. In the late thirties bones start to lose calcium at a greater rate than can be replaced. Additionally, our body's ability to absorb calcium from the food we eat is diminished as we age—this is another reason for the loss of bone density.

So, alas, the skeleton, built of these very active bones, may become brittle in the golden years. The bones thin and sometimes begin to lose their strength. When this happens, fractures are more common and recovery may be slower. Fractures may reoccur even after healing has taken place.

Osteoporosis is generally considered to be the result of an acceleration of the normal aging process. Varying degrees of osteoporosis are present in the bones of one out of every four women over the age of forty-five and nine out of every ten women over seventy-five.

Exercise and Osteoporosis

Even if you have been diagnosed with osteoporosis, you are *not* powerless. You can participate in your own treatment and improve your situation. Weight-bearing exercise—for example, walking, using a StairMaster, jumping rope, or jogging slowly—is the best treatment for osteoporosis. A reasonable and consistent exercise routine is a major component of the battle to keep osteoporosis at bay. Although non-weight-bearing activities like swimming are great exercise, they are less effective in fighting osteoporosis than a brisk walk. Your bones need to be resisting gravity for exercise to help in the prevention of bone loss.

Don't laugh, but if you want to avoid a broken hip in the future, start pumping the iron now. Recent information from the Human Nutrition Research Center on Aging at Tufts University in Boston published in the *Journal of the American Medical Association* shows that postmenopausal women who worked intensively on exercise machines twice weekly for a year built up their bones, increased the size and strength of their muscles, improved their balance, and reduced their risk of spine and hip fractures. So it makes sense that if you make your muscles stronger—and your muscles attach to bone—then your bones will get stronger too.

Fractures caused by osteoporosis strike 1.5 million Americans every year. Most of these are women. And a broken hip or leg is only the first part of the problem. When elderly people are hospitalized and immobilized, they can start a slow spiral downhill, with pneumonia and death being the outcome.

Toning, stretching, and strength building should be a part of your exercise program as you age, since keeping your joints healthy and staying limber are both important in defending yourself against the wear and tear of aging on the bones, joints, and muscles. I love free weights. Not only do they make muscles fit, but since they also strengthen bones, posture improves too. The weights don't have to be heavy and you don't have to worry about adding bulk to your frame. For most women the best ones to use are two, five, seven, and ten pounds. There is ample evidence that if you lift weights, no matter what your age, your muscles will get stronger, which will help ward off osteoporosis.

Hard Bones and Calcium

A calcium supplement cannot increase bone density once bone mass has been lost. However, this does not mean a woman should dispense with a supplement. On the contrary, recent studies have found that Americans in general do not get enough calcium. Calcium supplements help women get enough calcium to hold their own against further bone density loss. If you take no other daily supplement, you should take calcium, aiming for 1500 mg per day of elemental calcium, which is usually available in combination. Good combinations that will help you get the most out of your calcium supplement are calcium carbonate and calcium citrate. The fact that calcium supplements help in the battle against osteoporosis is indisputable. Many postmenopausal women should consider taking estrogen to ensure the absorption of calcium—but this is an individual decision that should be discussed with your doctor.

Coffee and Calcium Loss

Yes, it is true that coffee helps strip the body of calcium, but recent studies have found that one glass of skim milk per day counteracts the deleterious effects of caffeine on calcium absorption. Why not mix hot skim milk with coffee to create your own healthy café au lait?

Parkinson's Disease

Parkinson's disease involves the degeneration of nerve cells in that part of the brain responsible for the control of muscle movement. These nerve cells produce dopamine, a chemical that is important in the transmission of signals from cell to cell within the brain. As the levels of dopamine fall, the disease progresses. Although much research has been done on Parkinson's, there is no cure and the cause is still unknown.

Early in the disease, symptoms may not be readily apparent. You may notice a dragging of one foot while walking or stiffness in a limb. Symptoms include shaking at rest, a masking of facial expressions, stiffness, problems in balancing, a shuffling gait, a low-pitched or monotonal voice, and difficulty in speech, chewing, and swallowing. Parkinson's disease may affect one side of the body or both sides. It may affect balance mildly or cause severe instability. Fully developed Parkinson's may require that a person be confined to a chair or bed. More than 1 million Americans suffer from Parkinson's disease, which usually affects people in the middle or later years.

If you develop a tremor, don't assume you have Parkinson's. It may be indicative of another disorder, such as a stroke or brain tumor. A tremor may also indicate essential tremor, the most common form of tremor and not a serious condition. Blood tests, a CT scan, or an MRI may be used to confirm a diagnosis.

While Parkinson's disease is a serious condition, remaining in good general health and exercising regularly can help slow the progress of the disease. Rest periods during the day will also help alleviate the tremor, which may be aggravated by stress and exhaustion. A medication called levodopa (L-Dopa) is usually used to increase levels of dopamine in the brain and thus improve movement and balance. Physical therapy is also helpful in alleviating stiffness and slowing the loss of physical mobility. Although there is no cure yet for Parkinson's, treatment with L-Dopa works well. This is another situation in which your own self-monitoring and careful attention to diet, exercise, and your body's need for rest can significantly improve your quality of life and slow the progress of the disease. Once again, early detection is key in Parkinson's, since there are many new drugs that can be used to slow the progress of the disease.

Raynaud's Disease

"I've come to accept Raynaud's disease—but it hasn't been easy. I really have to be careful during the Pittsburgh winters and make sure I park close to my office building. I rarely go out in the winter if I don't have to."

Hollie Davidson (age 50)

IF YOU SUFFER from Raynaud's disease, your fingers and toes will often turn white upon exposure to cold. There is stinging pain, and the skin often turns blue or red before recovering. It is normal for blood vessels in the extremities to narrow upon exposure to the cold, but in

Raynaud's disease, this response becomes exaggerated. The condition results from changes in the circulation in the hands and feet, and it is four or five times more common among women than among men. The first episode usually occurs before the age of forty.

For most, Raynaud's disease is more of a nuisance than a disability. The best way to avoid the aggravation of this malady is to dress intelligently and protect the entire body—including head, hands, and feet—from the cold.

Seizure Disorders

You can have a seizure and not have a true seizure disorder. I know: I had a seizure a few years ago in my doctor's office. The story is comical now, but at the time threw me for a loop.

I was sitting on my gynecologist's exam table after having a pelvic exam. As we discussed the treatment options about an ovarian cyst that was being problematic, I felt myself getting faint. I knew this was silly and decided to fight it. (An intelligent person would have just put her head down. But . . . no! I decided I could will this away.)

As the blood drained out of my head and away from my brain, I fainted. Normal enough. But when my brain didn't get the circulation it needed and the oxygen dropped, I also had a grand mal seizure. I was so out of it I don't really remember much. But my doctor does! Fortunately, it hasn't happened since.

Seizures may have any number of causes and a single seizure need not mean that you have a seizure disorder. Repeated seizures are indicative of a seizure disorder and fall into two main categories: grand mal seizures and petit mal seizures. Petit mal seizures occur mainly in children and rarely begin after the age of twenty. In the past, seizure disorders were referred to as epilepsy, a word that tends to stigmatize rather than inform. Now, the preferred diagnosis is seizure disorder.

Grand mal seizures involve loss of consciousness and convulsions. Once consciousness is lost, the muscles are rigid for about twenty seconds and then a period of violent and rhythmic convulsions occurs. This lasts for between one and two minutes and is followed by a short period of sleep before consciousness is regained. A person who has such a seizure has no memory of the seizure. Such a seizure is caused by abnormal electrical activity in the brain. These seizures tend to be random, but some women with seizure disorders find that seizures may be triggered by menstruation. Less often, the seizure may be caused by a stimulus such as light or sound. Medication is effective in controlling or reducing seizures in more than 75 percent of cases.

Sinus Problems

I wish I had a dime for every older women whom I have seen in my office with the complaint of a sinus infection or postnasal drip. Occasionally, this diagnosis turns out to be true. But more times than not, what is perceived as an infection is just thick secretions that linger in the back of the nose and throat. The nose, sinuses, and throat are like any other mucosal surface in the body. They dry as our estrogen levels drop and they are very sensitive to dehydration. So when you don't drink enough water, this is one of the first places you'll notice it. Patients are astounded when I assure them that there is no infection or tumor. I then ask them to be religious about drinking at least eight glasses of water a day. In fact, I tell them that they will be urinating like a racehorse but that this simple therapy will work. This is one case that if you just give mother nature a hand, she can do the rest.

Stroke

> *"I was talking with my grandmother when she started slurring a couple of words and then jumbled up her sentences. It was nothing more than that. But I recognized the significance."*
>
> Tanya Emerson (age 34)

THE BRAIN USES 20 percent of the heart's output of blood and about the same amount of the blood's supply of oxygen and glucose. If the blood flow to the brain is disturbed for even a few seconds, dramatic consequences occur in the functioning of the brain.

A stroke is a lay term for a cerebrovascular accident (CVA)—an interruption of the blood flow to the brain. Just as such an interruption in the heart causes a heart attack, here it causes a stroke. The interruption can happen in one of two ways: a blood vessel can become blocked, depriving an area of the brain of blood, or a blood vessel can rupture and flood an area of the brain with blood. Stroke, the third leading cause of death for women in the United States, is a catchall name for the types of disorders that occur when this blood flow is interrupted; it also includes situations in which the flow of blood to the brain is just slowed, causing a transient ischemic attack (TIA).

A cerebrovascular accident can also refer to blood clots that put pressure on parts of the brain. Whether these clots lie on or under the dura mater (the thick, canvaslike layer of tissue that surrounds the brain) makes a difference in nomenclature and symptoms. An *extradural hematoma* lies between the skull and the dura. A *subdural hematoma* lies between the brain and the dura. These clots usually result from a fall or severe bump on the head. In an older person, they may be hard to diagnose because the symptoms may be gradual. An elderly person who is increasingly forgetful, confused, or drowsy should be checked with a CT scan or an MRI for this abnormal collection of blood under the skull. A *subdural hemorrhage* is an accumulation of blood between the dura and the brain with a subsequent compression of brain tissue. Classic symptoms include headache, seizures, drowsiness, or confusion after a head injury (even something as minor as a bump on the head). An *extradural hemorrhage* is a collection of blood between the skull and the dura. The symptoms may be the same as those for a subdural. In addition, look for nausea, vomiting, dizziness, or an enlarged pupil. In most cases, the treatment is surgical removal of the clot.

An *aneurysm* is a ballooning of the wall of the blood vessel due to a weak spot in the muscle layer in the blood vessel. The weakness may allow blood to leak from the vessel gradually or it can blow dramatically and cause sudden death. The congenital condition *arterial-venous malformation* (AVM) is an abnormal connection between a high-pressure system in the arteries and a low-pressure vein. These malformations can also bleed, resulting in a stroke.

A stroke that injures a part of the brain will produce symptoms that reflect the area of the brain where the damage occurs. Symptoms can include sudden headache, numbness of the face, blurred vision, severe vertigo, the inability to speak or recognize words, or loss of consciousness. A stroke may also affect the motor system, causing weakness or paralysis in an arm or leg. The symptoms may occur over minutes or hours. No matter what the time frame, this is considered a medical emergency and a person should be taken to the local emergency room immediately.

If a serious stroke has occurred, intensive care will be required, including life-support mechanisms. The severity of a stroke depends on the extent of the bleeding and the location of the injury. It also depends on whether other areas of the brain can carry on the functions of the damaged area. The recovery process varies in relation to the seriousness of the stroke. Recovery, which can be partial or complete, may take up to a year or more and involve physical therapy. If little neurological damage occurs, less care will be required and recovery will be a more rapid, less complicated process.

A stroke is serious, but depending upon how quickly help is obtained and blood and oxygen supplies restored to normal, full recovery is possible. Again, recovery depends on the location and the extent of the damage. Many strokes result from preexisting conditions such as high blood pressure, atherosclerosis, and other forms of heart disease.

While neurological disorders are often beyond a patient's control, stroke is a disease where atherosclerosis and high blood pressure are very accurate warning signs, which should be heeded and controlled. In many instances, these problems can be altered ahead of time by dietary changes, not smoking, moderate exercise, and medication. If you do have high blood pressure, an elevated cholesterol level, or another form of heart disease, you should be monitored closely by your physician and take measures to control these maladies. Know your family history: if other family members have suffered from vascular problems, you may be at risk.

Transient Ischemic Attack

I remember having a conversation with my maternal grandfather when I was little. He worked on the Union-Pacific Railroad as a young man and still remembered train schedules down to the minute. I would listen intently as he told stories of the hoboes who would hitch rides across the Missouri plains. One day, as I sat captivated, I noticed that his words suddenly didn't make sense. Some were slurred or dropped altogether and he seemed to lose his spot in the story. I remember being scared and confused. But no sooner had I noticed something wrong than he was back on track, picking up where he left off. This was a classic transient ischemic attack (TIA).

The symptoms of TIA are similar to those of stroke, with one very important distinction: they are transient, gone within twenty-four hours, and there are no lasting sequelae. TIA is most often a result of atherosclerosis, but it also may occur if you have high blood pressure, if you smoke, or if you have diabetes. The risk of TIA increases with age. TIA should be considered as a warning sign that a stroke may follow. If you have suffered a transient ischemic attack, you should discuss with your doctor ways to minimize the possibility of a future stroke.

The newest diagnostic technique to tell a patient with TIA that a stroke is looming is color ultrasound of the carotid arteries and the arteries in the brain. This is a noninvasive technique that can zero in on an artery that is blocked or appears weak. If it is blocked, it can be treated with medicine or surgery. If the arteries look clear, your doctor may recommend aspirin to keep the blood from clotting too readily.

Varicose Veins

Varicose veins *are* unsightly, but they can also be painful and they are not always harmless. Varicose veins are enlarged veins, usually in the legs and ankles. Easily seen beneath the skin and appearing swollen and twisted, they tend to become increasingly prominent over time. Women are almost twice as likely to have varicose veins as men, and varicose veins affect about one in ten Americans. That women are so much more prone to the condition is often attributed to pregnancy, though varicose veins also run in families.

A varicosity occurs when the valves in a vein begin to malfunction. Usually, valves help propel blood to the heart. If a valve is stretched or damaged as the result of pregnancy, a congenital condition, obesity, phlebitis, or some other cause, the valve can no longer close properly and blood begins to pool in the vein. This causes the vein to enlarge and become varicose.

Because varicose veins are usually visible to the eye, a diagnosis is easy. Superficial or obvious varicose veins are generally dark blue, twisted, and quite dilated. You may experience an aching or swelling in your legs if deeper veins are affected. Sometimes skin ulcers form, usually at the ankle. These are the result of the increased pressure of the blood within the vein, which causes a "waterlogging" of the surrounding tissues.

Self-help is essential in the treatment of varicose veins. You want to avoid being in one position—sitting or standing still—for a long period of time, so try to move around. Whenever possible, elevate your legs, at least twelve inches above the level of your heart—this is particularly helpful at the end of the day. Support stockings help to relieve the pressure on the damaged veins and give added support. Put your stockings on first thing in the morning, before you even get out of bed. While you want to feel noticeable pressure in the lower portions of your legs, they should not be tight at the calf or groin. A reasonable and consistent exercise routine that includes walking is also recommended.

Surgery is often for cosmetic reasons, but also can be necessary in certain extreme cases. The results of stripping or removal of the problem vein can be quite good. In one study, 85 percent of patients who had had the surgery were doing well ten years later.

My parents have already told me that the golden years are not for sissies, and from my work with patients, I would add that the golden years are also not for the uninformed. Tough as it is to hear what symptoms and future problems are involved with any long-term disease or chronic condition, the more you know, the more control you have over your life and course of treatment.

I don't by any means want to suggest that attitude is everything. The best people in the world with the most positive, healthiest attitudes may suddenly be stricken by a life-threatening disease that saps their strength. Bad things can happen to good people too. It's a roll of the dice of fate. But by the same token, the more you know, the more prepared you are, and the better your underlying health—the better your chances of surviving any medical challenges that will be thrown your way.

PART 6

AGING AND THE BODY

"I can't tell you I'm thrilled with the aging process—but it beats the hell out of the alternative."

Maggie Grieschel (age 84)

I N ORDER TO practice informed self-care, you need to know what to look for and where to look. The parts of the body that are most sensitive to the aging process are the digestive tract, your skin and hair, your bones and joints, and your cardiovascular system. All of these parts of the body manifest aging through subtle but distinct changes.

As you age, your entire digestive system slows down, as does the swallowing motion of the esophagus. These changes may be slight, but combined with the rigors of the digestive process, they may take their toll. For example, your body becomes less efficient in absorbing the nutrients it needs, so if you do not already take a vitamin supplement, you may want to add one to your daily health regimen. Because this is an area of the body you will want to monitor closely, you should pay particular attention to changes in bowel habits, such as periodic constipation or diarrhea, and consult your doctor about such changes. Early diagnosis—the best way to ensure a positive outcome in battling any disease—depends on you.

Your hair and skin record the aging process before your own eyes. Your skin becomes slightly thinner and less elastic as time goes on. Some wrinkles and a certain amount of drooping or sagging are inevitable. The skin also becomes drier. (If you have been prone to acne all your life, this is a blessing in disguise.) If you don't use a moisturizer, you should start using one; and if you already do, you may want to change to one that is richer in natural oils. The two most important things regarding skin care are:

1. Protect it against the sun.
2. Watch for any changes in existing moles and any new growths on the skin.

If you notice any changes or suspicious marks, you should see your doctor.

Your hair also changes as you age. By the age of fifty, 50 percent of people have gray hair. Your hair also becomes thinner and drier as you age. You should vary the shampoo you use every now and then, and use products suitable for drier hair. Having your hair trimmed regularly will also help keep it healthy. If gray hair seems dull rather than distinguished to you, coloring your hair is a safe, if time-consuming option.

As mentioned earlier, the bones of women are more susceptible to osteoporosis after menopause. All women over thirty-five should take a calcium supplement. If you have young daughters, you should encourage them to take a supplement as well, while they still have a chance to build bone mass.

Also as you age, your joints begin to stiffen. In fact, osteoarthritis is often referred to as a disease of use. It usually begins in the larger joints—the hips, knees, and spine—that bear your weight. In the case of osteoporosis and arthritis, if you are overweight, you should try to lose weight. And weight-bearing exercise will help strengthen the bones and muscles in general. The sooner you incorporate a sensible exercise routine and a healthy diet, including calcium, in your life, the fewer age-related changes and problems you will have.

Your heart is the muscle of life, and as time goes on it becomes less elastic and less efficient, as do your blood vessels. It is perhaps in caring for your heart that you may have the most positive effect on your health later in life. Although in the world of medicine the results of all studies may be debated, there is no debate regarding the beneficial effects of diet and exercise. There is much to be said for the need for more studies that seek to understand the hearts of women. But what we do know is that a healthy, low-fat diet and moderate but consistent exercise can help the health of your heart.

We are, as a culture, almost morbidly conscious of death because of our focus on cancer and AIDS, and yet heart disease kills more women and men than these other diseases combined. In a world where control often seems elusive at best, we would do well to concentrate on that area of our health care where we can make a significant difference—the heart. A healthy heart improves your chances for a healthy life. Have your blood pressure and cholesterol level checked regularly. Lower your fat intake and raise your activity level.

Let's admit it—the prospect of aging meets with some resistance in all of us. Few of us are pleased with the changes in our body as we begin to notice them. But, instead of being disheartened by the signs of aging, you may want to think of them as street signs and warning signs on the map of life and remind yourself that the most important thing is to heed the directions and take the right turns to ensure your good health.

THE SKIN

"How come I never really paid attention to my skin when
I was in my twenties? I wish I had some of that time
back."

Kathryn Schneider (age 41)

I REMEMBER ONE DAY last year when I was flying across the country and went to the bathroom. As I was washing my hands, I looked in the mirror and saw a middle-aged woman staring back at me. It wasn't the first time I saw the blush of youth gone. But this time it was a shock. My face looked dry and tired and I felt like I was looking at someone who looked ten years older than I felt. That was it! I was determined not to let this opportunity slip away from me. It was time to take better care of my skin—so I have.

The Sun and the Aging Process

"When I was in college I used to cut classes in the late
spring so I could start working on my summer tan. In
those days we smeared our bodies with baby oil and glis-
tened in the noonday sun. Today the tan is gone—but I
have the wrinkles as a reminder."

Anne Bachman (age 42)

I WAS GOING THROUGH family snapshots the other day and found one from my days in Little Rock, when I would ride my horse five to six times a week. I would spend every Saturday and Sunday outside—no hat, no sun protection. And the picture showed it. I honestly looked ten years older then than I do now. And it was all due to the sun. I knew about all the risks. But I also loved the look of a tanned face. My skin has recovered to some extent—but I have also paid the price for those days. That's the funny thing about the sun. It always leaves a calling card and is not very forgiving. I took my skin for granted and now, in my forties, work to curb age's effects as much as possible.

289

The one thing I didn't do was smoke. I grew up in a nonsmoking doctor's family and always knew cigarettes were bad for me. Smoking is one of the worst things you can do to your skin. I also didn't drink eight glasses of water a day—but I do now.

As I got older, I not only got wiser, I also became more careful. When I started working in television, I became even more careful. Now I cleanse my face twice a day and use a moisturizer morning and night with a sunscreen with a sun protection factor (SPF) of 15. Besides my eight glasses of water a day, I get facials, which I regard as a real treat. Between the wear and tear of my schedule, the grit and grime of city life, and the amount of air travel I log, I've come to see my facials as more of a necessity than a luxury, not only for my skin's sake but also for my mental health.

A suntan has been fashionable ever since Coco Chanel shocked sophisticated circles, shed her creamy, pale complexion, and led thousands into the sun-worshiping fad. One of Chanel's legacies is that we have yet to give up our love of the sun and the golden effects of tanning. While I knew about her role in creating one of America's favorite pastimes I also grew up with a mother who never baked her skin. She would sit under a tree while we were at the pool or walk on the beach with her face covered by a wide-brimmed hat. In my youth I never understood the wisdom of that. Today she is living proof that by simply taking care of yourself you don't have to look or feel your age. Her face is radiant—no special potions or plastic surgery. Just the intelligence to save her skin from the sun.

We all know we probably got too much sun as kids, and some of us still indulge in sun worshiping even after having been inundated with the facts about sun damage. In addition to the damage the sun does cause, recent studies have shown that the improved quality of sunscreen products is both a blessing and a curse. Ironically, these products may be contributing to the rising rate of melanoma because they allow people, especially fair-skinned people, to stay out in the sun for longer periods of time without burning. In fact, studies show that men who use sunscreen actually have a higher risk of melanoma. The bottom line is stay out of the sun. If you go in the sun, wear protective clothing and a hat in addition to using a strong sun screen.

The UV (ultraviolet radiation) index is now going to be part of many local weather forecasts, which will give you an opportunity to take extra precautions against overexposure to the sun when the index is high.

The index is based on satellite measurements and reports the UV strength at various locations nationwide. The measurements are taken at high noon. Here's a list of exposure level and the corresponding index value.*

Exposure Level	Index Value
Minimal	0–2
Low	3–4
Moderate	5–6
High	7–10
Very high	Over 10

A Skin Story

Your skin is the largest organ of your body, and as such it is a perfect reflection of the aging process. In addition, the muscles in your face are about the only ones attached to the skin. Your facial muscles allow you to display thousands of facial expressions, and every single one registers on your skin.

Inevitably, time writes its story on your skin. As you begin to grow older, the fatty layer beneath the skin that gives your face contour begins to grow thinner. Your skin also produces less collagen, the spongy protein that gives the skin its resilience, as you age. What collagen your skin does produce in later years begins to become more inflexible. In addition, the fibers in your skin called elastin begin to weaken, like old rubber bands used once too often, and they do not snap back after a smile or a grimace as quickly as they used to. In short, the skin on your face begins to fit more loosely on the bones and to carry the evidence of your facial expressions in wrinkles that refuse to fade.

No one with any common sense expects or wants to look like a twenty-year-old at fifty, but we all want to look good at any age. And we certainly don't want to look older than we are! Your twenties and thirties are the time to begin to use sunscreen all year-round and to use

*Taken from the *UC Berkeley Wellness Letter*, August 1994.

a moisturizer if you don't already. Tell everyone you know—daughters, sisters, friends—to use sunscreen and start yourself.

You may also want to consider using an exfoliant. Exfoliants get rid of dead skin cells on the surface of your skin, which in turn stimulates the cells underneath to divide more rapidly. This process of irritation draws more fluid to the area, which makes the skin temporarily appear to be smoother and more even in tone. You may also want to talk to your doctor about using Retin-A, which is particularly effective in improving sun-damaged skin. Retin-A speeds the cycle of skin cell production. It also increases the collagen in your skin and can turn precancerous cells back to normal. But Retin-A also weakens your skin's outer layer, the one that protects against sunburn, so you must be conscientious about using your strongest sunscreen and avoiding the sun as much as possible. Retin-A is also useful in removing age spots. Age spots also may be removed with liquid nitrogen or prescription creams that contain hydroquinone, which can bleach those age spots away.

Over-the-counter alternatives to Retin-A are the hydroxy acid preparations. These work as mild exfoliants and most are safe. However, you must follow the directions carefully and not overuse them. If you have sensitive skin, try them cautiously or check with your doctor.

There are many ways, short of surgery, to improve the appearance of your skin. But the most important thing you can do for your skin is to protect it from the sun. As we age our skin gets thinner and drier. Be sure to drink your water and use a good moisturizer. Moisturizers not only hold moisture in the skin but plump up lines and wrinkles and give the skin a smoother appearance.

Self-Examination of the Skin

As you age, you may notice new skin tabs, blotchy areas, and other changes. Most of these changes are not indicative of dangerous conditions. But you should also make note of any moles or freckles that seem to be changing. The easiest way to remember the warning signs of a skin cancer is this acronym:

A—Asymmetry   C—Color

B—Bleeding   D—Diameter

SUN TIPS

- Never stay in the sun for long periods of time.
- Avoid exposure when the sun is most intense, between the hours of 10:00 A.M. and 2:00 P.M.
- Always use a sunscreen, even if you will only be in the sun for a matter of minutes. (In addition, I recommend using a moisturizer with an SPF of 15 every day.)
- Choose a waterproof sunscreen with a SPF of 15 or more. Keep reapplying it throughout the day, especially if you are in and out of the water.
- Choose a sunscreen that protects against UVA and UVB radiation.
- Apply sunscreen a half hour before going into the sun and after swimming.
- Protect your lips as well as your skin. Use an opaque sunblock containing zinc oxide, which protects against UVA and UVB radiation.
- Keep babies in the shade and cover their heads with a cool hat or bandana.
- Never, ever, use a sunlamp or frequent a tanning parlor.
- Use the same strength sunblock during the winter that you use in the summer—even on overcast days.

See page 122 for the ABCD method of staying on the alert for dangerous changes to your skin.

Adult Acne

While many people suffer from acne only as teens and in their early adult years, a significant number of people are plagued by their sebaceous glands all their lives. Scientific studies in the past fifteen years have shown that it is not diet but heredity that determines the predilection for this skin condition.

Acne is caused by plugged hair follicles. Because it causes highly visible pimples, cysts, whiteheads, and blackheads, it is easy to diagnose. The oral medication Accutane is helpful in alleviating acne, but should not be taken if you are pregnant or if you are trying to conceive. Also taken orally, tetracycline is helpful in the treatment of acne, but once again should not be taken if you are pregnant or could become so because you are not using birth control. If you have chronic acne, you should consult your physician because it is a condition that can easily be helped.

Psoriasis

Psoriasis is a common skin condition characterized by reddened, cracking patches of skin that itch and may bleed periodically. These patches occur most commonly on the elbows, knees, scalp, or torso. Psoriasis is caused by a genetic predisposition that involves the acceleration of the life cycle of skin cells. The normal cycle of skin cell production is approximately a month, but in people with psoriasis, the process of cell production is accelerated and takes only three or four days. Flare-ups may occur after cuts, burns, or insect bites. They may also be caused by a viral or bacterial infection, by certain medications, or by drinking too much alcohol.

Psoriasis may be mild or severe and sometimes chronic. Three million Americans have psoriasis and approximately 100,000 of these cases are severe. It is common in fair-skinned people; first episodes usually occurs between the ages of fifteen and thirty-five. Coal-tar soaps, ointments, and shampoos may be used to relieve symptoms. In severe cases an anticancer drug called methotrexate may be taken orally to slow the production of skin cells.

SKIN TYPES

Skin may be oily, dry, normal, balanced, or combination skin. In oily skin the sebaceous glands, which produce the oil, are overactive. Oily skin is more susceptible to acne, but less susceptible to wrinkling. Dry skin is caused by underactive sebaceous glands and the environment. And regardless of your skin type, skin will become drier with age. Although there is little chance of acne with dry skin, wrinkling is common. Balanced skin has few problems, but it too will become drier with age. Combination skin, which has oily patches and dry patches, must be cared for differently. Use a moisturizer for the dry areas and an additional cleanser for oily patches.

If you do not know what type of skin you have, you should discuss your skin type with your doctor or a cosmetician and determine the cleaning regimen and soaps and skin products for your kind of skin.

When you wash your face, never use hot water and use a mild soap or skin cleanser appropriate for your skin type. If you have dry skin, apply a bath oil to damp skin after bathing.

Moles and Skin Tabs—What to Ignore, What to Pay Attention To

"I thought I knew my skin. But now that I've turned forty, I keep finding new things all the time—and none of them are very attractive!"

Brenda Comstock (age 41)

WITH EXPOSURE TO sun and weather and the rigors of pregnancy, a woman's skin begins to show the inevitable signs of aging. You may notice that you have more freckles or moles as time goes on. You may also notice tiny skin tabs at your neck or on another part of the body. Most of these changes are not dangerous. Nonetheless, it is important to examine your skin frequently so that you are aware of any significant changes in moles or other growths— changes that might indicate a more serious problem.

Almost everyone has moles, which are benign, pigmented skin lesions. They may contain hairs and are usually mixed brown and black in color. Sometimes they become wrinkled and even fall off in old age. Mole are generally harmless, but they may become cancerous and should always be monitored. If a mole becomes itchy, inflamed, changes color or size, or bleeds, you should see your physician immediately.

Skin tabs are tiny tabs of skin that protrude from the body and are harmless in most cases. They develop with age and sometimes fall off on their own. If a skin tab becomes itchy or red and irritated, you should consult your doctor, who will probably remove it in a simple procedure.

What is most important when it comes to skin care is that, once again, you have more control than you think. While you don't want to become paranoid, you do want to monitor any moles and skin irregularities and inform your doctor of any changes, so that early diagnosis and treatment are possible.

Liver or Age Spots

The spots that occur on the face, arms, and hands are more appropriately called sun spots, since they are usually caused by exposure to the sun over the years and are generally not dangerous. Sometimes, however, liver spots occur from other, unknown causes. Generally they begin to occur after the age of fifty-five. To help avoid liver spots in the future and maintain the health of your skin in general, wear a good moisturizer with an SPF of 15 and avoid prolonged sun exposure.

ELECTIVE OR COSMETIC SURGERY AND THE "PRICE" YOU PAY

"If I had known how much it would hurt, I would have thought twice."

Samantha David (age 43)

NO MATTER HOW you slice it (no pun intended), women get a raw deal from society as we age. The older man is described as "distinguished," while the older woman is left out in the cold.

Women over forty are changing all that just by being so natural. There are beautiful examples everywhere we look—from movies and television to business and finance to sports and even to motherhood. They are role models who have taken care of themselves and prove it by the way they look and live. Women like Lauren Hutton, Jaclyn Smith, Hillary Clinton, Mary Steenburgen. Cybill Shepherd launched a new sitcom and bragged that she was over forty. Fifty can look like forty or even thirty, without any artificial aids or cosmetic doctoring. The sky may not be the limit, but more and more how well we age is up to us, and there's an open season on looking good at any age.

Face-lifts, Chin Tucks, and Lid Lifts

"I knew I wanted a face-lift. I gave it a lot of thought
and did my homework to find a good surgeon. I didn't
expect it to change my life—but in some ways it did. I
love how I look and feel more confident than ever."

Jennifer Cranson (age 44)

To GET A FACE-LIFT or not to get a face-lift. It's not the only question, or the most important question, but it is certainly one of the most often asked questions by women as they grow older. A friend of mine once said, "Everything shows on your face," and the older I get, the more I believe she is right. I'd like to think the joy shows as much as the hardships, but there's no denying a wrinkle's a wrinkle, whether you got it laughing or crying. There is no right way or wrong way to look at yourself in the mirror. How you look at your wrinkles is up to you. Some women barely notice their wrinkles. Other women, whose self-esteem may be directly tied to their physical beauty, have great difficulty accepting their wrinkles. Women usually begin to have concerns about starting to look older in their mid- to late thirties, concerns that lead many to consider plastic surgery.

The word "plastic" comes from the Greek *plastikos*, which means "that which may be molded." Obviously, plastic itself has little to do with the advanced synthetic materials used in plastic surgery today. Plastic or reconstructive surgery is a surgical specialty devoted to improving the physical appearance or function of a specific body part. Reconstructive surgery is often necessary after injury or disease, but the majority of women (and now men too!) seek out plastic surgery for cosmetic reasons. In fact, every year more than half a million people in the United States have some form of plastic surgery, and the number is growing. The number one area on which plastic surgeons are asked to work is—what else?—the face. After all, the face is the first part of us that people see, the part that usually makes the first impression. It makes perfect sense that when we are thinking of improving ourselves, we often think of putting our best face forward.

The most common facial surgeries are the rhytidectomy or face-lift, and the blepharoplasty or lid lift. A chin tuck is usually incorporated into the face-lift. You should be forewarned that many surgeons expect payment in advance. In most cases, insurance does not cover cosmetic surgery.

The Rhytidectomy

Besides the abuses from the sun, cigarettes, and dehydration, gravity plays a role in how our skin ages. When you look at someone and the skin is sagging and you can see jowls, it's all a matter of gravity. The jowls are caused by pockets of fat that sit over your cheek when you are young. But with aging, the fat moves south, giving the face that saggy, older look. A face-lift removes excess or saggy skin from the face and neck and removes or relocates those fatty areas.

There are many variations when it comes to the procedure itself. The standard lift involves an incision that begins at the hairline above the ear and extends down into the crease in front of the ear. It continues around and behind the ear and proceeds back into the hairline, where excess skin is excised. Liposuction is used many times to remove fatty deposits along the jaw and under the chin and a separate ¼-inch-long incision may be made for this under the chin. Sometimes a brow lift is performed along with the face-lift. This raises and tightens the skin of the forehead. In this case a separate incision is made just behind the hairline of the brow.

A face-lift cannot make you look twenty years younger or change your basic looks. If you smoke, a face-lift cannot repair or conceal the skin damage that smoking causes. If you continue to smoke after a face-lift, the improvements you notice after surgery will disappear more quickly and your doctor may warn you that your result may not be as good as that of a nonsmoker. What a face-lift can do is make you look "good" for your age and in so doing have a positive effect on your self-esteem. The benefits of a face-lift last for about ten years if you maintain good health habits, including eating a healthy diet, drinking plenty of water, and not smoking.

Blepharoplasty

Your age and habits may leave the most evidence on the skin around your eyes. One day you may notice creases and bags around your eyes and not like it at all. Others find such changes to be signs of character and wisdom. In addition, bags and pouches under and around the eyes can take a physical as well as a cosmetic toll on your looks: excess skin and fallen pockets of subcutaneous fat may impair peripheral vision and cause chronic eye discomfort. (If this is the case for you and you want surgery, you will probably be able to get your insurance carrier to cover the cost, since here there is a physical need.)

There are a variety of options when it comes to eyelid and eyebrow surgery. The principle in each case, however, is the same—excess skin and soft tissue are surgically removed and the remaining tissues are then sewn back together, layer by layer.

Most eyelid surgery is done on an outpatient basis. A local anesthetic is used and the time spent in surgery may range from about 1¼ hours for two lids to 3 or more hours if all four lids are done. When the sedation has worn off, you will be able to go home. Once home you may be instructed to use ice packs for up to 72 hours. This early recovery period may be a little unsightly, but it is rarely painful. Your bruises will fade in one to two weeks and disappear in three weeks. You'll want to be extracautious about protecting your eyes from the sun during this recovery period. It's inevitable that some nerves are disrupted by the surgery, which may cause your eyelids to feel numb. Sensation will usually return in about six to eight weeks.

While it may be called "elective" surgery, it's still surgery, and as with any surgery there can be complications. The most serious complications of eyelid surgery involve bleeding. Bleeding can increase the amount of bruising and may interfere with healing enough that excess scarring can result. Very rarely, blood can pool behind the eye and permanently affect the vision. It is extremely important to monitor any changes in your vision in the first 48 hours after surgery, and also to discuss all possible complications with your doctor *before* deciding to have elective surgery.

One other note: lid surgery may keep your eyes open, but you'll need to have your metaphorical eyes open beforehand, because a blepharoplasty will not remove crow's-feet, laugh lines, or deep wrinkles. It also will not correct any overall asymmetry of your face. You should discuss what you can realistically expect from the surgery with your doctor before going ahead, and you should also consider getting a second opinion.

Chin Tuck

The chin tuck is often part of an overall face-lift. It can also be done as a separate procedure for women whose big concern is the doubling or sagging that takes place in the chin area with age. The procedure involves a single small incision under the chin and the removal of excess fat with liposuction.

Peels and Dermabrasion

"I wasn't ready for surgery but I also wasn't ready to accept the lines around my mouth as 'me.' I talked to a doctor about a chemical peel and checked with a few people who had gone to him. The solution stung a little— but I sure look better."

Pamela Dixon (age 55)

IF YOU HAVE fine lines, crow's-feet, or wrinkles due to too many years in the sun, these cannot be removed with a face-lift. In this case your doctor may recommend a chemical peel or a dermabrasion for removing the finer lines in your face.

A chemical peel involves applying a mild acid solution to your face. This causes the superficial outer layers of the skin to slough and "rejuvenates" the skin. Done as an outpatient procedure in your doctor's

300

office, it's an excellent way to control the fine lines in the face. The strength of acid solution and the number of times it can be applied depends on the texture of your skin, the strength of the solution, and the wisdom of your doctor. Most people report that the solution stings when first put on the face—but that quickly goes away. The solution is kept on the skin for a few minutes and then washed off. Your face will be red where the acid was applied and you will need to avoid being in the sun while your face heals. The results can be excellent.

Dermabrasion is good for deeper lines. Dermabrasion is like using sandpaper to smooth out rough areas. It is usually done when a person is sedated and can be combined with one of the surgical procedures. The face usually looks like it has had a sunburn. You need to stay out of the sun while your face heals. Again, the results can be excellent when it comes to removing creases and pits that a face-lift does not affect.

Liposuction

Many women are tempted by the notion of sucking out those excess pounds from their hips or other pouchy places, but the truth is that liposuction is effective only if you are just a few pounds overweight. It is meant to recontour the body, but it is *not* going to remove the twenty extra pounds you've been carrying around. What liposuction can do is remove diet- and exercise-resistant fat deposits. It is most effective when used on the lower abdomen, buttocks, and thighs.

The surgery starts with a small incision in the area where the fat deposit is located. A blunt, tubular instrument then removes the fat by suctioning it out under high vacuum pressure. If you have this procedure done on your lower abdomen, you may be required to wear a girdle for two months or more to encourage the skin shrinkage process. You will also have to exercise to tighten up the skin in the affected areas.

Liposuction will not flatten your stomach when excess skin is present. In this case it may produce an uneven effect with rippling of your skin and some sagging. If you are considering liposuction, you should interview your doctor and find out how much experience he or she has with the procedure. Make sure you are dealing with an expert.

Breast Augmentation and Other Cosmetic Breast Surgeries

"After nursing three babies, my breasts sagged so much
I felt like they would one day reach my toes! My husband
thought I was silly, but I had my breasts done anyway—
and I love the result."

Erica Piel (age 43)

BREAST AUGMENTATION, or breast enlargement, is one of the most popular cosmetic surgery choices among women—even with all the recent controversy regarding breast implants. This probably reflects the constant turmoil of how we feel about our breasts and the societal pressure to be forever sexy and "perfect." Although breasts certainly serve the primary role of nourishing our young, they remain an integral part of our sexuality. But what exactly are perfect breasts: the ones in the magazine? the breasts of a twenty-year-old? or the breasts of a woman who has had children?

If you want to have breast augmentation surgery, you should be realistic about what to expect; discuss your expectations with your doctor beforehand. Once you have had breast implants, you should make sure that your mammograms are read by someone who specializes in reading mammograms after breast augmentation surgery.

There are many different approaches to breast augmentation surgery. There are also different types of breast surgery, including mastopexy (a breast lift) and reduction mammoplasty (breast reduction surgery). Silicone-filled implants are no longer available for purely cosmetic cases—only for reconstruction following breast cancer surgery. Saline-filled implants are used for cosmetic surgery.

THE TEETH AND GUMS

*"I floss my teeth twice a day for a good reason. I would
like to keep them!"*

Lillie Sallenworth (age 91)

GINGIVITIS AND PERIODONTITIS are the most common gum disorders associated with aging and can be combated with good dental hygiene.

Dental Care

Tooth decay is a bacterial disease that is the most common cause of tooth loss. Ranked just behind the common cold as one of the most common disorders of the human condition, tooth decay affects children and young adults most frequently, but can remain a problem throughout life. Tooth decay is the result of the interaction of a vulnerable tooth surface with sugar and bacteria. In the process of digesting food, bacteria help convert some of the sugars or carbohydrates you eat into acids, which then become part of what is referred to as dental plaque. Plaque is most common in the pits and fissures at the junction of the teeth and gum, as well as at the sites of cavity fillings. The decay-producing acids in the plaque begin to attack the hard outer enamel of the tooth's surface. Once the enamel has been penetrated, the softer dentin beneath is attacked. Tooth decay in adults takes one or two years to develop.

The best preventive measure is consistent and extensive dental hygiene with frequent dental checkups. For example, adult women who still get cavities should see a dentist for checkups at least twice a year. You should also discuss your dental hygiene regime with your dentist to see if there is any room for improvement. In addition, if you smoke or if you drink heavily, you should see your dentist more frequently, since you are at greater risk for tooth decay and gum disease.

Periodontal Disease

While tooth decay is the major cause of tooth loss, after the age of thirty-five periodontal disease can become another frequent cause. Often referred to as gum disease, periodontal disease actually occurs in the periodontium, which includes the gums (gingivae), the periodontal ligament, and the tooth sockets or alveolar bone. Together these structures support your teeth.

Almost everyone experiences some degree of periodontal disease in the course of a lifetime. It is a disease that does not occur in one day, nor can it be cured overnight or cured in the sense that it will never reappear. Periodontal disease is caused by bacterial plaque, which is found in everyone's mouth. The result of the disease is weakened tooth support. Gingivitis is the less severe form of the disease; periodontitis is the more serious condition.

Gingivitis

Gingivitis is an inflammation of the gums that is caused by deposits of plaque. Mild forms of gingivitis are common in adults. Pregnant women and people with uncontrolled diabetes are prone to gingivitis. Symptoms include reddened, swollen gums that bleed easily.

Healthy gums are pink and firm. If they are swollen or tender or if you notice that they bleed when you brush your teeth, you should consult your dentist. The earlier the disease is treated, the less damage is done to the soft tissue supporting your teeth.

Treatment involves a process called scaling in which your dentist or periodontist will remove the plaque and calculus (a chalky substance composed of mineralized plaque and often called tartar) through a deep cleaning with dental instruments. It may be painful because of the swollen and tender gums. If you have gingivitis, scaling will probably become part of your dental maintenance routine; you will have to pay more attention to your own dental hygiene at home. You should brush your teeth at least twice daily. Some dentists recommend brushing after every meal. You should also floss at least once a day. Electric toothbrushes have not been found to be more effective than ordinary brushes in the removal of plaque, but if your dexterity is impaired, they may help you brush. WaterPiks also do not add to plaque removal, although the irrigation they provide can minimize the harmful effects of plaque.

Periodontitis

When gingivitis goes untreated, periodontitis may develop. Additional symptoms of periodontitis include a bad taste in the mouth, bad breath, pain when eating hot, cold, or sweet foods, a dull sound when you tap a tooth, or an actual loose tooth. Not only the gums are infected, the periodontal ligament and tooth sockets are also infected. Plaque-filled pockets form between the teeth and gums. Over time, the gums begin to gradually detach from the teeth. Pus may form as infections develop. Yet, despite the seriousness of this condition, it is often painless. Therefore, if you notice any changes in your gums, a bad taste in your mouth, or bad breath, it is extremely important that you see your dentist. If the condition is caught early, you may be able to avoid surgical treatment.

The first steps in treatment for periodontitis are the same as those for gingivitis. Your dentist will clean your teeth and their root surfaces by scaling and instruct you on a meticulous routine of dental hygiene that will include flossing and extensive brushing. If your gums do not improve, your dentist may evaluate you for any orthodontic problems, which may have caused teeth to crowd or overlap, resulting in increased plaque deposits.

If yours is an advanced case, surgery will be recommended. Procedures include a gingivectomy, which involves trimming the gums and therefore the pockets where plaque and calculus gather, and a "flap" procedure in which the gum tissue is lifted so that the area around the bone may be thoroughly cleaned and recontoured. The gum is then sutured back into place.

In all cases of periodontal disease, prevention is not only the best treatment, but achievable. (However, as we age, a certain increase in plaque is almost inevitable, since we must eat to live.) Get in the habit of brushing your teeth two or three times a day and flossing twice a day. A WaterPik will also help in removing smaller, more inaccessible food particles and in massaging the gums. Prevention also includes twice yearly visits to your dentist where you can be screened for gingivitis and periodontitis.

HEADACHES

*"I didn't have a worry until I turned thirty. Then it's an
ache here, a creak there, and an occasional headache.
God, somedays I think I'm about to detonate!"*

Michelle Toner (age 35)

HEADACHES DON'T NECESSARILY get worse with age. But if you have spent a lifetime suffering from them, they might not get better either. Everyone has experienced some kind of headache at some time. The most common headache is the tension or "everyday" headache. These headaches aren't caused because you are tense. In fact, a headache results when blood vessels to the brain, after constricting, suddenly dilate and flood a part of the brain with blood. This blood congestion is what causes the discomfort. The pain is usually over the forehead, temples, or over the back of the upper neck.

A tension headache may have many causes—including excessive use of alcohol or tobacco, hormonal changes like those in PMS, and stress—or, as in many cases, no recognized trigger at all. Such headaches are easily treated with aspirin, acetaminophen, or ibuprofen. If your tension headaches occur more than two times per week for more than a month, they are considered chronic (this often happens in midlife). These headaches may occur at any age and in persons of either sex.

Talk to anyone who suffers from migraine headaches and they will describe very particular symptoms that recur. Migraines are usually preceeded by an "aura"—flashing lights or a change in sounds. This aura is a warning that the pain is soon to emerge. The pain can be quite severe and cause nausea and vomiting. Classically, all a person wants to do during one of these attacks is lie down in a dark, quiet room. For many patients these headaches recur.

At present, fluctuations in the level of serotonin, a neurotransmitter that is produced by nerve cells, are considered to be responsible for migraine headaches. Migraines, which are also referred to as vascular headaches, are considered to be a chronic disorder for which there is no cure.

Analgesics, such as aspirin, acetaminophen, or ibuprofen, may provide some relief in the case of a mild migraine, but those who suffer from severe migraines usually find over-the-counter medications to be of little help. Taking medication at the first sign of the aura provides the best chance of getting relief. Some people report that large doses of caffeine in combination with an analgesic also provides relief. Other drugs used to treat migraines are ergotamine and isometheptene. Ergotamine is one of the most widely used medications for migraine and, again, works best when taken at the first sign of the aura. A new injectable drug, sumatriptan succinate, known by the trade name Imitrix, is now on the market. After receiving the first injection in your doctor's office, you can then inject yourself at the first signs of an attack. It's now in pill form and both work well.

If you suffer from migraines, it is wise to keep a diary that includes what you eat and your sleeping habits. If you can trace an attack to a certain food, such as chocolate or cheese, you can avoid that food. If oversleeping triggers attacks, you might try avoiding sleeping in on weekends. Many women report attacks are more severe when taking oral contraceptives—an association that may prompt changing to another type of birth control.

Unrelieved headaches of any kind for six months or more are considered chronic. Head pain or a continuing or chronic headache may indicate another, more serious, underlying condition, such as a brain tumor, and should not be ignored. When consulting a physician, a good description of the headache and any other symptoms is essential. Use a diary to keep track of:

- Time of day of onset of symptoms
- Frequency and pattern of recurrence
- Type of pain and any other distinguishing characteristics
- Approximate duration
- Any accompanying symptoms
- Personal method of treatment for relief

THE BONES AND THE JOINTS

The human body is composed of 206 bones, which has always been an astonishing number to me. They range in size from the femur (the thigh-bone), which is the largest bone in the body, to the incus, a tiny bone found in the middle ear that is smaller than a pencil eraser. Bones are made up of cells, proteins, and minerals like calcium and phosphorus. Bones are continually depositing and withdrawing calcium and phosphate. Bone marrow, the soft inner core, is responsible for manufacturing blood cells.

Arthritis and Other Joint Disorders

Arthritis is a joint disease. There are many kinds of arthritis, the most common of which is osteoarthritis, which has been part of the medical lexicon for centuries. Living life, with the resultant wearing down of the joints over time, is the major cause of osteoarthritis. When affecting small joints like the fingers, many areas may be debilitated; whereas if a knee or hip is affected, that may be the only joint involved.

The chief symptom is pain that may be worse in the morning after the joint has been relatively immobile during the night. With a little warm-up in the morning, much of the stiffness and pain abates. Sometimes a change in the weather is enough to trigger discomfort or joint swelling. Bony lumps called Heberden nodes may form at the end of the fingers; these are generally only of cosmetic concern. Aspirin, ibuprofen, or other pain relievers with anti-inflammatory properties allow some relief for those who suffer. Regular, but moderate, exercise may help to keep the pain from worsening.

The less common rheumatoid arthritis is the most debilitating form of arthritis. Usually it occurs between the ages of twenty and fifty. (See page 257 for more information.)

Lupus

Systemic lupus erythematosus is an autoimmune disease where the body literally turns on itself and attacks the connective tissues. (See page 267 for more information.)

THE BACK

The back is composed of more than thirty bones, running from the base of the skull to the tailbone. During a lifetime, a great deal is expected of these bones, yet often very little attention is paid to the maintenance of the back until pain is present and back problems have begun in earnest. In the past, doctors thought that the back ought to be a certain way—as straight as possible, without knobs or bumps. But, of course, backs are as human as the rest of us and just as individual as we are.

Back Strains and Spasms

I learned respect for my back when I was a teenager. One day I did what everyone did in the days before electric garage door openers: I merely leaned over and lifted the garage door. Did I bend my legs? Of course not. I did it wrong and paid the price with a sprained back. Fortunately the pain went away, and I'm lucky that I've never had a problem since—but I still remember the pain and stiffness.

Back pain can occur at any point in the spine, but the lower back is affected most often. An injury can result from what appears to be an inconsequential movement, like lifting that garage door or swinging around with an object while your feet are planted in one spot. And I have known more than one nurse who has ruined her back moving a sedated patient off an OR table. It can also happen to any weekend athlete who has dreams beyond her physical capabilities. Don't count out stress as a contributing factor. About nine out of ten people never know the exact cause of their initial back pain.

Symptoms include pain and stiffness in the area. Sometimes there can also be pain radiating down one leg. Treatment with analgesics and ice initially, followed by heat and rest, will usually take care of the problem, although recurring bouts of discomfort are common. Relaxation techniques should also be used when recovering from a back injury and may prove to be one of the best therapies available.

Prolapsed Discs

Discs cushion the bones or vertebrae of the back. They are the soft cushiony pads between one vertebra and another. A disc is composed of a jellylike substance encased in a fibrous skin. A prolapsed disc is a disc that has ruptured, thus reducing the cushioning layer between the bones and putting pressure on a spinal nerve. Prolapsed discs occur most often in the lower back, but any disc may be affected—including ones in the neck. Discs in the lower back are referred to as lumbar discs and those in the neck as cervical discs. The risk of having a prolapsed or herniated disc increases with age.

Symptoms of a prolapsed disc in the neck include pain over the area, with radiation of the pain possible down one or both arms and numbness or weakness in an arm or hand. Similarly, a prolapsed lumbar disc may cause pain in the lower back, which may go down one or both legs and may be accompanied by numbness or weakness in the buttocks, legs, and feet. In addition, when you cough or sneeze, you may feel a shooting pain down your back, and usually you will find that one arm or leg is affected more than the other.

If your doctor suspects a prolapsed disc, after a thorough history and medical examination, she or he will probably obtain a CT scan or an MRI to ascertain the location and the amount of the damage. In isolated cases, myelography will be performed. In this procedure, dye is injected into the spinal column, outlining the area of the injury, and then an X ray is taken.

The most important point to make regarding a prolapsed disc is that in many cases it can repair itself. This process usually takes two to six weeks and involves getting the proper rest (which may include complete bed rest) and practicing relaxation techniques. Such a commitment is a great deal easier to make if you consider that this investment may help you avoid back surgery—a far more costly, time-consuming, painful, and chancy prospect.

There have been several innovations available to patients instead of rushing into conventional back surgery. For instance, endoscopes, which are surgical telescopes, can be used in some cases to remove only the portion of the disc that is herniated and leaving the healthy part of the disc in place, where it can still serve its role as a cushion. One alternative to surgery is injecting an enzyme called chymopapain into the disc. Chymopapain is derived from the papaya tree and causes the disc to shrink. This reduces the pressure on the affected nerve and often eliminates the pain. Another choice is percutaneous discectomy, a procedure that allows an injured disc to be removed via a large needle, much like the needle used to inject chymopapain. When nerve compression cannot be relieved by either of these techniques, conventional surgery may become the only option.

There is a growing school of thought that all these ways of treating lower back pain may be terribly archaic—even if they do represent the best that modern medicine has to offer. More and more patients are turning to relaxation techniques, hypnotherapy, and stress reduction—with the assumption that the majority of back patients are in pain because of stressful and difficult elements in their lives. Many people find that when these extraneous problems are minimized or eliminated, the pain subsides.

Caring for Your Back

"I came to the realization that I couldn't carry my baby,
a bag of groceries, and open the front door all at the same
time without something giving."

Michelle Norris (age 36)

THE BACK IS an area of your body that will benefit greatly from enlightened self-care. From how you lift heavy objects to how much you weigh, how you stand, and how you sleep at night, you have a great deal of control over the health of your back.

Speak to your doctor or chiropractor about a simple routine of back exercises to relieve pain and strengthen the muscles of your back. The most commonly recommended exercise is to lie flat on your back with your knees bent and press the small of your back to the floor ten times, squeezing your buttocks as you do so. Another very simple way to alleviate stress in the back is to shrug your shoulders now and then during the day and take a few big, deep breaths. Hold the air for a second and repeat.

There are many books on care of the back and back exercises. If you have back problems, investing in a book or in an appropriate exercise program is quite worthwhile. Another reminder: strong abdominal muscles are a great defense against a bad back, so do those sit-ups!

The cardinal rule when lifting anything, from a baby to a box of books, is to bend your knees and not your back. When picking up a baby, whether from a crib, bed, or a changing table, stand as near the crib, bed, or table as possible before you bend your knees. When you lift from any distance, you are obviously straining your back more than you would if you were closer to the object that you are lifting.

You should also try to avoid stiffness in your back whenever possible. If you drive a great deal or work seated at a desk for hours, you can help avoid muscle fatigue by breaking up your routine with repeated walks to stretch your back. Stop your car periodically for a brief walk, or get up from your desk and walk up and down the hallway now and then. A small pillow at the base of your spine may also help relieve undue pressure on your back when seated. To the uninitiated, these seem like small measures that can hardly make much difference, but in essence, what you do when you take a break from your routine is to give your back a rest from the very taxing job of keeping your body upright.

You may even keep your back from experiencing unnecessary stress and strain while sleeping. Make sure your mattress is firm enough. Do not sleep on your stomach, unless you put a pillow under your abdomen to keep your back from sinking toward the mattress. The best sleeping position for your back is on your side with your knees drawn up toward your chest. Remember how you slept with a pillow between your legs when you were pregnant? Well, you may want to do it again. A pillow between your legs may keep your back from twisting while accommodating the position of your legs. If you sleep on your back, a pillow under your knees will relieve the pressure on your back.

Finally, if you are overweight, you are straining your back unnecessarily. While there are many good reasons for losing weight, preventing unnecessary back pain may be one of the most convincing. (See page 271 for more information on weight loss.)

THE FEET

"I'm convinced that high heels are a diabolical male plot against women's feet."

Cynthia McCoy (age 39)

W E DEMAND A GREAT DEAL of our feet and often give them very little in return. As women we have been trained to torture our feet in the name of beauty and, perhaps, because of the goal of adding an inch or two in height. Our feet carry us everywhere. We owe them the best possible care as we pound toward our goals and dreams and into middle age.

If the Shoe Doesn't Fit, Don't Wear It

The worst thing we can do for our feet is wear shoes that don't fit. That may make sense to you, yet a surprising number of us still do this. Comfortable, properly fitted shoes will help avoid many foot problems, including corns and calluses. If you must wear high heels, try not to wear them for a long period of time and stick with two-inch heels. Wear a walking shoe on your way to work or to a special occasion and put on your heels after you arrive. Always keep a spare pair of shoes in your office, in case the ones you are wearing begin to feel uncomfortable. Some women report that after a pregnancy their feet seem to be larger. If you feel this might be the case, buy new shoes—don't try to fit into your old ones. The pain of ill-fitting shoes is one pain that is entirely possible to avoid.

Foot Problems

Bunions

A bunion is a bony protrusion at the base of your big toe. It may be painful and may limit the motion of that toe. A bunion is sometimes caused by an inherited condition called hallux valgus, which is responsible for the tendency of the big toe to overlap another toe. But the

313

usual culprit is a poor-fitting shoe—especially a high heel with a pointed toe, which keeps pushing and squeezing the big toe into the other toes. Bunions are a common, but minor problem and occur at least twice as often in women as in men (because of high heels, of course).

The best treatment is prevention: avoiding high heels and wearing comfortable shoes. Foot pads may be helpful. In extreme cases, surgery may be required.

Corns and Calluses

A corn or a callus is the result of constant pressure or friction on a certain area of the toe or foot. A callus is a thickening and hardening of the skin; it usually appears on the outside of the big toe or on the bottom of the foot. A corn is smaller than a callus and usually appears on a toe, particularly the little toe.

The best way of treating corns and calluses is to eliminate the cause—usually an improperly fitting shoe. If you don't change your footwear, your corn or callus will remain, and you will probably develop more. Wear soft leather shoes or sneakers and make sure your shoes are not too tight. In some cases, if the problem persists, a podiatrist, or foot specialist, will remove the tissue surgically. However, it is probably not worth having the procedure unless you eradicate the cause—that painful shoe.

Hammertoes

A hammertoe, also known as a mallet toe, is a toe that has become clawlike in appearance. Any toe can become a hammertoe. Hammertoes may be caused by pressure from an ill-fitting shoe, but they also occur in people who have had long-term diabetes and suffered muscle and nerve damage as a result. The best treatment is to correct your footwear. However, if the hammer is severely painful and limiting the motion of your foot, surgery may be required.

Ingrown Toenails and Fungus

An ingrown toenail occurs when the sharp edge of the toenail grows into the skin of the toe. Redness and swelling may occur and the toe may be painful to the touch. The best way to avoid an ingrown toenail is to cut your toenails straight across and avoid cutting too close to the nail bed. If the tissue around the toe has become infected, your doctor will prescribe an antibiotic. Soaking your feet in warm water and applying a topical antibiotic may also be helpful.

A fungal infection is caused by fungus spores that attach themselves to the bed of keratin cells that make up your nails. You may contract a fungal infection by walking barefoot in public or as a complication of athlete's foot. Fungal infections can persist indefinitely. If the nail is involved, it may thicken and become detached. Unfortunately, there are no satisfactory treatments for fungal infections of the nails. Creams and ointments may help in controlling the fungus in the surrounding tissue, but they do not penetrate the nail itself. Oral antifungal drugs have side effects and are usually not recommended for treating an isolated fungal infection of a nail. Once again, the most successful treatment is prevention—do not walk barefoot in public places, treat athlete's foot immediately, keep your nails clean and trim them carefully, not too close to the nail bed.

THE HANDS AND FINGERS

Carpal Tunnel Syndrome

"I put off seeing a doctor for a long time. But then the pain in my hands just kept getting worse. My doctor said I had carpal tunnel syndrome and it was probably from my work in the grocery store."

Marsha Brandenstradt (age 47)

THE CARPAL TUNNEL is a passageway in the wrist. When the fibrous tissue that makes up the tunnel compresses the underlying nerves and tendons that extend into the hand, you may experience pain and a numbness or tingling in your fingers and hands. The telltale sign that separates carpel tunnel syndrome (CTS) from other conditions is that the little finger is not included in this numbness and tingling.

315

If you work at a computer, at a computerized checkout stand, or as a carpenter, assembly line worker, violinist, or butcher, you are at risk for this malady. The injury stems from repetitive movements that tax this portion of your hand and wrist. Also, pregnant women may be at higher risk for CTS, particularly if they gain a great deal of weight. Diabetics are at risk as well. Treatment includes resting the joint, wearing a splint to aid in this process, and, in some cases, medication. If medication is advised, it is usually given in the form of a steroid drug, such as cortisone. Sometimes surgery is necessary, which involves cutting the fibrous sheath and relieving the pressure on the nerves and blood vessels.

Tenosynovitis

If you have difficulty in straightening a finger or thumb, this may be a sign of tenosynovitis, an inflammation of the sheath surrounding a tendon. Certainly, such a symptom will demand a visit to your doctor. Other symptoms of tenosynovitis include a crackling sound when you move the finger and tenderness or pain in the finger. While tenosynovitis may occur in the shoulder or wrist, it is quite common in one or more fingers. The deformity that results is sometimes referred to as trigger finger, because the sheath that protects the tendon of the finger becomes inflamed and therefore it becomes difficult to straighten the digit. This condition is most prevalent in women over fifty. It is generally not serious, and rest may produce a complete cure, but it should be attended to.

If the cause is an infection, as opposed to constant overuse, an antibiotic may be necessary. If the infection does not respond to antibiotics and pus is building up in the internal spaces in the finger, surgery may be required to alleviate the buildup of pus and keep the infection from spreading. In most cases, trigger finger is not serious. However, if you do find that you cannot straighten a finger, you should consult your doctor as soon as possible.

THE EYES

"I was devastated. I realized that I was holding the news-
paper farther and farther from my eyes. I remember
watching this happen to my mother when I was a girl—
and somehow I just never imagined it happening to me."

Sandra Blakemore (age 44)

A N OLD PROVERB has it that the eyes are the windows to the soul. They are also our windows on the world. The eyes provide us with an ever changing three-dimensional movie of the world in extraordinary detail. The eye records in an instant what a dozen cameras cannot begin to film.

Parts of your eyes age differently. For instance, as you age, the lens begins to accumulate more fibers, which makes it less elastic. This accounts for the fact that by middle age focusing on objects nearest to you becomes difficult.

Cataracts

A cataract is a clouding of the lens of the eye. This clouding of the lens decreases the transmission of light that gets in and consequently vision is obstructed partially or completely. A cataract may begin in one eye, but eventually, in most cases, both eyes are affected. Over twenty million people worldwide have gone blind as a result of cataracts and nearly half a million cataract surgeries are performed in the United States alone each year. While these numbers may seem alarming, cataracts are actually one of the least serious, if most common, form of eye disorders because *the loss of sight can almost always be restored with surgery.*

Symptoms include blurred vision, seeing halos around lights, and generally impaired vision. As we age, we all develop some clouding of the eye lenses, and by the time we reach sixty most of us have cataracts to some degree. Certain diseases also contribute to cataract formation, particularly diabetes mellitus (page 244). If you are taking corticosteroid drugs for rheumatoid arthritis or if you have been exposed to ultraviolet

317

radiation from sunlight over a period of years, you are at higher risk for the formation of cataracts. This disease is one reason to wear sunglasses year-round to limit the exposure of the eye to any ultraviolet light.

Often the first stages of the clouding of a lens are so gradual that you won't notice anything in particular until, say, you take a vision test to renew a driver's license and fail for the first time. You may also begin to have problems with night vision or notice a general clouding of your sight. At the first sign of any change in vision, you should see your ophthalmologist or optometrist for a complete exam, and after forty, this should be part of your maintenance routine (see "Eye Care over Forty," page 322). Your doctor will give you a complete eye exam with an ophthalmoscope. If the cataract is so opaque that the ophthalmoscope cannot look through it, ultrasonography may also be used to check for other abnormalities. Ultrasonography is a technique that uses sound waves to create an image of an interior area of your body. A transducer, a device that resembles a wand, sends and receives high-frequency sound waves inaudible to the human ear (ultrasound). The image is then displayed on a video screen and photographed for purposes of examination.

Cataract surgery is one of the most successful operations performed today. The procedure is performed under local anesthesia. It is usually done in a hospital on an outpatient basis and takes about an hour. The clouded lens is removed and replaced with an artificial lens called an intraocular lens implant. An incision is made at the outer edge of the cornea. The lens is removed through this incision, and the new lens is inserted. Fine sutures are used to close the incision. The procedure is considered to be painless, though you may experience a dull discomfort in the area for a few days after surgery. Acetaminophen or ibuprofen may help relieve the discomfort. You may also want to talk to people who have had the surgery beforehand to hear firsthand accounts, learn how much their eyesight improved as a result of the operation, get advice regarding how to prepare for the surgery, and learn what to do afterward to make your recovery as easy as possible. Alternatives to surgery include thick-lensed eyeglasses and contact lenses.

Glaucoma

"I thought the test for glaucoma would feel weird and be uncomfortable. I was surprised that I couldn't feel anything at all—and relieved when the pressures were normal."

Joyce Gladstone (age 45)

GLAUCOMA IS THE leading cause of blindness in the United States. Two million people, or about 3 percent of those over sixty-five, are affected. Of these two million people, at least 60 percent are legally blind. If glaucoma is detected and treated early, blindness or severe loss of vision can be avoided.

Glaucoma occurs when the pressure within the eyeball increases. The result to be avoided is progressive pressure on the optic nerve, with damage to that delicate structure. The increased pressure within the eyeball stems from the lack of drainage of the aqueous humor—the fluid that circulates behind the iris (the colored portion of the eye) through the pupil (at the center of the colored portion of the eye) and then into the space between the iris and the cornea. Produced constantly, this fluid must also drain constantly. When the fluid cannot drain properly, pressure builds within the eye. The greater the pressure, the greater the damage to the optic nerve. Blind spots or patterns begin to develop as the optic nerve deteriorates. If glaucoma is not treated, total blindness will result.

There are two kinds of glaucoma, acute and chronic. The chronic form of glaucoma is most common, affecting 95 percent of those who suffer from glaucoma.

Chronic Glaucoma

The major symptom of chronic glaucoma is gradual loss of peripheral vision. Because this loss may be so gradual, chronic glaucoma may not be detected for years. There are no early warning signs for chronic glaucoma, and your central vision—what you count on generally—will remain intact until the final stages of the disease, by which point your chances of avoiding loss of sight have greatly decreased. The risk of glaucoma increases with age, and thus, to catch chronic glaucoma at an early stage, it is imperative that you have regular eye examinations after the age of forty.

The earliest sign of chronic glaucoma is increased pressure on the eye, which may be detected by a tonometry test—a painless, inexpensive test that determines the pressure within the eye. If your eye pressure is increased, further tests will be performed to determine if you have glaucoma. A physician will examine your eye with an ophthalmoscope, which will allow her or him to look directly at the optic nerve and assess its health. Your peripheral vision will also be tested.

If there is no damage to the optic nerve, the condition will be treated with eyedrops that decrease the pressure in the eye. Other drugs, such as beta-adrenergic blockers or acetazolamide, may have side effects, and you should discuss your choices in detail with your physician.

When medication is not a viable alternative, surgery may be necessary. One surgical option involves using a laser to open the blocked drainage channels in the front chamber of the eye. If the situation is more advanced, a procedure called a filtration process will be recommended. It involves creating a drainage passage surgically, which will relieve the pressure within the eye.

As with so many medical conditions, early detection is the next best thing to prevention. Here are four risk factors to pay particular attention to when considering chronic glaucoma:

- If you are over forty, your chances of developing chronic glaucoma increase.
- Glaucoma is hereditary—about 20 percent of those who develop glaucoma have more than one close relative with glaucoma.
- If you are African American, your chances of developing glaucoma are significantly increased.
- If you have diabetes, your risk of developing glaucoma is three times greater than the average risk.

Acute Glaucoma

Acute glaucoma occurs most often among the elderly, but is far less common than chronic glaucoma. The symptoms are far more obvious and include halos around lights, blurred vision (most often in one eye), pain, and redness in the eye. Acute glaucoma often develops suddenly and may demand emergency treatment. Attacks of acute glaucoma occur most frequently at night. The pain may be extreme and can cause vomiting. If you have any of the above symptoms, you should contact your ophthalmologist immediately or go to the emergency room of your local hospital.

The surgery for acute glaucoma is usually an emergency operation called an iridotomy. An iridotomy creates a drainage hole in the iris to relieve pressure. The advent of laser surgery allows this drainage hole to be made without making an incision in the eye. If your situation is not an emergency, laser iridotomy may be performed in a doctor's office, which will allow you to resume normal activity within a day or two, depending on your general health.

Macular Degeneration

Macular degeneration is another major cause of blindness in the United States and primarily affects the elderly. The macula lutea lies at the center of the retina and is responsible for your central vision. In the early stages of this disease deposits form and blood vessels grow in the macula. If these vessels leak plasma or blood, the cells in the retina become damaged. When that occurs a scar forms and a portion of the vision is lost. This disease typically affects both eyes.

If you develop macular degeneration, you will notice difficulty reading small print and seeing distant objects like street signs. Fortunately, side vision is preserved so you will still be able to walk around unaided. It is important that macular degeneration be diagnosed early if treatment is to be successful. You doctor can examine the macula easily with an ophthalmoscope. The best treatment available is laser surgery to seal the leaky blood vessels.

EYE CARE OVER FORTY

If you have no eye problems, you should have your eyes examined about every three years once you reach forty and every year after the age of fifty. Forty is the age when your eyes naturally begin to change. Usually, about this time in life, people tend to become more or less presbyopic (unable to focus on objects at close range). Over fifty, you should have your eyes checked more frequently for signs of glaucoma or other eye diseases.

Symptoms of presbyopia include eyestrain, which may leave your eyes feeling tired and weak, and a decreased ability to focus on objects close to you. If you were already farsighted, you may begin to need stronger corrective lenses. If your vision has always been good, but sometime after your fortieth birthday you begin to have difficulty reading, sewing, or doing other close work at a normal distance from your eyes, you should have your eyes examined. The ophthamologist will probably prescribe reading glasses for you. You will probably need new stronger lenses about every year after then until you are sixty-five, at which point changes in your prescription will be necessary less frequently.

The importance of conscientious eye care over forty cannot be overestimated. By going for regular eye exams, you can ensure that almost all eye conditions—including cataracts and chronic glaucoma—will be caught and treated early. Having your eyes checked regularly will do nothing less than help ensure good vision for the rest of your life.

THE EARS, NOSE, AND THROAT

"Why is it that we think nothing of wearing eyeglasses,
but consider a hearing aid a sign of old age?"

Melanie Natrone (age 64)

THE EAR IS marvelously complex and is responsible not only for hearing but also for balance. Disruptions in either of these two functions are the most common ear problems encountered with aging.

As you grow older, a certain amount of hearing loss is almost inevitable. Almost one third of the population over sixty-five has some significant hearing impairment. Severe, age-related hearing loss is called presbycusis, from the Latin *presby* (old) and *cusis* (hearing). This condition occurs more often in men and is the result of changes in the inner ear and the nerve of hearing. Hearing that has already been damaged by loud noise (remember the times your ears hurt at a rock concert or you cranked your Walkman up to the almost uncomfortable level?) will get worse when presbycusis sets in. Age-related hearing loss is also called sensorineural hearing loss.

Sensorineural hearing loss preferentially affects the upper frequencies, where children's and women's voices fall. So older people typically complain that they have difficulty hearing voices in crowded environments. That's because the louder, lower frequencies of background noise drown out the higher frequency voices. Sitting at a table for eight in a noisy restaurant can make communication hell. And ringing in the ear, known as tinnitus, may accompany this kind of hearing loss.

If close friends or family members begin to notice that you are not hearing as well as you used to, you should see your doctor. After an audiogram, a standard hearing test, your doctor may suggest a hearing aid, since a sensorineural hearing loss is not treatable medically or surgically. While more than 25 million Americans could benefit from using hearing aids, only one fifth of this number use them regularly. Unfortunately, there is still a stigma about wearing a hearing aid, even though most of us seem to have gotten over the stigma when it comes to glasses.

Vertigo or dizziness has many causes, but in the older population it is usually related to sluggish changes in blood flow to the inner ear. The underlying disease is usually atherosclerosis. Depending on your history and the severity of symptoms, your doctor may be able to prescribe a medication that will make the inner ear less sensitive to sudden movements. Some physicians believe that an aspirin every other day will decrease the stickiness of platelets and keep the blood running to the inner ear more efficiently.

THE KIDNEYS AND URINARY TRACT

Cystitis

Cystitis is an inflammation of the bladder. It often occurs as a result of sexual activity. During sex, bacteria may be introduced into the urethra and then into the bladder. In the bladder, the bacteria multiply. When the body cannot rid itself of these bacteria through urination, cystitis occurs. Cystitis is more common in women than in men, particularly because the anus is so close to the female urethra and because the female urethra is so short. Cystitis is usually caused by a type of bacteria called *Escherichia coli*, commonly found in the rectal area, but it can also be caused by other agents like chlamydia. Cystitis is most common among sexually active women between twenty and fifty years of age and also occurs among women experiencing menopause.

Symptoms of cystitis include frequent or urgent urination, a burning sensation during urination, pressure in the lower abdomen, strong-smelling urine, and, less frequently, blood in the urine. If you have the symptoms of cystitis, your doctor will do a urinalysis. If the bacterial count is abnormal, a seven-day course of antibiotics will probably be prescribed. Symptoms usually disappear within twenty-four to forty-eight hours. If cystitis occurs more than twice within a six-month period, a prophylactic dose of antibiotics may be prescribed.

One thing you can do to help prevent this problem is to urinate after sexual intercourse. This will help clear any bacteria that have recently entered the urethra or bladder.

Stones and Cysts

"I couldn't believe the pain. I thought I was going to die. In fact, at the time, I thought that was a reasonable alternative. My husband got me to the hospital and they put me on morphine until I passed this little rock."

Loralee Davis (age 59)

324

THERE ARE BLADDER STONES and there are kidney stones—all in different sizes and shapes. Ninety-five percent of all bladder stones occur in men. They usually pass without medical intervention and cause no lasting damage.

Kidney stones are relatively common in both men and women. By age seventy, 10 percent of men and 5 percent of women will have had at least one stone. Talk to anyone who has ever had a kidney stone and you'll hear a tale of excruciating pain. Some women say that the pains of childbirth pale in comparison to passing a kidney stone.

Early symptoms include pain in the flank, which then moves to the groin and vulva, a constant need to urinate, and blood in the urine. If you have a family history of stones or have had stones before, you are at higher risk.

Calcium stones, which account for approximately 85 percent of all kidney stones, are more common in men than in women. Uric acid stones occur more frequently in men as well. Cystine stones occur equally in men and women and are the result of a hereditary disorder. Struvite stones, formed mainly in women, are the result of a urinary tract infection when bacteria that produce a specific enzyme are present. These stones can cause kidney damage by obstructing the urinary tract.

If you have symptoms of kidney stones, your doctor will want a chemical analysis of your blood and a twenty-four-hour collection of urine. This means that you take samples of your urine every time you void during a twenty-four-hour period. If you are in severe pain, you may be in the process of passing the stone, and your doctor may ask you to urinate through a strainer to retain the stone for analysis. It is important to determine the composition of the stone so that proper treatment can be administered (treatment varies according to the type of stone). Surgery is sometimes necessary.

There is one rule that holds true for everyone who suffers from kidney stones. If you have had a kidney stone or have hereditary risk of having one, you should drink six to eight glasses of water a day, including one at bedtime and one during the night. Water dilutes urine, which inhibits crystals from forming in the urine. This is good advice under any circumstances.

Urethritis

The most common urinary ailment is urethritis. Urethritis is an infection of the urethra. Because of the proximity of the urethra to the vagina, sexually transmitted diseases may also be present. Symptoms include frequent urination, pus in the urine, and pain during urination. Urethritis should not be ignored, particularly because it may be sexually transmitted and ultimately caused by a chlamydia infection or another sexually transmitted disease. If you find you have urethritis, you should also inform your sexual partner. Treatment involves antibiotics. If the urethritis is caused by gonorrhea, penicillin will be prescribed. (For bladder cancer, see page 116.)

THE DIGESTIVE TRACT

Esophageal Reflux or Heartburn

Who hasn't had heartburn? A burning sensation in the chest or upper abdomen is its first sign, and this is one of the most common complaints among adults. The problem increases with age. I used to pride myself on the fact that I could eat anything with no sequelae. Well—no more. Heartburn occurs when the acidic contents of the stomach are regurgitated back into the esophagus. This is such a common problem that usually a simple discussion with your doctor will lead to a diagnosis.

I thought heartburn was the hardest part of being pregnant. That expanding abdomen can displace the stomach and there may be hormonal influence at work on the sphincter. The result? Until I was a few weeks away from delivery and the baby dropped, I slept on two or three pillows. I can't tell you the number of bottles of Maalox and Tums I went through. But, with the delivery of my children, I was able to say good-bye to this problem.

Most cases can be treated with a few preventive measures. Avoid alcohol, especially for several hours before bedtime. Don't smoke—cigarettes increase stomach acid and cause the sphincter between the stomach and the lower esophagus to open, allowing food and gastric juices to back up into the chest. Limit your intake of chocolate, alcohol, coffee, fat, and—believe it or not—peppermints. Medications such as birth control pills, antihistamines, and heart medications may aggravate heartburn. Try sleeping on an extra pillow, since gravity will help keep those gastric juices in your stomach where they belong.

One final note: as you are leaving your favorite restaurant, resist the temptation to grab that chocolate mint. It's the worst thing you can pop into your mouth after a big meal. It will increase stomach acid and relax the sphincter, paving the way for a most uncomfortable night.

For mild cases grab one of the over-the-counter preparations, but if your symptoms persist, see your doctor. You may be someone who needs a stronger, prescription medication.

Hepatitis

Hepatitis is an inflammation of the liver usually caused by a virus. Hepatitis A, the most common form, is usually transmitted by fecally contaminated food or water. The symptoms are much like those of the flu, although jaundice may also occur. Most people with hepatitis A recover completely within one to two months. If you are older or have other health complications (such as diabetes mellitus or a heart condition), recovery may take longer. Chronic hepatitis does not develop from hepatitis A. There is no specific treatment for hepatitis—the best treatment is avoidance. That means making sure that everyone who handles food washes hands beforehand. This disease is a threat to anyone who travels to underdeveloped countries. Depending where on the globe you plan to visit, you may be encouraged to get a shot of gamma globulin, which will protect you for about six months.

Hepatitis B is transmitted by exposure to contaminated blood and can be caught through sexual intercourse with an infected person. While the symptoms are much the same as for hepatitis A, this is the more serious type of hepatitis, which can lead to chronic hepatitis and sometimes liver failure and death. (See "Viral Hepatitis," page 176.)

A vaccine is available for hepatitis B. If you are a health-care practitioner, you may want to consider getting the vaccine, depending on your exposure to bodily fluids in the workplace. If someone you are intimately involved with has hepatitis B, you should practice safe sex or be immunized. The vaccine, which consists of three separate injections and provides lasting protection, is now recommended by the American Academy of Pediatrics for infants. This is one vaccination that can actually save your life.

Non-A, non-B hepatitis cannot be detected through a blood test and thus is often transmitted via a blood transfusion. It may also be sexually transmitted and it too can cause chronic hepatitis. With this form, you may feel run-down for months and complain that you just don't have the energy you used to. It may resolve itself on its own with rest and no other specific treatment.

Polyps of the Colon

It is generally assumed that two out of three Americans over the age of sixty have some sort of growth or lesion in their colons. For those of us with a family history of cancer of the colon or polyps, this problem may start a lot sooner. Such polyps are, for the most part, harmless. While polyps are not considered to be hereditary, they do tend to occur in several members of a family. Familial colonic polyposis is a rare disorder in which polyps appear throughout the colon in large numbers, up to one thousand or more. Gardner's syndrome involves the appearance of multiple colonic polyps or other nonmalignant tumors in other parts of the intestines. It is believed that cancer of the colon originates in polyps, so with these hereditary conditions, measures should be taken to screen for colon cancer at an early age and throughout life. (See "Colon and Rectal Cancers" page 89.)

THE FEMALE ORGANS

Vaginitis

Considered to be the most common gynecological complaint among women, vaginitis is simply a vaginal infection or inflammation of the vagina. Symptoms include itching and burning, unusual discharge from the vagina, pain during intercourse and sometimes in the lower abdomen, and occasionally vaginal bleeding. If you have any of these symptoms, you may have vaginitis or you may have a sexually transmitted disease (see pages 172–180). If you have vaginitis, you should tell your sexual partner that you are being treated for a vaginal infection.

The three most common types of vaginitis are trichomoniasis, yeast infections, and nonspecific vaginitis. Trichomoniasis is caused by a parasite and generally transmitted through intercourse (although you can get trichomoniasis from a wet towel or bathing suit or a toilet seat). There are generally no symptoms, but in some cases a frothy, greenish discharge may develop. Treatment is with oral antibiotics.

The main symptom of a yeast infection is irritation and itchiness, but you may have a discharge that resembles cottage cheese. Yeast infections are common in pregnant women and diabetics. If you are taking an antibiotic, you may also develop a yeast infection, since the antibiotic can change the pH and the normal flora of the vagina. One way to help prevent a yeast infection while taking antibiotics is to eat yogurt containing the live acidophilus culture. Yeast infections may also occur when you are taking the pill or if you have an iron deficiency. Recurrent yeast infections can also be a sign of HIV. If you have had multiple sex partners or if you are an IV drug user and have recurrent vaginitis, you should be tested for AIDS. Treatment for uncomplicated cases is straightforward, using over-the-counter Mycostatin suppositories.

Nonspecific vaginitis is frequently referred to as bacterial vaginosis. It is caused by different organisms, one of which is *Gardnerella vaginalis*. Usually there are no symptoms, although some women develop a fishy smelling discharge that also coats the vaginal walls.

Vaginitis may be annoying, particularly because it often recurs, but it is usually not serious. Just one word of advice: check with your doctor the first time you have an infection before you treat yourself with a cream or suppository from the drugstore.

Fibroids

Fibroids are benign tumors that develop within the uterine wall or attach to the uterine wall. They are a common complaint of women and the incidence of fibroids increases with age. They range from minute to the size of a grapefruit or small melon.

Twenty percent of women over thirty-five have fibroids, which are sometimes the "cause" of hysterectomies, even though a myomectomy—removal of *only* the tumors—is now possible and often recommended. A myomectomy, however, is considered a more complicated procedure than a hysterectomy, and thus the latter procedure is sometimes recommended simply because it is "easier." If you have fibroids and a hysterectomy has been recommended, you should get a second opinion.

Symptoms of fibroids include pressure and sometimes pain in the lower back or abdomen and heavy or long periods. When there is sharp pain in the abdomen, it is considered an emergency situation. However, in many cases, there are no symptoms.

If you have fibroids, you usually have more than one, but fortunately they generally grow slowly. They may grow rapidly during a pregnancy, however, or if you are taking the pill, because they respond to higher levels of estrogen. Since they are estrogen sensitive, fibroids often shrink or disappear after menopause, unless you are taking extrogen replacement therapy.

Fibroids are often identified during a routine pelvic exam, when they are felt by your doctor. A sonogram or CT scan may be ordered to confirm the diagnosis. Often, if you have no discomfort, treatment is not necessary. If you have not had children yet and wish to, a myomectomy may be advisable, since large fibroids may interfere with conception and pregnancy.

Loss of Pelvic Support and Prolapsed Organs

*"My doctor told me it's the price I paid for having five
children. I wish all these tissues hadn't become so weak
and loose. But the kids were still worth it."*

Maureen Boyd (age 44)

UTERINE PROLAPSE RESULTS FROM the stretching of the ligaments that support the uterus. Prolapse may also result from a weakened pubococcygeal muscle. This is the muscle that supports the pelvic floor. The best defense against prolapse is to do Kegel exercises, and do them regularly. However, doing your exercises will not always prevent prolapse.

In first-degree prolapse, the uterus has descended into the vaginal canal, but has not descended into the vaginal opening. In second-degree prolapse, part or all of the cervix appears outside the vagina. Third-degree prolapse, which is considered complete prolapse, is most common in women over seventy. In a complete prolapse, the whole uterus has descended so that it shows outside of the vagina.

If your prolapse is such that you do not notice it, you will not need surgery. Some women also avoid surgery by using a device called a pessary, which is inserted into the vagina and helps to hold the uterus in place. When a prolapse is complete, a hysterectomy is usually performed, although uterine suspension surgery is sometimes recommended for younger women as an alternative to complete hysterectomy. The latter surgery lifts the uterus back into its normal position and secures it by shortening the ligaments holding it in place.

Ovarian Cysts

Ovarian cysts are fairly common and most go away of their own accord. It should be noted, however, that women who develop such cysts between the ages of fifty and seventy are at higher risk for ovarian cancer. Since most cysts are felt during a routine pelvic examination, this is one more excellent reason to see your gynecologist on a yearly basis before, during, and after menopause. Whereas a tumor is a solid lump, a cyst is a sac that is filled with fluid. If a cyst is large, it may cause abdominal pain, interfere with hormone production, and cause irregular bleeding from the vagina. A cyst may also cause pain during intercourse and swelling of the abdomen that is firm, but painless. Emergency symptoms are rare, but may occur if the cyst ruptures and bleeds; these include vomiting and sudden and severe abdominal pain and require immediate medical attention.

Surgery is usually necessary if a cyst does not disappear within two or three menstrual cycles or if there are complications. If you are over forty and the cyst is more than two inches in diameter or if you are postmenopausal, you should have the cyst removed surgically. If the cyst is small, the ovary may be left intact, but if the cyst is large, the ovary and sometimes the fallopian tube may also be removed.

(For ovarian cancer and other cancers of the gynecological organs, see pages 100–107.)

Genital Warts and Chlamydia Trachomatis

See "Sexually Transmitted Diseases and AIDS," page 171.

SLEEP AND HEALTH

". . . It has long been known that total sleep deprivation is 100 percent lethal to rats, yet, upon autopsy, the animals looked completely normal. A researcher has now solved the mystery of why the animals die. The rats develop bacterial infections of the blood, as if their immune systems had crashed."

Sandra Blakeslee, *The New York Times*, August 3, 1993

A T THE TIME OF THIS WRITING, I have just resumed sleeping through the night for the first time since my son, Charlie, was born. He started sleeping through the night at seven months. I can't tell you how good it feels to have my batteries recharged. Charlie had me on his schedule and my sleep deprivation was well-worn. Of course, I know there is no substitute for a good night's sleep. In the modern world, we work hard to live life to the fullest, cramming as much as we can into our waking hours, assuming we'll catch up on sleep later. But the reality is—you can't catch up on sleep. Once it's gone, it's gone. Trying to make up for lack of sleep on the weekend is a poor strategy that usually backfires in a bout of insomnia on Sunday night. This is not hearsay, but simple biological truth. Sleep is a daily need and should be treated as such. As much as food is fuel for your body, so is sleep. A regular schedule is the goal. The more your sleeping schedule on the weekends resembles your weekday sleep schedule, the better your sleep will be. Just as with bingeing and dieting, it doesn't work to deprive and then indulge yourself.

I remember interviewing a sleep specialist on *Good Morning America*. His angle was that we are all sleep-deprived, we just fool ourselves. He insisted that we need eight hours of sleep a night to keep our bodies running in tip-top shape. I scoffed and told him I needed only five to six hours of sleep a night (this was two years before Charlie!). I bragged that my days were full and I fell asleep the moment my head hit the pillow. His eyes widened and he laughed. "It's not normal to fall asleep that quickly," he told me. "That is a classic sign of chronic sleep deprivation." The only person I was fooling was myself. I believe him now—but I would be a liar if I told you I have changed completely in the interim.

> *"I get eight hours of sleep every night. But now it's
> an hour and then I'm awake. Another hour and I
> go to the bathroom. Another hour and I'm planning
> the next day. But I'm sure it adds up to eight
> hours!"*
>
> Florence McMurtry (age 86)

A S WE AGE, our daily need for sleep changes, from an infant's sixteen hours to a teenager's eight or nine hours. Sleep patterns in adults vary widely, but as we age we all begin to get less deep sleep and somewhat less overall sleep. We also spend more time awake in bed and begin to take longer to fall asleep. We may make more trips to the bathroom so sleep gets interrupted. These changes begin as early as thirty, but may not be obvious until we are much older.

While many Americans get seven hours sleep a night or less, recent studies have found that we thrive on as much as nine hours sleep a night. So, if you keep saying to yourself, "Why am I so tired, I got seven hours sleep last night?" the answer may still be that you are not getting enough sleep.

> *"I never had trouble with my sleep until I turned
> forty. I had gained thirty pounds having children*

and had never taken it off. All of a sudden I was diagnosed with sleep apnea. I was tossing and turning all night and not getting enough oxygen. I've lost the weight and am sleeping well again. And the craziest thing is that I'm having dreams after years of not remembering what a dream was like."

Madeline Crossett (age 51)

ONE SURVEY BY the American Cancer Society has shown that sleep disturbances increase over time. Of women in their thirties, 14 percent were found to have nonspecific sleep disturbances. By the time women hit their early eighties, 31 percent had sleep disturbances. The reasons for this may include nervous system degeneration and sleep-wake clock disturbances, but also physical problems, such as frequent urination and the chronic pain of arthritis, or other conditions associated with aging.

One of the most serious sleep disturbances is sleep apnea, a condition where you literally stop breathing at night. Associated with snoring, it is more common in men than in women. A significant weight gain may cause a "crowding" of the structures of the throat and neck, blocking off the airway during sleep. Over time, when the body is constantly deprived of rest and oxygen, the heat and lungs can wear out. This is considered a serious medical problem.

Treatment may consist of weight loss, the elimination of alcohol and other drugs, a device called CPAP that supplies positive pressure to the airway during sleep, or surgery.

NATURAL SLEEP AIDS

The first natural sleep aid is one you're not going to want to hear about any more than your kids want to hear about it: *set a regular bedtime and try to stick to it as much as possible.* In addition, note the following:

- Get regular exercise, but do not exercise right before bedtime. Try to exercise at least three hours before you plan to go to sleep.
- Avoid stimulants such as coffee before bedtime; if you do drink coffee, try to confine your intake of caffeinated coffee to the early morning hours.
- Do not have more than one to one and a half alcoholic drinks in an evening, and do not have an alcoholic drink late in the evening.
- Take your calcium supplement in the evening. There is some information that suggests that we digest calcium better in a sleeping state and that calcium may have a positive effect on sleep.
- If you are interested in herbal remedies, consider valerian root as a calmative remedy and discuss further possibilities with your herbalist.
- Drink lots of water during the day, taper in the evening, and don't drink any right before you go to bed.
- Have a cup of camomile tea before bedtime.
- If you wake in the night, do not read in bed. Have a glass of skim milk and try to return to bed and to sleep. If you must read, read in a comfortable chair in another room, so that you do not begin to associate bed with wakefulness.

PART 7

HEALTHY MIND, HEALTHY BODY

"If the qualities and experiences associated with the female role were regarded as the norm (or at least being normal) in this society, our interpretations and treatments of 'mental disorders' would be different."

Carol Tavris, *The Mismeasure of Woman*

OUR MENTAL HEALTH is just as important to our well-being as is our physical health—maybe more so, since our state of mind inevitably influences how we take care of ourselves. Just as there are physical diseases and conditions that women over forty are more likely to develop, there are mental disorders and conditions to which women over forty are more susceptible. It's even more important to be aware of these problems and pressure points, because they can be harder to recognize and diagnose. A lump in the breast is a recognizable problem, but symptoms of depression can be clouded or hidden in the guise of personal routines and habits, such as the inability to get out of bed and go to work or becoming isolated from friends and family. It's important to be able to recognize these problems so that you can get help when you need it—before a problem reaches crisis proportions. In the case of mental health, a woman needs to know enough to be able to recognize when things are awry and when it might be time for meditation, therapy, a support group, hypnotherapy, or medication.

It's also important to recognize some of the myths that go along with mental health:

Myth: Psychiatric problems affect women more than men.

Myth: Depression increases with menopause.

Myth: Depression increases when you are busy and have many things to handle.

Knowing the myths helps clear the way to the truth and help.

Seeking Help When You Face a Crisis

"Frankly, I was very hesitant to get help. I've always considered it a badge of honor to work hard and be self-reliant. My body was strong and I always assumed my mental health would keep up. Then one day I realized I

had nothing else to give—and it was time to give something back to me."

Iona Long (age 53)

W E'VE ALL HEARD the old phrase "If it doesn't kill you, it will make you stronger." But it's also true that getting help when you need it will make you stronger. In fact, asking for help is a sign of strength. There are crisis points in everyone's life and having difficulty managing them is normal, even logical. If you think you can't get through a particular event or transition in your life without help, you're ahead of the game.

Here are some of the crisis points for which many people seek help:

- Death of a child
- Loss of a spouse
- Loss of a parent
- Catastrophic accident
- Divorce
- Postoperative depression
- Menopause
- Loss of a job
- The empty nest syndrome (children leaving home)
- Moving
- Retirement
- Illness (yours or a loved one's)
- Accepting and treating a drug or alcohol addiction
- Caring for an elderly parent and an infant—one at a time or simultaneously

In the course of life, we all experience some of these crises. As we deal with them, all our energy is focused on the situation—that's how we survive. And yet, as we focus on getting through, the rest of life is put on hold. It's as if we hold our collective breath until the crisis has passed. These are the times when we need to pay particular attention to our mental health as well.

You are only as good a caregiver to someone else as you are to yourself. If you are experiencing one or more of these problems you should be particularly careful to fight against the tendency to isolate yourself from friends, family, and the outside world. Get fresh air. Go for a walk and let your brain go into neutral. Try to maintain a healthy diet and exercise plan, get enough sleep, and ask for support from your family or friends. If they don't seem to understand what you're going through, consider professional help like therapy or counseling. All of this is, of course, easier said than done. But one thing is certain: if you find that you are unable to cope with the stress you are under, consider it an obligation to yourself to get the help you need.

Knowing When to Seek Help

"You tell me why I don't feel better about myself. I'm
attractive, a successful attorney, and I have good friends.
From the outside I'm the envy of everyone. And inside I
feel like I'm slowly rotting away."

Emily Rison (age 41)

IF YOU FIND that now that you're in your forties and your previous battles with low self-esteem, depression, or anxiety seem to be bigger and take longer to win, you are not alone. For a variety of reasons, women forty or older who've handled bouts with such problems successfully in the past may find themselves felled by what had been relatively easy to conquer a decade ago. A woman in midlife whose job might be on the line may find herself unable to cope with the anxiety of the situation. A woman whose children have left home may find that her self-esteem has plummeted to regions heretofore unrecognizable to her. A woman in the throes of a nasty and heartbreaking divorce may find that she cannot shake the depression that has settled on her like a shadow. (It is particularly noteworthy that a study by the Joint Commission on Mental Health and Illness found that divorced and separated females reported a feeling of "impending breakdown" more than any other group of either sex. Divorce, then, is a time in a woman's life when she should be particularly aware of her mood swings and seek help if necessary.)

You are your own best mental-health barometer. You know yourself, and you know what mood swings are normal for you. If you find yourself unable to shake a gloomy mood or a deep, persistent sense of fear and anxiety and you know this is not like you, ask for help. One woman's debilitating lack of self-esteem may be another woman's ambition-free contentment. What's important is knowing yourself and keeping yourself on a healthy mental course despite life's bumpy detours and side roads. Checking up on your own mental health should be as important and as routine as seeing your gynecologist and getting your annual physical. If you are concerned about depression, you should feel as justified in seeking help as you would going for a mammogram because you found a suspicious breast lump.

One other thing: if you are going through a tough time, a divorce, a newly empty nest, a job shift, a family illness, and your doctor knows about this, don't let him or her pooh-pooh your physical complaints. Just because you're under stress or suffering emotional turmoil doesn't mean your physical complaints aren't real and shouldn't be taken seriously. What you're feeling physically is always very real, and you are the best judge of your body. There is a tendency to correlate the physical complaints of women with their mental state. We can all help to change this attitude by insisting that our medical complaints be taken seriously and addressed immediately. Such insistence is a good sign of mental health.

What Is Depression?

"Major depression is more than an anguished mood or the loss of the capacity to experience pleasure."

Dymitri Papolos, M.D., and Janice Papolos, *Overcoming Depression*

EVERY ONCE IN A WHILE I can feel a wave of the blues upon me. I can rarely pinpoint a cause—and, in fact, I no longer search for one. What used to throw me I now welcome as a normal fluctuation of my psyche. I feel comfortable welcoming it because I don't expect it to stay. Perhaps if I had ever battled severe depression, I wouldn't be so unalarmed about this. But over the years I've come to recognize these short-lived periods, and use them to slow down and indulge myself—in short, to be a little selfish, spend time on myself, and spoil myself when I otherwise might not. It takes time to allow the indulgence, and it's not always easy with work and the kids, but I now consider these episodes way stations and I think they make me healthier in the long run.

Moods are part of life and are often effective in causing us to make life-enhancing decisions and changes. The person who is depressed because she does not like her job and finds a new job that is more satisfying is using depression as a catalyst for change—as a signal that something isn't right. Thus, there are times when depression is a normal and appropriate response. Such depression, however, does not last. It comes, you embrace it, figure it out, and move on. Life goes on in all its joy and turmoil. A person suffering from clinical depression, however, has no such relief. The line has been crossed from normal mood swings to a clinical depression.

There are many types of depression, and many people suffer from depression. In fact, whatever the name assigned to the condition—affective manic-depressive illness, recurrent mood disorders, unipolar or bipolar depression—depression or mood swings have been affecting human beings throughout history.

How Does It Feel to Be Depressed?

"I don't like being depressed. My children always tell me
I look so sad, and that makes me feel awful, and guilty,
and then I just get more depressed."

Amanda Eppison (age 38)

A PERSON WHO IS depressed may characterize her mood as one of sadness and hopelessness. She may feel irritable, have bleak prospects for the future, or even be unable to think about the future. She may feel that she is dragging herself through the day. She may feel unmotivated. Simple tasks may take longer to complete and accomplishing such tasks may give her no satisfaction. Ideas may come more slowly, and she may feel generally isolated from the life going on around her. Some people also experience a state of persistent agitation when they are depressed.

In addition, depression may be accompanied by severely disturbed sleep patterns and loss of appetite. Food has no taste, and sleep may be elusive even when one is exhausted. The opposite may also occur. Eating may be seen as the only relief; and although the majority of depressed people report some degree of insomnia, 15 to 30 percent report the need to sleep more than they normally would and report never feeling rested, even after sleeping twelve to fourteen hours.

Treating Depression

Before the advent of lithium and antidepressants, psychotherapy was the main method for the treatment of mood disorders. As the good word spread regarding the success of these drug treatments, psychotherapy was viewed by many as unnecessary. To categorize these mood disturbances as solely physiological, however, is an oversimplification. A number of complex psychological and biological factors are involved in the onset of an episode of depression or mania and the aftermath.

The basic strategy for treatment of depression is an integrated treatment approach that involves relieving painful symptoms with the appropriate medication (see "A Note on Prescription Drugs," page 353) at the same time that the patient and her family are educated regarding the nature of the problem and plans for treatment. Relieving your symptoms is definitely not a cure, and ongoing therapy is usually recommended in order to avoid recurring bouts with depression.

At the same time that it is necessary to continue with therapy, it is also important to take your medication. Sometimes a patient may think, I feel fine. I'm well. Time to throw away the pills before I have to kick the habit. Abandoning medication before your doctor thinks prudent may trigger another episode and leave you right where you started in the first place.

I have a colleague who was diagnosed with depression in his forties. Once this occurred, he recognized that the symptoms had really been with him for years. His doctor put him on Prozac—with miraculous results. He no longer snapped at co-workers, his work was top-notch, and he professed to be quite content with his life and relieved that the paralyzing fog of depression was lifted. At the same time he hated being on a medication with no "finish line" in sight. So after a year of staying on the medicine, he stopped. He didn't clear it with his doctor—he just stopped. His rationale was that if he felt better the drug would linger in his body long enough and he would be able to feel the symptoms encroaching again. When he stopped, the mood swings came back; but he didn't see them—his co-workers did. It took someone close to him to urge him to check in with his doctor again.

I do not tell this story to lecture that you should never try to get off medications. Instead, it should serve as a reminder that it is not wise to stop or start such serious medications without checking with your doctor first. This scenario also reminds us that depression can be so insidious that it can sneak up on a person, who may be the last to recognize that he or she is struggling.

I am also aware that for many people the idea of taking a medication to alter one's mood or psyche is unpalatable. In such instances you might be more comfortable with therapy, hypnosis, or support groups. But there is growing evidence that chemical imbalances in neurotransmitters may be an underlying cause in many cases of depression—and that's where medications play a role. The bottom line? Check with your doctor and make sure you understand the pros and cons of any route you choose.

Suicidal Thoughts

"When I was six years old I found my mother in her car in the garage, dead from carbon monoxide. When my mother was a child, she was the first one to find her mother dead from a sleeping pill overdose. I have been haunted ever since by whether this is something I will be unable to escape."

Debbie Rongahm (age 43)

THE CONTEMPLATION OF SUICIDE may be human, but persistent thoughts of suicide are a warning sign that something is very wrong. Some people contemplate suicide because they think it will be a means of extricating themselves from a terrible situation, such as a bad divorce, bankruptcy, or the death of a beloved. Others consider the act a means of relief from a relentless, clinical depression. And there are those who talk of suicide, and even attempt it, in a desperate cry for help, never really meaning to take their own lives. None of these possibilities can be taken for granted. Anyone who talks of suicide or just gradually drops the subject should be taken seriously and found help.

If you find yourself drawn to thoughts of suicide, you should seek immediate professional help. If you know someone who keeps discussing suicide as a possible solution to her or his problems, you should encourage that person to seek help. A person plagued with suicidal thoughts is often best treated in a hospital on an inpatient basis, at least for the initial diagnosis and observation (see the next section).

Psychiatric Hospitalization

"Dying is an art I do very well."

Sylvia Plath

IN SOME CASES when depression is severe and thoughts of suicide predominate, inpatient treatment is advisable at least in the initial stages. Psychiatric hospitals have not been portrayed positively in books, in real-life and fictional accounts, or in movies, but times have changed and most are greatly improved and offer real hope for patients. Notwithstanding the Nurse Ratched phenomenon, hospitalization for psychiatric evaluation and treatment can be a positive and lifesaving experience in many instances. In general, the care in psychiatric hospitals is compassionate and personal. In addition to intensive therapy, there are many choices of activities. Facilities are adequate, visitors are encouraged, and those who are voluntarily admitted are always free to leave. If you or someone you know has had any of the following thoughts, hospitalization may be the best way to get treatment.

- I need to be safe from myself. I don't know what I might do to myself if left alone.

- I feel the need to be separate and isolated from the world for now.
- I am very afraid that I will commit suicide.
- I can't function in my life.
- I need to be around people who will understand.

These days most psychiatric hospital stays last from two weeks to thirty days. The hospital serves as a temporary way station where a person can be closely observed and quickly diagnosed. If medication is necessary, the proper dosage can be quickly determined through observation. In most cases, once discharged, the patient resumes a normal life.

Anorexia Nervosa and Bulimia Nervosa

"When I was in college I was anorectic. After two years in therapy I resolved the problem. Two years ago, my husband lost his job. We were in terrible financial difficulty. I was under tremendous pressure, and I stopped eating. I knew what I was doing to myself—trying to control something when I felt so out of control—and so I went back into therapy. In therapy, I realized how depressed I was about my situation. Things are much better now, and I'm enjoying my meals."

Katie Minnoran (age 47)

OFTEN ANOREXIA AND BULIMIA are referred to as disorders common to teenagers. While adolescence is definitely a high-risk period for both, there are many women who, having experienced one or the other condition in adolescence, either continue to suffer with the condition in adulthood, but keep it hidden, or relapse into old ways at crisis points.

Unfortunately, I've known women who have battled both of these eating disorders. They are still dealing with the repercussions as adults. I had a college roommate who was a wonderful ice skater. One year after Christmas vacation her coach made a comment about a rival skater, that she was tall and thin and graceful. That was enough for Lisa to interpret the comment as an insult and she stopped eating. By the time we graduated she was down to sixty-seven pounds and hospitalized. I saw her not too long ago. She was married but infertile. Her doctors told her that until her nutrition improved, her inability to conceive would likely persist.

Anorexia is generally diagnosed as self-induced starvation. A woman who is anorectic wants to be as skinny as possible and expresses an aversion for food. The desire to lose weight becomes an obsession. No matter how thin a woman suffering from anorexia may get, she always thinks she is too fat. She literally has a distorted body image. The most obvious danger with anorexia is death by starvation, but there are other risks involved. A woman who has been anorectic for a number of years stands at much higher risk for osteoporosis and gastrointestinal disorders, among other conditions.

My encounter with bulimia was with a wonderful nanny we had working for us. For several months I was stumped about why our groceries weren't lasting as long as they should have. We were going through loaves of bread and potatoes and I couldn't figure out how my daughters could have consumed that much food. Then I started paying attention to the other signs—the fine film in the toilet bowl, the fact that my nanny rarely ate with the rest of us, her poor teeth, and the fact that she always let it be known that her mother considered her overweight. By the time I put it all together, she knew her secret was out. Attempts to get her help failed. She moved to another part of the state—shamed, but not better.

Bulimia, which may occur in tandem with anorexia, is an eating disorder that involves bingeing and purging. The bulimic cycle involves eating extreme amounts of food and then desperately attempting to get rid of the food by vomiting, taking laxatives, and/or exercising excessively. While the anorectic is usually grossly underweight, the bulimic may be of average weight. As with anorexia, bulimia can put a woman at risk for many conditions, including osteoporosis and gastrointestinal disorders.

The important thing to remember is that age does not protect a woman from eating disorders. If you feel you may have an eating disorder, or know that you do, you should consult your doctor for recommendations in seeking therapeutic help. These eating disorders are not simple: they are very serious psychiatric problems and can easily follow a woman into middle age. They should not be ignored. Psychiatric help with someone who is well versed in anorexia and bulimia is the best first step.

The Shape of Grief

*"Every moment, every hour of my day is spent mourning
Sarah. Why would God allow her to die when she was
just nine? Don't tell me to get over it. I'll take this grief
to my deathbed."*

Melissa Atherton (age 41)

G RIEF, LIKE PAIN a subjective experience, involves the feelings and emotions a person experiences after a loss—for instance, the loss of a loved one to death or the end of a relationship or a divorce. Mourning is the process by which we express and resolve our grief, and mourning is different for every individual.

The stages of grief, as outlined by Elisabeth Kübler-Ross, are:

- Denial and isolation
- Anger
- Bargaining
- Depression
- Acceptance

You may experience these stages while dealing with the prolonged illness and eventual death of a loved one or upon the sudden death of someone dear to you. You may also experience the same stages when learning of your own diagnosis with breast cancer, heart disease, or another life-threatening illness, or upon being fired from a job, upon your children's departures for college, or upon being informed by your husband that he wants a divorce. The degree of the response will vary, but the stages are almost invariably the same.

The exception to the rule is what is referred to as an absent grief reaction. We live in a world that lionizes the take-charge, no-nonsense attitude. "Pick yourself up and start all over again" is an approach that we as a culture admire. We salute those who are serene in the face of great loss or pain, those who are resolute and undaunted. But what we do not include in our observation and admiration of those who seem unmoved by events of great sorrow is the aftermath of such stoicism. Everybody grieves, and those who do not grieve at the time of their loss inevitably express their grief in other ways over time. On the anniversary or birthday of the person who has died, someone experiencing absent grief reaction may exhibit erratic behavior or mood swings that inhibit a normal life. Or this postponed grief (because absent grief is really the postponement of grief) will be displaced onto trivial, otherwise insignificant losses, like the loss of a glove or a phone number, losses whose consequences are relevant only when considering the recent bereavement.

Grief is a natural part of life. And just as it is important to accept the joyful experiences of life, it is also important to experience your grief. Postponing grief isn't good for your mental health. It's generally been assumed that the initial experience of grief takes a full year, but it is also normal to experience signs or symptoms of your grief long after a year has passed. Keep in mind that the most important component of healthy mourning is proceeding from recognition of your loss to acceptance of your loss. The time period for this process differs based on the circumstances and the individual. If someone you love is suffering from an incurable chronic condition, you will probably have experienced a period of anticipatory grief, knowing what is coming, which may make the eventual loss less of a shock. If, however, you are experiencing the death of a child, no amount of anticipatory grief will prepare you for your loss. This is normal, and it's normal to need help getting through this period of mourning.

In the case of grief, time and counseling do help. Talking to a therapist, counselor, or member of the clergy may be particularly helpful, since it will allow you to reflect upon your relationship with the person you have lost and in this manner share your grief.

Sleep Disorders

See "Sleep and Health," page 332.

Anxiety

"One day I realized I couldn't make myself open the front door and walk to the car. I was paralyzed with fear. It's now been years since I've been outside."

Ruth Goldstein (age 65)

ANXIETY IS JUST another way of describing nervousness. Anxiety can be a positive influence on your life: controlled anxiety is what mobilizes people to get the job done, whether that means finishing a great painting or getting your child to the emergency room. Sometimes, however, anxiety can become a problem. A woman who is extremely anxious may have trouble sleeping, eating, or enjoying sex. She may find it difficult to relax and often has trouble going about her daily life in a constructive manner. Anxiety may be manifested in many different ways, including:

- Jitters
- Trembling
- Shakiness
- A sensation of a tight band around your head
- A sensation of muscles jumping under the skin

Anxiety can manifest itself as a phobia. A simple object may produce anxiety, such as a cat or snake or mouse or even a door, and when this anxiety response becomes habitual, this is considered a phobic reaction. One of the most well-known phobias is agoraphobia, or the fear of being in open places. Agoraphobia is most common among women. In some severe cases of agoraphobia, women retreat completely into their homes in order to avoid such anxiety attacks. Phobias are best treated with psychotherapy—sometimes in combination with medication.

351

Women sometimes experience anxiety as a reaction to a drug they are taking (such as diet pills or blood pressure medication), caffeine, or alcohol. If there is no medical reason for your anxiety, your doctor will probably begin to explore the possible psychological reasons. Anxiety is often caused by a recent event, such as moving or divorce.

If you think you may be suffering from anxiety caused by psychological reasons, you should talk to your doctor. Your doctor may want to prescribe a tranquilizer to be taken for a short period of time and, if you are going through a difficult period in life, may also recommend counseling. Tranquilizers belonging to the benzodiazepine group and called minor tranquilizers (including Valium, Xanax, Librium, Halcion, and Ativan) are most commonly prescribed for anxiety. They differ mainly in duration of effect, but their clinical effects are nearly identical. These drugs have a calming or sedative effect and are therefore often characterized as "downers." Like alcohol or barbiturates, tranquilizers work as central nervous system depressants. They are classified as sedative-hypnotics, which means that at low doses they produce minor sedation (giving a feeling of relaxation) and at higher doses they produce hypnosis or sleep. The minor tranquilizers are far and away the most widely prescribed psychiatric medications, and 65 percent of minor tranquilizer prescriptions are for women.

If you are depressed as well as anxious, certain tranquilizers including Valium can cause your depression to deepen. Thus, you should discuss all aspects of your condition with your doctor before taking tranquilizers.

Tranquilizers can be addictive and their effect for women may vary widely at different times of the month, depending on the hormone levels in your system. If you are taking other medications, you should discuss all of these with your doctor before beginning to take a tranquilizer. You should also abstain from alcohol because both alcohol and these medications may interact and be more toxic to your system than either one can be alone. They are also metabolized by the liver and combining them can damage your liver over time.

Tranquilizers are potent and they need to be taken with care, respect, and caution. In fact, addiction to these drugs may go unnoticed for long periods of time, since there may be no apparent symptoms of addiction. All the more reason you should be cautious if you choose to take such medication and be honest with yourself in analyzing why you are taking it and how dependent you are on your medication. Plan to use them as a short-term bridge—not a long-term solution.

The fear, obviously, is becoming a chronic user of tranquilizers. So try developing other methods of managing your anxiety, such as:

- Keep a record of when you become anxious so that you can begin to identify the causes of your anxiety.
- Review your daily habits and patterns to see what might be adding to your anxiety and what you might be able to eliminate from your diet or change in your lifestyle—such as excessive caffeine intake, lack of exercise, chronic sleep deprivation.
- Tell friends about your anxieties; expressing your fears may help lessen them, and others may help you achieve a sense of perspective regarding what is bothering you.
- Monitor your anxiety to see if it's tied to your menstrual period. If you think it is, avoid salt consumption before your period and try to exercise more in the days prior to menstruation. Both strategies can help lessen anxiety and other symptoms associated with premenstrual tension.
- Look into relaxation techniques and meditation. Yoga, meditation, and stress reduction programs are available in almost all communities or on tapes that you will be able to find easily in your community library or local video store. Treat yourself to a massage.
- If you feel that you suffer from chronic anxiety, consult your doctor, who will be able to help you find a reliable psychotherapist.
- If you have trouble finding a therapist, consult your local mental health association, local health department, or community health center for further assistance.

A Note on Prescription Drugs

"I know there's a stigma to taking an antidepressant. But after my husband died, it was the only thing that helped me get through the transition."

Esther Colton (age 68)

WHEN YOU NEED a medicine for a problem like manic-depression, it's like taking penicillin for a strep throat. You need the medicine and depend on it to carry on a normal life. It's not an addiction. At other times prescription drugs are addictive, which is one reason that it is so necessary to always let your physician know what you are taking. No matter what the case, treat all prescription medications with respect—whether they are classics like penicillin or the newest medicine on the block.

The most common new "miracle" drug is Prozac. It was introduced in 1988 as one of the latest in a new generation of antidepressants. It is sometimes referred to by therapists as the "P vitamin," and has been called the "pill of the year" by patients, doctors, and the press for the last few years. It now has FDA approval for treating depression, anxiety attacks, and certain eating disorders, and for aiding in weight loss. The particular excitement involving Prozac hinges on the drug's selectivity for serotonin—a chemical in the brain that triggers the pleasure center. This has led many to speculate that Prozac is less likely than other antidepressants to produce dangerous side effects. However, in some studies Prozac has been found to produce paradoxical reactions in patients. In these situations Prozac affects the individual as though it were a stimulant, such as cocaine or amphetamine, and it may be this quality that makes Prozac so popular. Prozac has also been linked with some dangerous side effects, including agitation, restlessness, and other signs of central nervous system disturbance. It should be treated with respect and not as a wonder drug or miracle cure.

If you are on a tranquilizer or antidepressant, such as Xanax, Valium, or Prozac, you should be under a physician's care and your use of the drug should be reviewed periodically. Long-term use of any prescription drug brings with it the possibility of addiction and may also make the drug less effective.

If you are experiencing personal problems and are considering medication, your doctor will want to ascertain whether your depression is chemical or situational in nature. If you suffer from a depression that has a physiological component, you may have to take medication in order to lead a normal life. If you and your doctor decide on temporary treatment of a situational depression (such as one caused by the death of a child or a particularly difficult divorce), you should consider this to be only a temporary solution. Remember that taking medication does not address the underlying problems, which may continue to trouble you unless you take the initiative to face your crisis. In addition, drugs can become part of the problem if they become a habit.

Women and Co-Dependency

"There is no evidence that co-dependent women are suffering from a disease. They are suffering from a lack of resources; they are embedded in a network of family and friends that makes escape very difficult."

Jacqueline Goodchilds, quoted in *The Mismeasure of Woman*

AS CAROL TAVRIS STATES in her enlightened book *The Mismeasure of Woman*, women are "crazy," while men have "problems." Nowhere is this more clearly demonstrated than in the diagnosis and treatment of the new, catchall condition "co-dependency." We live in a society in which "blame" and "illness" are associated with dependency or co-dependency, but not with extreme independence or hyper-independence—a trait quite common in many men. This is because we live in a society in which there is only a single standard of behaviors indicative of mental health, the male standard. Thus, women are more likely to be diagnosed as co-dependent simply because they are putting others first—as one must often do, for example, when raising children.

There are both good and bad ramifications for women in the development of the notion that the partners of those who act self-destructively also suffer. What is positive is that the partners too can get help. What is not so great about labels that designate behavior as aberrant or "sick" is that in this case thinking of yourself as sick is an entirely self-defeating way to begin to go about solving your problems and improving your life. Beware of suggestions that you are co-dependent and seek a second opinion. If you feel that co-dependence is really a problem for you, there are twelve-step programs geared to the issue of co-dependency. Consult Al-Anon or Alcoholics Anonymous in your area for recommendations regarding a program that is right for you.

If you are not sure that this is your problem, remember that co-dependency may be the most overused and least understood buzzword of the decade, and you should beware of anyone who wants to ascribe this term to you too readily.

Women and Self-Esteem

". . . There is really nothing innate or God-given about
self-esteem. It has to be learned along the way."

Linda Tschirhart Sanford, *Women and Self-Esteem*

MEN AND WOMEN both suffer from low self-esteem at one time or another. They just deal with it differently. But it is women who are routinely labeled as clinically "suffering" from low self-esteem. The *Diagnostic and Statistical Manual of Mental Disorders* (the equivalent of the *Physicians' Desk Reference* for mental illness) actually labels the condition as "self-defeating personality disorder." Self-defeating personality disorder and co-dependency are the two newest, most common, and indiscriminately applied labels used to describe the psychological complaints of women. A great deal of the description of this disorder would seem to describe a woman fulfilling her traditional roles well and for many would not seem to be an "illness" at all. It's important to remember that the diagnosis of mental illness is sometimes arbitrary and often subjective because so many of the descriptions of healthy personality adjustment depend upon male models. What matters is whether or not you can function creatively and constructively in the life that you have chosen for yourself. Thus, you are the best judge of whether or not you are chronically unhappy or unable to cope with the demands of life. Functioning well and being happy are the linchpins of a positive mental outlook. You know best when life isn't "working" for you and when you need help.

"Everyone thinks I'm the Rock of Gibraltar and I
really feel like a Fabergé egg."

Author

I DON'T HAVE one friend who hasn't confessed to feeling hit with a wave of low self-esteem at one time or another. For me it was when I was in my late thirties and recovering from a divorce, having moved to a new job and a new city and facing economic pressures. I put on my game face every day and pushed ahead—but inside I thought I would burst into tears if somebody looked at me cross-eyed. It was different from being depressed. I really questioned whether I would be able to keep up with the rest of the world. The fear of being left behind was enough to keep me going, but I knew that would last only so long. One day I realized that I couldn't separate the physical from the emotional exhaustion. I knew I needed help. I found a wonderful therapist and started working from the ground floor up. I also underwent a few sessions of hypnosis, which I credit with my successful turnaround. I don't think my story is unusual. In fact, I suspect my story is rather typical. And I'm sure I wouldn't be as content today if I hadn't sought help then.

Here are six key complaints of women who experience real problems regarding self-esteem:

1. The experience of the self is minimal. Women experiencing this lack of self seem to have difficulty describing themselves and often end up declaring that perhaps there is not much of a self there.

2. You dismiss yourself by saying, "So what if I'm a good person?" A woman who describes herself as a wife and mother, a kind and caring person—society's standard for a "good woman"—but doesn't feel good about herself may have chronic problems with self-esteem.

3. You discount what you are capable of by saying, "Sure, I can do that, but here's a list of everything I can't do and haven't accomplished." Women who judge themselves this harshly tend to have extremely high standards for themselves—standards that are so high they sometimes preclude the enjoyment of very real accomplishments.

4. You berate the accomplishment itself by saying, "Well, if I can do that, it can't be very hard or important." (This is the woman who, when told she is an excellent teacher, says, "Oh, well, teaching's easy.") By denigrating what you have accomplished, you take away the feeling of confidence and accomplishment from yourself.

5. You say to yourself and others, "Oh, you should have seen me ten years ago" or "I'm not really successful. I'm just lucky." This kind of undercutting of the self is often referred to as self-concept dislocation or the impostor syndrome. Somewhere along the line you convince yourself that your accomplishments are not earned—just due to luck. Such a situation may occur when a major event in a woman's life (such as divorce, a major illness, or the kids leaving home) forces a reevaluation of herself. This crippling kind of self-doubt often occurs after the loss of a loved one.

6. You experience a crisis of self-esteem by saying, "I used to know who I wanted to be, but now I'm not sure anymore." Many women raised with one standard of achievement have to reorganize how they see themselves in midlife and reexamine their priorities because they find themselves living in another world.

"Self" Improvement

Therapy is often helpful in addressing the issues that may be causing or adding to your low self-esteem, but therapy alone will not change your self concept. Only you can be responsible for your own individual growth. Whether this includes contemplating a career change, adding an exercise routine to your schedule, improving your diet, taking up a hobby, or simply reevaluating your expectations for yourself is an individual decision. The point is that improving your self-esteem is up to you.

Abuse and Domestic Violence

"You better get this straight. A man who hits you doesn't like you."

Annette Burin (age 57)

ANY WOMAN—old or young; tall or short; fat or thin; Asian American, African American, Caucasian, or Native American—can find herself battered by the man she thinks loves her. Women who are battered need help. They need to know there are people that they can talk to. They need to know that there is help available and that what has happened is not their fault and not something that should be kept secret.

If you are a battered woman (or know someone who is or might be), here are some facts about domestic violence that I hope will help you seek and find the help you need. I also hope they will bring domestic abuse out of the closet of hearth and home and into the bright light of public debate, intervention, legal restraint and appropriate rehabilitation.

- Domestic violence is the leading cause of injury to women.
- Domestic violence causes more deaths than muggings, rapes by strangers, and car accidents combined.
- Almost four million women are beaten by their male partners every year.
- Twenty-five percent or more of the women who are beaten every year in the United States are beaten while they are pregnant.
- When there is a complaint, police are more likely to file a report when the offender is a stranger than when he is an intimate.
- Every year at least three million children witness acts of domestic violence.
- The children of abused mothers are 50 percent more likely to abuse drugs and alcohol and six times as likely to attempt suicide.
- Over half of the women who are abused go on to abuse their own children.
- At least 50,000 women in the United States seek restraining orders every month.
- The majority of men who are abusers will not go voluntarily to batterers' programs.
- Despite the growing awareness of abuse, doctors and other health-care workers diagnose the situation correctly less than 5 percent of the time.

Here is the message: Domestic violence is a crisis in the United States. And perhaps the worst fact of all is that even with increasing public awareness, the situation itself does not seem to be improving. If you are a victim of domestic violence or know someone who may be, contact your nearest women's shelter. They will be able to help you figure out where to turn and how to get control of your life.

Rape

"When I was raped, it wasn't the degradation or humil-
iation that haunted me. I knew rape was a crime, not a
sexual act. I knew it wasn't my fault. And I fought hard
to keep from blaming myself and won. But what I
couldn't change or overcome with logic, love from my
true friends, or therapy was the fear. It took more than
a year for me to get over the feeling that every day I was
going to die."

Name withheld

THERE ARE MANY PLACES in a book on women's health where rape might be covered. Rape is a violent act; the physical damage a woman sustains may be great. But when a woman is raped she also suffers mentally. In fact, after a woman is raped she is at greater risk for all mental disorders except schizophrenia, and studies have found rape to be second only to military combat in terms of the psychological trauma that the victim suffers afterward. As we all know, rape is the only crime for which the victim is sometimes blamed. While such antediluvian attitudes are changing, this prejudicial view is yet another burden heaped on the woman who is recovering from a rape. Thus, because of the profound psychological toll that rape takes, it seems appropriate to focus attention on the subject within our section on mental health.

When it comes to women and rape, just enough progress has been made so that we are able, as a society, to see just how much *more* progress must be made in dealing with preventing this crime and helping survivors to recover and thrive. Rape involves a sexual act, but it is a crime of violence. Even though a rape victim is injured physically, she is also wounded psychologically—and wounded deeply. As with the survivors of disasters and wars, those who survive rape have their identities threatened at the very foundation. When a woman is raped, her autonomy is taken from her. Rebuilding that sense of autonomy becomes one of her

360

most difficult tasks. The recovery must involve not only physical but also psychological healing.

Rape has traditionally been defined as forced sexual contact with a stranger; date rape or acquaintance rape are the terms now used to cover forced sexual contact with someone you know. The facts regarding how many women have been raped are unclear. However, most studies on the incidence of rape indicate that approximately one fifth of all women experience at least one rape attempt in their lifetime.

We were shocked and outraged to find out what an epidemic breast cancer is among women. We need to apply the same strategy now when facing the statistics on rape: rather than fearing them, we need to move from shock to outrage and use our anger to spur efforts to prevent this crime.

Coping with Rape

"I did everything wrong. I felt so filthy and violated. I couldn't wait to get home and wash every part of him off me. I must have been in the shower for forty-five minutes. My skin was red I scrubbed so hard. I called the police about an hour later. They were nice but to the point. There was nothing they could do. I had washed all the evidence away."

Name withheld

IF YOU HAVE been raped, call the police or have someone make the call for you; or if you are not severely injured, go to the police station to report the crime. Also ask the police at once for the number of the nearest rape crisis center. Telephone the crisis center and request that someone meet you at the police station or hospital emergency room.

If you are at home, your first instinct may be to strip off your clothes and shower—but don't. Do not bathe or shower, because that will destroy the evidence of the rape. A careful examination and the retrieval of semen is necessary in order to provide DNA evidence against your attacker.

If you have concerns about birth control, discuss them with the rape crisis counselor and the doctor that you see. "Morning after" contraception is available at most urban or university-affiliated hospitals for rape survivors, and the spermicide Nonoxynol-9 may help prevent transmission of HIV. Since sexually transmitted diseases (STDs) sometimes do not have obvious symptoms, you should also be tested for these immediately and then have follow-up testing done to double-check for STDs. Because HIV can be transmitted during a rape you will need to be tested for the virus. It takes several weeks to six months for the virus to produce enough antibodies to be detected so a blood test should be performed a couple of times over the following months (some experts suggest being tested after one month and a second test after six months). You should also make plans to see a rape counselor for at least a six-month period after the rape occurred.

If you are raped, your sense of security is altered forever. Walking down a street, even in daylight, can be an agonizing experience, and riding an elevator alone with a stranger can seem an almost insurmountable task. For all rape survivors, dealing with the fear that rape breeds is one of the hardest tasks; it often seems impossible. A woman may feel that fear has become a permanent part of her makeup. But time and counseling will help—as long as you make your psychological recovery as important as your physical recovery. If you have been raped, it is as important to see a rape counselor or therapist as it is to see a medical doctor.

More and more therapists—including Mary Koss, Ph.D., of the University of Arizona, one of the country's leading experts on rape—compare the aftermath of rape to the post-traumatic stress disorder (PTSD) suffered by Vietnam War veterans. The symptoms associated with PTSD and rape recovery include nightmares, jumpiness, extreme anxiety, and difficulty sleeping. Just as combat veterans reexperience their trauma through flashbacks, nightmares, and unwanted images that may erupt in the mind at any time of the day or night, so rape victims may experience the event in this manner, years or decades after the event. Whatever the label, it should be clear to every rape survivor and her family and friends that the rape must be dealt with afterward: this is an essential aspect of the recovery and healing process.

Years ago, rape was a crime that was hidden in the closet. A woman who was raped suffered twice—first at the hands of her assailant, then in silence for long afterward. That silence was the fear of humiliation, for society taught that a woman who is raped will be ostracized. Thank goodness, this is no longer the case. If you have been raped, ask for the loving support of friends and family and the community and take pride in the fact that you survived. When rape happens to you, it isn't only your problem; it's society's problem too. Share your story, and you will help others.

Here are some suggestions that may help facilitate recovering from rape:

- Surround yourself with loving friends and family.
- See a rape counselor or therapist.
- Join a rape support group.
- Donate your time to a rape crisis center. Helping others will help you in your recovery.
- If you live alone and you are having trouble sleeping, arrange to spend nights with a friend for a week, two weeks, or more, until you begin to feel more comfortable.
- If you were raped in your home or apartment, consider the possibility of moving.
- Walk away from any situations that spell danger to you—do not feel compelled to prove you are brave. You've already proved that.

Pressing Charges

You do not have to make the decision to press charges right away, but if you do decide to press charges, you will need medical evidence to prove that you were raped. This is one reason that you should request that your initial physical examination be done by a physician who is trained in treating rape victims.

Pressing charges can be a grueling process, and some women feel that it would be too traumatic to do so. Others feel it is important to press charges, both for their own sense of justice and also to try to keep their attacker from attacking someone else. Nevertheless, those women who do press charges can feel as if they have been victimized twice, once by a criminal and then again by the criminal justice system. If you do decide to press charges, be prepared to be treated as if you were in some way an accomplice to the crime and be prepared for a lengthy questioning process that may feel like a cross-examination. (You may already have been through this phenomenon when you reported the crime.) These days, police officers do undergo sensitivity training, but it is still the case that people often feel uncomfortable around rape victims. Be prepared to encounter an unsettling experience and try to make sure a supportive friend accompanies you when you do press charges.

Coming to Terms with Blame

*"Deep down inside I knew the rape wasn't my fault. But
I kept yelling at myself that I shouldn't have been walking
to my car alone."*

Erica Damon (age 37)

RAPE IS A CRIME. The person who commits the crime is to blame, not the victim. True as this is, when it comes to the subject of rape, blame is not all that simple. Women may blame themselves because they are subtly (or not so subtly) held responsible or even accused by society. ("She shouldn't have been walking late at night," "She shouldn't have been wearing that outfit," "She shouldn't have been drinking in a bar" are all nothing less than veiled accusations.) Self-blame may play another role in a woman's recovery after rape. In some cases, women blame themselves in an effort to regain the all-important sense of autonomy that has been taken from them. To have a sense of autonomy, we must have some sense of control. For some women, blaming themselves gives them at least a reason (if a false one) for what happened. This helps restore the idea of the world as a safe place, and helps to restore equilibrium—but only initially. It's a false recovery.

If you've been the victim of rape, the best thing you can do (in addition to seeking help from a rape crisis center) is to tell yourself the truth: "A terrible thing happened to me, and it was not my fault." Telling yourself this will help you believe in yourself. Believing in yourself will help you during the recovery process. You must also place the blame where it belongs—on the perpetrator of the crime.

Preventing Rape

In most communities there are rape prevention lectures or courses or information that is provided through a local women's center. Here are some general rules for minimizing your risk.

If you are in your car:

- Lock the doors at all times.
- If you have car trouble, raise the hood of your car, then get back in your car, lock all doors, and wait for the police. Don't accept help from a stranger.
- At night, park only in well-lighted areas.
- Consider installing a phone in your car, especially if you are out a lot at night.

If you are at home:

- Keep the doors locked at all times.
- Use a peephole on your front door and don't let in anyone you don't know or who is unexpected (for example, a service or repair person you have not called for).
- Use initials on your mailbox, not a first name.
- Leave a radio and a light on when you are gone.

If you are on the phone:

- Do not give out personal information or your phone number to someone you don't know.
- Do not leave a message on your answering machine saying you are not home.
- Never leave a message on your answering machine indicating your name or that you live alone. It's better to leave a message like this: "You have reached 555-2985. Please leave a message and one of us will get back to you."
- Report any obscene phone calls.

Other preventive tips include:

- Don't be alone with someone on a first date. Meet in public places until you build up a level of trust.
- Don't walk or jog at night unless you are in a well-lighted, well-populated place.
- Carry Mace, if your state's laws permit it, pepper spray, or a whistle.
- Don't give out personal information—such as your address and phone number—to someone you have just met.
- Take a self-defense course. One is probably being taught in your community at this time.

Mental Health and Aging

"When I am old I shall wear purple."

Jenny Joseph, "Warning"

IT'S BEEN SAID in various ways, but "the golden years take stamina" says it well. I wish I could say it's a picnic growing older, but in fact it's hard work to do it well. One thing that helps is keeping your positive mental attitude intact. Attitude isn't everything, but it is one major component of the big picture. Taking care of your mental health, both at the crisis points in your life and in between, will help you take good care of your physical health; and taking care of your physical health by eating well and exercising regularly will in turn help keep your mental attitude a positive one.

There are times in life when a positive attitude is hard to come by and takes a lot of work to maintain, but it's worth it. When all else fails, just remember, the deck is *still* stacked against women, which is sometimes enough to drive you crazy. Well, don't let it. Remember, we're all in this together, and the more we challenge the dealer, the more we'll ensure a fair hand for all women when it comes to our mental well-being.

PART 8

THE BEST REVENGE IS BEING A HEALTHY WOMAN

"I hope Shirley MacLaine is right and we all get a crack at living life again. But just in case she's wrong, I'm not going to consider this a dress rehearsal."

Joy Snyderman (age 69)

Caregiver, Heal Thyself

"I carve out an hour or two for myself every week. This is sacred time. It's not for running errands or catching up on work. It's for me. It's quiet time. It allows me to be introspective and in that way I think it makes me a better person."

Melanie Jones (age 43)

A BOYFRIEND I WAS once crazy about said, "You can always rest when you're six feet under." That may be true but I've come to appreciate that if you don't rest sometimes, you'll probably end up six feet under sooner than you would like. I suspect I work as hard as anyone, but I've always played hard too. There's time for both in this life.

Have you found yourself saying any of the following?

- "I'm having too much fun to slow down."
- "I'll rest when I'm eighty."
- "When the kids get better, then I'll get sick."
- "I don't need a vacation, I like what I'm doing."
- "I don't have time for a relaxing bath, I only take showers."
- "What with getting the kids to and from afterschool sports and activities, I just can't fit exercise into my schedule."
- "Eating healthy takes too much time."
- "My husband would flip if I didn't serve desserts."
- "My husband smokes, so I smoke."
- "There's too much to do to sit down."
- "I actually don't like peace and quiet, I have to have the TV on all the time."
- "I'm not happy unless I'm busy."
- "Therapy [or massage, facials, pedicures, relaxation techniques . . . you fill in the blank] is self-indulgent."
- "I don't have time to go to the doctor."

If you think you've never uttered one of these paeans to giving care and not taking care, think again. You're not a normal, red-blooded American woman if you haven't uttered at least one of these verbal avoidance pills to keep yourself going. What, after all, is our superwoman but a kind of ultimate, universal caregiver? It's not enough to take care of a family, a small patch of land, and a job; you have to take care of the world—better yet, the universe.

I don't know about you, but I've found myself uttering a couple of those phrases over the years. I'm a working mom like everyone else— and I mean moms who work inside and outside of the home. I have a husband and three children. We women all look at one another's lives and imagine that someone else is living a more glamorous, a more controlled, a more fun life. But, actually, all of us juggle the fun stuff with the more mundane. I love my life, but I do admit to taking less than perfect care of myself some of the time. So every now and then, I stop and say to myself, "Hey, if you want to live to be eighty and *enjoy* being eighty when you get there, you'd better slow down." Then I sit down and breathe, literally. I take ten slow deep breaths and plan how to squeeze a little more time for myself and my family out of the next few days. It's always a struggle to figure out how to get enough work done during the day, preserve the family sit-down dinner, and keep enough energy and patience for bedtime stories. These are the balls in life that might not bounce back if I drop them once too often and that is always in the back of my mind. But also in the back of my mind is the ball signifying my physical health and peace of mind. I know that if I drop that once too often, it might not come bouncing back either. Like any mother, if I fall apart, so does a big chunk of my family.

> *"I've always considered it my role as a wife and mother to take care of my husband and children and to put their needs before mine. That's the reality of how I have defined myself. Does that mean that sometimes I've put my own health needs on the back burner? Sure. But that comes with the territory."*
>
> Rhea Myers (age 56)

D ON'T FORGET, real, substantial, lasting change occurs little by little and over time, not all at once or overnight. Some days work and some days don't. Life won't necessarily get easier if you start to take care of yourself, but it will get better. One thing I've found as a doctor, a mother, and a spouse that is puzzling, but true, is that it's easier to take care of someone else than it is to take care of yourself. Nonetheless, we women are the health-care providers of our families. We glean new medical facts, listen to our doctors, and get mates and children to their medical appointments. In the meantime, we struggle to make sure we don't fall through the cracks. So, I work on it constantly, because I expect be around and kicking up my heels a lot when I'm eighty.

I'm Not Dying, I'm Just Aging

"Women these days are in crisis because we're not in control of our health. But we can be in control. I snapped into it at thirty-nine. Now I realize the whole game isn't about being perfect. It's about being perfectly fit."

Joan Lunden

I N OUR CULTURE, we think of the normal aging process as a dreadful disease. However, the truth is that to age is human, and to enjoy it is divine, and the best way to ensure enjoying growing older is to take steps to stay healthy. To stay healthy, you have to take responsibility for your own health maintenance, even in an imperfect system. This includes practicing prevention before prescriptive medical measures are necessary. The cornerstone of prevention is surveillance, which includes appropriate screening measures for your age group and risk factors. The building blocks of maintenance include adequate and comprehensive nutrition, regular exercise, getting enough rest and sleep, minimizing your stress levels, and enhancing your health with other healthy habits and personal health care. While we need to improve our present health-care system, we also need to take advantage of what is right with it, and not allow ourselves to make a lot of poor excuses for not taking care of ourselves.

SELF-CARE MANTRAS

Here are some reminders for yourself, so that you'll devote enough time to take care of your own needs.

- I'll sit down while I drink this tea.
- I'll put my calls on hold while I eat my lunch.
- I'll walk home from work.
- I'll walk just to take a walk.
- I'll remember to breathe.
- I'll go to the gym instead of the movies.
- I'll go to the movies instead of the corner store for ice cream.
- I'll listen to classical music instead of the news.
- I'll take a bath and let my husband feed the kids.
- I'll drink herbal tea instead of a cup of coffee.
- I'll drink a glass of water on my coffee break.
- I'll aim for at least eight glasses of water a day.
- I'll skip the second glass of wine.
- I'll leave the company picnic early.
- I'll serve fruit for dessert.
- I'll hire a baby-sitter and plan to do *nothing*.
- I'll ask my husband to take the kids to the park and go get a massage.
- I'll call Mom, Dad, a special friend, a child away at school to say hi before they call me.
- I'll spend a little time dreaming.
- I'll like myself.

Checking Up on the Yearly Checkup

"I'm lucky. I have no family history of breast cancer, hypertension, or heart disease. But, while I might be ahead of the game, I know that's not enough and I still need to take care of myself."

Kathy Harreld (age 45)

WHEN I TALK to women around the country, I'm always surprised at how few actually see their physicians on a regular basis. I'm not a big believer in the annual exam where blood is drawn for every conceivable test, unless you have specific risks factors that make this essential. But I am a believer is having an established relationship with a doctor and being vigilant about diseases that you are at risk for. This approach to your health is better than a visit to the emergency room for a complaint that you might have been able to avoid by dealing with the problem earlier. I can't make you see your doctor. I know it's a drag to wait and wait and wait. I know he or she probably doesn't have time to answer all your questions, even when you are organized enough to bring your list and are ready to ask and listen. But I firmly believe that the relationship you have with your doctor is one of the most important relationships you can have in your life. And it is this constant connection that will help you monitor and correct aspects of your lifestyle that may damage your health as you grow older. There is nothing like a good witness.

How often to have a physical exam is a debatable issue. And who you should see is up to you. My gynecologist serves as my primary physician and I make sure that tests from other physicians are always sent to her. But you may decide on a family practitioner or an internist. As we age there are more reasons to see the doctor on an annual basis than there might have been when we were younger. Certainly if you have certain conditions—high blood pressure, a high LDL cholesterol level, diabetes mellitus, anemia, Lyme disease, arthritis, colitis, ulcers or other digestive disorders—you'll know what kind of schedule you should be keeping. Your yearly conversation with your doctor can also be used as a form of self-monitoring regarding your habits and lifestyle. This is one of the most important conversations you can have.

> *"Most of us take better care of our cars than we
> do our bodies."*
>
> Loralee Mathison (age 49)

I KNOW THERE ARE some things all of us would just as soon not know, even if they might do us some good. Some of us avoid seeing the physician because we're wary the doctor will find something wrong.

In short, we skip it because we are afraid. And some of us avoid physicians because we've been conscientious, had clear checkups for a couple of years, and see this year's checkup as a waste of time. The point of an *annual* physical examination is that it *is* annual. Consider it time to rotate the tires and check the oil. Think of it as your 40,000-mile checkup. Time-consuming as this may be, having a yearly record gives your doctor the most information regarding your health and the greatest chance of diagnosing any condition as early as possible.

Screening: The Key to Early Diagnosis and Successful Treatment

"I was thirty-six when my mother died. I have a family history of heart disease, cancer, lupus, and arthritis. So I'm constantly reminded about the importance of preventive care."

Melanie Jones (age 43)

IN THE MODERN medical world, screening tests are the first line of defense in terms of early detection and monitoring of disease. There are many kinds of tests that qualify as screening tests, from clinical breast exams, mammography, Pap smears, to exercise tests, invasive procedures, and imaging tests.

If you are forty and you have not already established an ongoing relationship with a doctor, you should. Your doctor will record your family history, risk factors, and past tests you are able to make available and decide what screening procedures are important for you to have on an ongoing basis. Now that you're over forty, you're going to want to stay current, not only on your Pap smears, but also other screening procedures that may pertain to your personal medical profile, such as:

- A first mammogram, if you have never had one.
- A yearly mammogram thereafter.
- A yearly pelvic exam with a bimanual evaluation—even if you have had a hysterectomy.

MAKING YOUR ANNUAL PHYSICAL WORK FOR YOU

Make your appointment for the morning, so that your doctor doesn't have as much time to run late.

Some questions should be asked when you make the appointment, or any time before the checkup. These include:

- What tests will I be given?
- May I eat breakfast?
- How long will the exam take?
- Will I be able to be reimbursed by my insurance company? (If you do not already know this.)
- When will you get my blood work back from the lab?
- What hours are you available for phone consultation, if I have questions?

Bring a list of your concerns with you so that you do not forget to ask the doctor about them. For example:

- I have joint pain in my fingers. Is this a sign of arthritis, carpal tunnel syndrome, some other condition?
- I've had periodic diarrhea over the past few months. Is there a test I should have?
- I've had an IUD through my thirties. Should I have my IUD removed? Change birth control methods? Keep using the same form of birth control?
- I have some moles that seem to be changing. Should I see a specialist?

Bring in a list of all the medications you are currently on or have stopped taking within the last month. List how often you take them and dosages. Remember to include over-the-counter medications, including aspirin.

If you are presently seeing other physicians, take along a list of their names, addresses, and telephone numbers.

- A test for colon cancer. This should be done yearly if you have a family history or any possible symptoms (if that is financially feasible). You should have this test periodically after the age of forty, since the risk for colon cancer increases.
- An annual or biannual cholesterol check, including the ratio of

HDL (good cholesterol) to LDL (bad cholesterol).
- A blood sugar evaluation, if you have a family history of diabetes or have had gestational diabetes.
- A periodic eye examination and, after the age of forty-five, yearly check for glaucoma.

Diet and Prevention: Making Food a Friend . . . Once and for All

"Never eat more than you can lift."

Miss Piggy

Food is not the enemy. Dieting may be. That airbrushed girl in the lissome pose (who doesn't really represent anybody anyway!) may be. Fried, processed, saturated, no-nutrient junk food may also be the enemy. But food is not the enemy. If you want to live well, you have to eat well. So, it's time to make friends with food once and for all.

I never said this would be easy. At least, it wasn't easy for me. I'm definitely a veteran of the food wars. Between medical school, my internship and residency, getting pregnant for the first time in my thirties and the second time in my forties, and doing live television, I've skipped every meal, eaten every meal twice, binged, dieted, and lived to tell about it. I lived on vanilla wafers and black coffee when I was doing my residency in pediatrics. I relied on graham crackers and peanut butter during my surgical training. I've been on liquid diets and protein diets—this week this diet, next week that diet. I've put on weight during pregnancy that was hell to take off. I've starved myself and pigged out. Add whatever you've done to this list, and I can say I would understand. And then I said, enough is enough. And I started making friends with food.

I started that process when I read an article about Martina Navratilova. After she immigrated to the United States her weight ballooned. She was in the dumps and trying to find the source of her unhappiness. According to the article, Martina made a list for herself: the things she liked about herself in the first column and the things she didn't in the second. Much to her surprise, she put almost all of her qualities in the plus column and only one in the negative column: her weight. So she set out to change it.

I did the same thing. I made my own list—and came to a similar conclusion. That was it. I knew that if I could accomplish all these other things in my life, I could conquer this too. So now I have an easy rule. I regard food as fuel. I eat foods I like—even some things that might not be so good for me. But I eat in moderation and exercise to keep everything in balance. Do I have the perfect body? Far from it— but I know I'm healthy.

Diet and Nutrition

"Do hamburgers, french fries, and ketchup count as three basic food groups?"

Rachel Snyderman (age 7)

In 1894, nutrition history was made and no one paid attention. William O. Atwater of the United States Department of Agriculture proposed guidelines for a healthy diet that are remarkably similar to what nutritionists are talking about today. He suggested that men who do "moderate work" get 33 percent of their calories from fat, 15 percent from protein, and the rest from carbohydrates. Somewhere his advice got lost and we were on our way to a diet that has become increasingly higher in fat and low on carbohydrates. It has not been a good trade-off.

Today Americans eat 37 percent of our calories from fat and we have the diseases to prove it. A high-fat diet has been linked to some of the leading causes of death, including heart disease, cancer, and stroke.

It was not until 1968 that Atwater's suggestions resurfaced; that year the American Heart Association suggested lowering fat consumption to 30 percent of total daily calories. Today, it has been suggested that even 30 percent is too high and that we should aim for 20 to 25 percent. Fat has become the scourge of the American diet. We need some, but not nearly as much as we consume.

Now we've revised things again with the food pyramid. Who hasn't heard of it? It's even in my daughter's Brownie handbook. Much to the chagrin of the Dairy and Beef Associations, it flip-flops what most of us have been doing. The pyramid recommends six to eleven servings of grains. For most women six servings a day is the target. (Reserve the eleven servings for your teenage boy!) But therein lies another problem.

377

What in the world is a "serving"? For the ice cream manufacturer, it may be half a cup of ice cream, because that makes the fat and calorie contents appear low on the nutritional label. But I might consider half a pint to be more to my liking. And when was the last time you really looked at the serving size on the box of cereal? It's a joke. If you eat what they recommend, you'll be ravenous by nine-thirty! This is the first place to start sleuthing. More on that later.

So let's start with the basics. What is fat? How much do we really need? And how in the world should we keep track of it? It may seem complicated, but with a couple of tools this is a slam dunk.

First, fat is fat is fat. You can talk about olive, peanut, or safflower oil, but each has 120 calories and 14 grams of fat per tablespoon. All oils are cholesterol free. With that said, some fats are better for you than others. Olive oil and canola oil have more monounsaturated fat than the others. Corn and safflower oil have more polyunsaturated fats. Why does this matter? Because using the right oils sparingly helps prevent raising low-density lipoproteins (LDL), the cholesterol that contributes to atherosclerosis (fat deposits in the arteries) and consequently contributes to heart disease and stroke.

Fat Facts

SATURATED FATTY ACIDS

These fats are the main culprit in raising LDL, the bad cholesterol. They are primarily found in meats and dairy products. Many of these foods also contain cholesterol. So try to limit your amount of beef, veal, lamb, pork, beef and poultry fat, butter, cream, milk (except skim milk), and cheeses and other dairy products made from whole milk. The other source of saturated fatty acids is from plants, including palm and coconut oils and cocoa butter.

The American Heart Association recommends that you limit your saturated fatty acid intake to less than 10 percent of total calories each day. The less the better.

POLYUNSATURATED AND MONOUNSATURATED FATTY ACIDS

Unsaturated fatty acids are often found in the liquid oils that come from vegetables. Common sources of polyunsaturated fats include sesame, sunflower, and safflower oils; sunflower seeds; and corn and soybeans and their oils. Monounsaturated fats come from avocados and olive, canola, and peanut oils.

Both polyunsaturated and monounsaturated fats are better than saturated fats, because they may aid in lowering cholesterol. But remember that they are still fats and should still be used sparingly.

The American Heart Association recommends that you limit polyunsaturated fats to no more than 10 percent of total calories.

Now I should admit to you that I have an ongoing love affair with olive oil. I love the taste and, since it is an unsaturated fat, it may play an ongoing role in keeping my LDL in check. Because it's so flavorful, I think one uses less. I use it for everything now—from salads to stir-fries. Get the extra-virgin oil and keep it next to your stove with the salt and pepper. You'll be surprised how much you come to depend on it.

The bottom line is that if you depend on olive or canola oil, you're ahead of the game—just remember to use them sparingly. You can also rely on vegetable sprays. But watch out for tricks. Remember that any oil that claims to be "cholesterol free" is trying to pull one over on you. *All* oils are cholesterol free, because they come from plants and plants don't have cholesterol. Watch out for olive oils that claim to be "light." They are light only in color and flavor. Calorie and fat content are consistent among the oils: 120 calories and 14 grams of fat per tablespoon.

The major vegetable oils include olive, canola, corn, safflower, sesame, soybean. They're low in saturated fatty acids and are the best to use. Olive and canola are the real standouts. Peanut oil has slightly more saturated fat, so it should be used only occasionally and sparingly.

DECREASING FAT IN YOUR DIET

Stay away from hydrogenated shortenings, since they are higher in saturated fats. And avoid lard, period. It's high in saturated fat and cholesterol and just not good for you.

California's Project Lean reports that while black and white women consume similar amounts of fat, they get it from different sources. White women tend to eat more cheese, butter, margarine, and nuts. Black women get their fat from fried fish and poultry, hot dogs, cold cuts, and whole dairy products. Hispanic women eat slightly more fat, with most coming from whole milk.

Fat is a high-calorie item. Each gram of fat is 9 calories; by contrast, a gram of carbohydrate is 4 calories. This means that gram for gram fat contains two and a quarter times more calories than carbohydrates.

The problem with fats is trying to keep track of what you put in your mouth. So I'll give you two ways to do it. First, the "real" formula, and then my way.

The formula really isn't that tricky. Figure out how many calories you need to eat in a day. For the average woman 1500 calories a day should do it. Multiply that number by 0.3 since 30 percent of your calories should come from fat. Then divide that number by 9 since there are 9 calories in each gram of fat. That will give you the total number of fat grams you should eat in one day.

So it works like this:

1500 cal × 0.3 = 450

450 ÷ 9 = 50

You should eat no more than 50 grams of fat per day.

It's okay to use 50 grams of fat as your absolute limit, but aim lower. Enough fat creeps into the diet anyway, so if you aim for 20 grams of fat it gives you some leeway if the number ends up closer to 30.

It's always good to keep a food diary, but I would be lying to you if I told you that doing so has worked for me. If you find keeping a written record cumbersome, try my way instead. Get a deck of cards. For every gram of fat you eat, peel off one card. If your limit is 40 grams you know you should have 12 cards left over at the end of the day. I know that on my most extravagant day I could spend more cards than are in that deck. Most days, I'm happy to have only counted out half of them. Of course, this requires that you know the fat content of the foods you are eating . . . and for the most part that is easy. There are small paperback books that can give you the calorie and fat content of most foods; the FDA-required labeling on commercially prepared foods makes the task simple.

Cholesterol

You can't have survived the last fifteen years without having the word "cholesterol" driven into your consciousness. It's everywhere and in some cases has been maligned. As with fats, some of it is good but too much can be a killer.

Cholesterol comes from two sources: foods and your liver. Foods that contain cholesterol include meats, dairy products, and egg yolks. Plant foods like fruits and vegetables don't contain cholesterol. Your liver has the ability to take some fats and convert them to cholesterol in your liver.

You need some cholesterol. This fatlike substance keeps your cell membranes intact, allows nerves to work, and plays a role in your hormones.

THE GOOD GUYS: HDL CHOLESTEROL

HDL is high-density lipoprotein. This type of cholesterol is produced primarily in the liver. It's believed that HDL tends to carry cholesterol away from the arteries and back to the liver, where it is removed from the body. HDL protects against heart disease and stroke. It's considered the "good" cholesterol because of its protective properties. A high level of HDL seems to protect against heart disease; a low level of HDL is considered a risk factor for heart disease.

THE BAD GUYS: LDL CHOLESTEROL

Low-density lipoprotein (LDL) is the primary carrier of cholesterol in the bloodstream and plays a role in heart disease and stroke. It is called the "bad" cholesterol because a high level predisposes a person to disease. A low level of LDL is what all of us should aim for. When there is too much LDL circulating in the blood, it clings to arteries and starts to form the plaque that can reduce blood flow to vital organs (especially the heart and the brain). This is atherosclerosis.

KEEPING TRACK OF CHOLESTEROL

Checking your total cholesterol level is a great idea but relatively worthless if you don't have it broken down into the HDL and LDL components. You could have a low cholesterol level with a high LDL count—this still puts you at risk for heart disease. Conversely, you could have a relatively high total cholesterol but find that a major portion of that is HDL, which protects you against heart disease. Here are the guidelines:

Total Serum Cholesterol	Classification
Less than 200 mg/dl	Desirable
200–239 mg/dl	Borderline
240 mg/dl or higher	At risk

LDL Cholesterol	Classification
Less than 130 mg/dl	Desirable
130–159 mg/dl	Borderline
160 mg/dl or higher	At risk

HDL Cholesterol	Classification
40–50 mg/dl	Desirable
Less than 35 mg/dl	At risk

Triglyceride Levels	Classification
Less than 200 mg/dl	Normal
200–400 mg/dl	Borderline high
400–1000 mg/dl	High
Greater than 1000 mg/dl	At risk

People with high triglycerides usually have low HDL and are at increased risk for cardiovascular and cerebrovascular disease.

The Role of Western Culture

The Western world has so many medical advances and has refined so many things in life. However, it's the fact that our diets are also refined that gets us into trouble. I remember a lecture in medical school given by an older professor who had traveled the world and studied how nutrition affects diseases. He showed a slide of a pile of grains and fruits and vegetables and an equals sign that led to a picture of a large bowel movement. The next slide showed meats and dairy products and an equals sign that led to a picture of a small bowel movement. His point? That we in the Western world eat refined diets with very little fiber and

roughage and that we have small bowel movements and a high incidence of colon cancer. Compare that with people in many third world
countries, where the basis of the diet is grains and the incidence of
colon cancer is very low. The premise is that large, bulky stools help
carry by-products and toxins out of the body, thus keeping them from
settling in the bowel, where they can trigger a cancer.

How we eat affects our risk for colon cancer, heart disease, and
perhaps other cancers, including esophagus, stomach, and breast. We
eat too much fat and too little fiber, and we lead lives that are too
sedentary. It wasn't always that way, but now those habits are part of
our profile. It happened gradually over the past few decades and now
we are paying the price.

From Paul Prudhomme to Dean Ornish

Dr. Dean Ornish took on the medical establishment and has proven
that a nonfat diet and an exercise program can *reverse* heart disease.
He has had his skeptics, but his patients are living testimonies to the
fact that what you put in your mouth has a direct effect on your
heart. Ornish suggests that if you stick with a nonfat vegetarian diet,
enough fat will slip in anyway to take care of your bodily needs and
at the same time you'll be lowering your risk of heart disease, stroke,
and cancer.

Unfortunately, I admit to having consumed the typical American
diet for too many years. I have also eaten according to Ornish's suggestions. For me the best route is somewhere in the middle. I try to eat no
more than 20 grams of fat a day. That means that some days I'll come
in lower, but it also allows me to splurge every once in a while and
know that I'll be able to make it up on another day. It also takes the
angst out of trying to be perfect. Averaging things out over a long time
is the best approach to sane eating habits for me.

I am not a vegetarian, but I do limit the amount of meat we eat in
our house. Our limits encompass not only the number of days we have
meat but also the size of portions. And this will be no shock to you, but
the portions we are accustomed to eating in the United States are too
big. Get out your deck of cards again. That deck is about the same size
as three ounces of meat, which is the portion size you should shoot for.
If you think your plate looks empty with a meat portion this size, do

what the Europeans do and eat off a smaller plate. For most of us, a salad plate is a better choice than a standard dinner plate.

The Hunt for Hidden Fat

Fat is lurking everywhere—in places where you would least expect it. Many food manufacturers don't make it easy on us. In fact, sometimes I think they are the root of the confusion.

Another important consideration is that fat tastes good. It gives our food depth and richness. Our bodies tend to crave it at times. And I'm a believer in indulging when the time is right.

The problem comes when we approach each meal as if it's our last! So remember, diversify. Sprinkle the not-so-good-for-you stuff through your diet. It's a lot like investing money. You wouldn't put all your money in one stock—you diversify. So do the same with your food— diversify. Have a sound basic diet and then enjoy the indulgences as they arise.

The grocery store is full of land mines. It will take a little longer to shop as a sleuth the first time, but once you know the pitfalls you'll find this hunt easy and fun. Soon, it will be second nature.

PITFALLS

- *Oils* that are labeled as "light" or "cholesterol free." One particular oil can't be any lighter in fat than another because they all contain 14 grams of fat per tablespoon. The only thing they'll be light on is color or taste. They're all cholesterol free, since they come from plants and plants have no cholesterol.
- *Fat-free foods* still contain calories and the serving sizes may be deceptively small. So read the labels carefully.
- *Cholesterol-free pronouncements* may not be telling the whole truth, since foods can be cholesterol free and still contain fat.
- *Packaged pasta* can sabotage any good eating plan. Beware of macaroni and cheese and prepared rice mixtures that can be loaded with fat and salt.
- *Muffins and croissants* can be deadly. This is a great time for you to do a little science experiment. Sacrifice one of those muffins. Put one in your hand and squeeze it. Really squeeze it between your fingers and then look at your hand. You'll be shocked to see how

RISK FACTORS FOR HEART DISEASE

Age over 55

History of premature menopause without estrogen replacement

Family history of heart disease

Smoking

Diabetes

High blood pressure

HDL cholesterol less that 35 mg/dl

the palm of your hand glistens with fat—the fat that was hidden in what you assumed was a healthy food. One additional note on muffins: a muffin has approximately 250 calories, while a *small* bagel has half the calories.

- *Crackers* can be loaded with fat and have very little nutritional value. Stick to bread, or look for the imported flatbread crackers that are low in fat and sodium.
- *Granola* sounds healthy but is usually top-heavy with fat and sugar. There are some fat-free varieties on the market but I think that's exactly what they taste like. My advice is to look for something else. Many of the presweetened cereals are okay if you want to use them as topping for ice cream, but they don't pack much nutritional value.
- *Avocados* are the exception to the rule that produce is your Garden of Eden. Two tablespoons of avocado has 4 grams of fat and about 45 calories! This is now one of those foods I usually avoid.
- *Dried fruits* can be good in a pinch but they can be high in calories— about 80 calories per ounce. Banana chips contain coconut oil.
- *Processed meats* contain some of the most deceptive labels around. Beware of "low fat," "lean," and "reduced fat." You will have to do your homework here and read the labels carefully. Each serving size

should get less than 30 percent of its calories from fat. You'll find this information on the nutritional label. And beware those turkey and chicken franks. They sound healthier but may contain gobs of fat. So, again, check the labels carefully. Stay away from organ meats, which are very high in cholesterol. Prepared seafood salads can be loaded with mayonnaise.

- *Dairy products* are notorious for hiding fat. We know we need calcium and that dairy products are a great source. The trade-off in fat may not be worth it, however. There is no reason to drink whole milk. Nonfat milk provides all the nutrients and calcium and none of the fat. Eight ounces of whole milk has the fat equivalent of two pats of butter.
- *Juices* are convenient and taste great but don't have the fiber of the original fruit. And the ready-to-drink juices may contain more water and sugar than fruit juice.
- *Canned foods* can be tricky, so read these labels carefully. Beware of lots of additives and extra sodium. When you can, buy fresh instead.
- *Mayonnaise* can have as many as 75 calories per tablespoon—and it's fat. If you like commercially prepared salad dressings, make sure you read how much fat is in a serving and remember that a serving size may be only 1 tablespoon.
- *Cookies* have become a hot item because of the onslaught of the nonfat varieties. Just remember that fat free does not mean calorie free.
- *Popcorn* that is prepackaged or microwaved can be loaded with fat, calories, and salt.
- *Frozen desserts* that profess to be "light," "low cholesterol," or "reduced fat" may not be any of these. Check calories and fat content very carefully and beware of any dessert bar that is dipped in chocolate.

BEST BETS

- **Pasta, Grains, and Dry Beans.** Forget all those crazy myths that carbohydrates are bad for you. These foods should be the mainstay of any good diet. They are not fattening and are loaded with nutrients and fiber; they also taste great. On the whole these foods are low in fat and calories and are filling (however fresh pasta and egg noodles have some cholesterol). Dry beans are the richest source of fiber. Keep eggless dry pasta on hand in all kinds of shapes and sizes. Brown rice is better than white rice, because it contains more fiber and more than three times the amount of vitamin E.

- *Bread, Bread, and More Bread.* I think bread is one of the greatest gifts on earth. It has been used by various civilizations for centuries and should be consumed with great joy. Bread is not fattening. It's what we put on it that does us in. It is the cornerstone of diets all over the world where obesity is rarely encountered. Today you can get fresh breads in cities and many smaller towns. If there's not a good bakery nearby, look for breads with at least 2 grams of fiber per slice. Whole-wheat pitas and breadsticks are terrific. If you like tortillas, corn tortillas are lower in fat and sodium than their flour counterpart. (Some people are more sensitive to carbohydrates than others and will need to adjust their bread intake accordingly.)

- *Cereals* can be an easy place to get good nutrition and still find something good to eat. The new nutritional labels make this hunt easy. Look for a natural grain cereal that is low-fat or nonfat. Oatmeal and cream of wheat are great.

- *Produce* is one area where you can do almost no harm. Try to eat five servings a day of fruits and vegetables, which have more vitamins and nutrients than any other food. Foods that are rich in vitamin C offer protection from cancer and help absorb iron from food. The best are broccoli, peppers, citrus fruit, strawberries, kiwi, cantaloupe, and tomatoes. Broccoli may be the perfect vegetable. It's high in vitamin C and may help prevent cancer. Members of the cruciferous family—including cauliflower, cabbage, and kale—are another great bet.

- *Seafood* is great, but if you're trying to watch your cholesterol, shy away from lobster, shrimp, and squid.

- *Fresh turkey and chicken* go without saying, but stick with white meat, of course.

- *Lean meat* should be the goal, so ask for the loin or round. Extra-lean ground beef is usually 15 percent fat.

- *Dairy products* are now responding to consumer demand. You can find healthy low-fat alternatives in your dairy case. Look for part-skim cheeses and nonfat yogurts. This is one place where the nonfat stuff tastes just as good as the real thing. However, watch out for low-cholesterol cheeses, which can be loaded with hidden fat and calories.

- **Juices** that are frozen or not reconstituted are the best. And any pulp will at least offer a little fiber.
- **Canned foods** are a great convenience. If you shop selectively, these can be healthy and good for you. Pick the canned fruits in natural juices instead of the heavy syrup. Canned sardines and salmon are good sources of calcium and protein.
- **Condiments** can add a lot of zest to your food. Start experimenting with mustards and fresh spices. You'll find your food will taste better.
- **Cookies** don't have to be avoided if you stick to fig bars, animal crackers, ginger snaps, or graham crackers.
- **Popcorn** is a great snack when it is air popped (which I confess I don't like) or popped with a scant amount of oil. There are a few good low-fat microwave popcorns on the market.
- **Frozen desserts** offer all kinds of options. The sorbets that are fat free are delicious. Some nonfat ice cream knockoffs are better than others. If you can't find a nonfat product you like, it's okay to occasionally give yourself a treat and eat a small portion of the real thing.

WISH I HADN'T DONE THAT . . .

How many times have you eaten something only to find out later the amount of fat and calories you put away? It's easy to consume much more than you suspect. So the next time you're reaching for a little something, keep these examples in mind.

- One-half cup of M&M's has 440 calories and 22 grams of fat. Imagine scooping two tablespoons of fat in your mouth—that's the equivalent.
- One avocado has 265 calories and 26 grams of fat. One avocado has the same amount of fat as eight strips of bacon. So the next time you're eating that guacamole . . .
- One-half cup of mixed nuts has 64 grams of fat. That's like putting 5½ tablespoons of Crisco into your mouth.
- Regular microwave popcorn contains 33 grams of fat per bag.

CALORIE COMPARISONS PER OUNCE

Vegetables	5–10
Fruits	15–20
Lean meats	25–50
Bread	75
Fat	200

Tips for Eating Out

Eating out is almost a national pastime. The average person eats more than one out of every five meals away from home. That translates into eating about 20 percent of total calories away from home. If you don't want to overdo it when you go out, have a low-fat snack before you leave to curb your appetite. If you don't know the restaurant, call ahead and ask if they can prepare low-fat options for you. Choose a restaurant that offers a variety of foods, and, if you're not sure how a dish is prepared, ask. In most cases you can ask for substitutions and have heavy sauces or butter left off. Be sure to make your choices clear to the waiter or waitress.

Not too long ago I was lucky enough to have dinner in Paris with Julia Child. Anyone who knows anything about Julia appreciates that she loves food with a passion—and that means the real thing, not low-fat and nonfat substitutes that so many Americans are devouring. So we had wine, which she fervently believes is good for the palate, the digestion, and, yes, the heart. And the four people at the table ordered a variety of food: I had chicken; Julia had lamb kidneys. I confess that Julia's choice would have never crossed my mind. Organ meats are rich and are high in cholesterol. But here's the catch: Julia ate only enough to satisfy her desire for the meat. She didn't clean her plate. She tasted and enjoyed. There's a lesson for all of us. Consider yourself done with a meal when you feel satisfied—not when you feel stuffed.

GOOD SUBSTITUTIONS

Start thinking and eating creatively. Ask yourself how you can get as much taste with less fat and fewer calories. Keep in mind that most produce is fat free and all fruits and vegetables are cholesterol free. If you're not sure about a particular food indulgence, ask yourself whether it's so good that it's worth wearing it! Here are some substitutions to consider.

- Mustard for mayonnaise
- Applesauce for oil
- Nonfat vanilla yogurt for topping
- Trail mix for granola bars
- Two egg whites for a whole egg
- Chilled, whipped evaporated skim milk for whipped cream

Why You Should Know How to Read a Label

You can't really figure out what you're eating if you don't know how to read a nutritional label. And finally the Food and Drug Administration has made it easier. Most foods in your grocery store have these labels and an ingredient list and now there's pressure to include them on those foods that aren't prepackaged, too. The labels are consistent and once you get used to reading them you'll find it unbelievably easy. Now foods can make certain healthy claims only if they fit these government criteria:

- Fat free means fewer than 0.5 grams of fat per serving.
- Low-fat means 3 grams of fat or fewer per serving.
- Lean refers to foods containing fewer than 10 grams of fat (4 grams of saturated fat) and 95 mg of cholesterol per serving.
- Light ("lite") means one third fewer calories, or no more than one half the fat of the higher-calorie, higher-fat version, or no more than one half the sodium of the higher-sodium version.
- Cholesterol free refers to foods that contain fewer than 2 mg of cholesterol and 2 grams or fewer of saturated fat per serving.

To make any inference about preventing heart disease, the food must be low in fat, saturated fat, and cholesterol. To make reference to being good for blood pressure and sodium, the foods must be low in sodium.

WHAT'S BIG TO YOU IS SMALL TO ME!

Always check the serving size before you begin calculating any of these nutritional numbers. If you don't know how much you are putting in your mouth, the process is worthless. Are you talking about two cookies or half the box? It sure makes a difference. Then look at the number of grams of fat. Fat is fat, so the overall number is important. But also note how much saturated fat makes up the total because this is the fat that clogs arteries. Then look at the percentage of total calories that the fat makes up. It should be less than 30 percent. Figuring out the percentage can be a little tricky so I always fall back on trying to limit the total number of fat grams. It's faster and easier.

HOW TO READ A LABEL

- *Serving Size.* Begin with serving size and make sure you understand what a half cup looks like. Make sure your serving size is the same as the one on the label, or all the information will be thrown off. If your serving size is twice as big you'll need to double the numbers.

- *Calories.* Figure this into your total caloric needs for the day.

- *Total Fat.* Look at this one hard and aim low. If you can, try for 20 grams a day, but never more than 50 grams a day. Look at the total and figure that into your daily allotment.

- *Saturated Fat.* This is the part of the total fat that contributes to heart disease and atherosclerosis. It is listed separately because it's the risky element. Nonetheless, count the total fat number when you are adding up your daily fat grams.

- *Cholesterol.* Eat less than 300 mg per day.

- *Sodium.* Salt or sodium—you can call it whatever you want to. It can play a role in high blood pressure and is something you should keep your eye on. Keep your daily intake low; 2400 to 3000 mg a day is a worthy aim, and less is even better.

- **Carbohydrates.** When you cut down on fat, you can eat more carbohydrates.

- **Protein.** Most of us get more protein than we need. Animal proteins are accompanied by fat and cholesterol. Aim for vegetable protein when you can.

- **Fiber.** Roughage or fiber—it's all good for your digestion. You really can't overdo it here.

- **Vitamins and Minerals.** Your goal should be to get 100 percent of these nutrients every day. Most of us don't. So supplement with a vitamin tablet and more calcium.

- **Daily Value.** This is intended to make the interpretation easier. I think it's confusing. The values are based on diets of 2000 or 2500 calories per day. I don't know many women who eat that many calories a day on purpose. So my advice is to look past this column.

My bottom line is to look at the serving size to make sure that's how much you want. Check the calories. Will the amount fit in to what you need to get along? Then look at the fat content and add the number of grams to what you've already consumed. Just peel off the correct number of cards and remember: you have only fifty to spend each day.

The Exercise Alliance

"Just do it."

Nike ad

YOU'VE HEARD IT all before, I know, and it does get monotonous. You've been practically brainwashed regarding the health benefits of a low-fat diet and consistent aerobic exercise. It goes without saying that exercise will never be as easy to take as a chocolate éclair and a good book (or whatever your favorite pleasure may be), but nonetheless we are going to have to get with the program. I'm sorry to say that many women still seem to be tuning out when the benefits of exercise are mentioned. I was startled when I read that no less than 34

Nutrition Facts

Serving Size $^1/_2$ cup (114g)
Servings Per Container 4

Amount Per Serving

Calories 90   Calories from Fat 30

% Daily Value*

Total Fat 3g	5%
Saturated Fat 0g	0%
Cholesterol 0mg)	0%
Sodium 300 mg	13%
Total Carbohydrate 13g	4%
Dietary Fiber 3g	12%
Sugars 3g	
Protein 3g	

Vitamin A	80%	• Vitamin C	60%
Calcium	4%	• Iron	4%

*Percent Daily Values are based on a 2,000 calorie diet. Your daily values may be higher or lower depending on your calorie needs:

	Calories	2,000	2,500
Total Fat	Less than	65g	80g
Sat Fat	Less than	20g	25g
Cholesterol	Less than	300mg	300mg
Sodium	Less than	2,400mg	2,400mg
Total Carbohydrate		300g	375g
Fiber		25g	30g

Calories per gram:
Fat 9   •   Carbohydrate 4   •   Protein 4

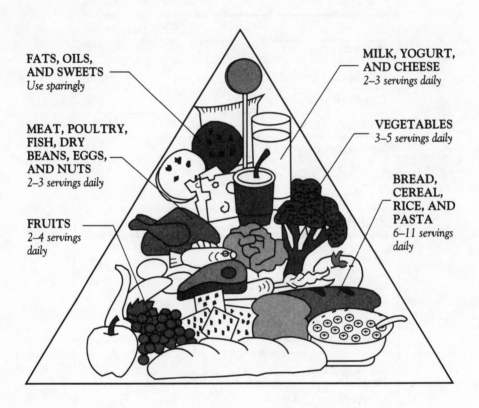

**FATS, OILS,
AND SWEETS** —
Use sparingly

**MEAT, POULTRY,
FISH, DRY
BEANS, EGGS,
AND NUTS** —
2–3 servings daily

FRUITS —
*2–4 servings
daily*

**MILK, YOGURT,
AND CHEESE**
2–3 servings daily

VEGETABLES
3–5 servings daily

**BREAD,
CEREAL,
RICE, AND
PASTA**
*6–11 servings
daily*

percent of women do *nothing* to keep fit and 50 percent of women consider themselves to be overweight. This isn't good, and we have to change it.

You don't have to join a gym. You don't have to become an aerobics fanatic. Just walk. Whenever possible avoid your car. Walk. Walk and breathe.

Training for the Second Forty Years of Life

"My daughter kept nagging me, until finally—at the age of seventy-two—I got on a bicycle. I hadn't been on one since I was a kid. I started slowly and worked up gradually. Now I ride almost every day. My energy level is the best it's been in years. There's nothing like it.

Natalia Shorenstein (age 73)

THERE'S A SAYING in karate that to make a friend of an enemy is a great victory. This may be the best way to approach aging. One way to begin to turn the aging process from foe to friend is through exercise.

The attitude to take is that it's never too late to get better at being yourself, and taking an active role in your body's aging process can give you a sense of control and inspiration as well as improve your health. If you're feeling overwhelmed by the prospect of adding an exercise program to your already hectic life and if you are feeling defeated by the years of inactivity you've already accumulated, don't say, "Oh well, I've lost that battle." Any amount of painless, non-weight-bearing exercise that you add to your daily routine at any age will help maintain your health and help minimize the risk of stress fractures and immobility. The research is clear—nothing improves life and life expectancy more than exercise. So do it, you'll feel better. Don't consider it a choice.

Personally, I love to hike and walk and do it every weekend with my husband and children. But during the week I can't always get away from the house. With the children here, I've had to figure out how to exercise at home—since I can't find the time in the day to run to a gym. So every year for the past few I've given myself a piece of exercise equipment for Christmas. I now have a stair machine, a treadmill, a stationary bike, and free weights. I admit I have a very short attention span—so I usually have the television and a magazine to keep me from getting bored. I find if the machine's right there, I avoid making excuses about not having enough time or not wanting to drive all the way to the gym. When it comes to exercise, I try not to give myself an easy way out. When I travel, I stay at a hotel or motel that provides a health club for its guests, and I use it.

> *"Do I have time for exercise? No—but I make time. I run first thing in the morning or I don't seem to get it in. I run because I feel better. I'm more resilient, more effective, and less testy. Exercise is a personal test of whether I have any control over my life. It is time for me—and I don't have to share it with anyone."*
>
> Diana Walsh (age 51)

SINCE I STARTED exercising regularly, I've felt better and had more energy—and you know what? If I skip exercising for more than a day or two, I miss it. If you had told me I'd miss exercising ten years ago, I'd have said, you're crazy, but now, I know better.

Do What Comes Naturally

I think what happens to a lot of people is that they regard exercise as something like climbing Mount Everest—you've got to get there first, you'll need a lot of equipment, and the goal is almost insurmountable and relentlessly time-consuming. Of course, nothing could be further from the truth. Exercise can be as simple and pleasant as a long, brisk walk on the beach or around the block. Ask yourself, "Do I need a car for this errand, or can I walk?" All you have to do is get out there and walk and keep up your pace. Or go to the gym and walk on the treadmill, listening to music. Don't be overwhelmed by all the media hype that might make you think you're not exercising unless you're playing professional basketball. That's not the point. The point is to keep your body moving, to get your heart to an aerobic level of activity at least three times a week for twenty to thirty minutes, and to make exercise a part of your life. Believe it or not, walking can do this. So can swimming, ice skating, using the machines at the gym, playing golf, and more . . . you've got a lot of choices. There is no good reason to say no. Put your mind in neutral and enjoy yourself.

Managing Obesity with Exercise

"Exercise can be as simple as giving up the elevator and taking the stairs. Whatever opportunity there is in our daily lives we should take."

Wanda Jones, M.D.

THE SCHOLAR ESTHER Rothblum, Ph.D., has observed, "In prehistoric times, goddess figures were both fat and pregnant, linking obesity with sexuality and fertility. In Victorian times, obesity in women was considered sexual. In poor countries, where large numbers of people die of malnutrition and infectious disease, thinness is not desired. Until the twentieth century, women in the United States were considered beautiful if they had large breasts and large hips—symbols of reproductive ability."

I think Rothblum's view—that the positive opinion of body fat that prevailed for centuries has been replaced in twentieth-century America by fat aversion—is right on target. However, at the same time that we realize there is too much societal pressure to look like a thin cover girl, there is also the reality that obesity in women is linked to heart disease, strokes, diabetes, and some cancers.

If you are overweight and trying to lose weight, exercise is a better ally than any fad diet you may be looking to for help; it should be part of your new lifestyle regimen. You need exercise to lose weight and keep it off. It's not about body shape or someone else's ideal—it's about being healthy. In the meantime, exercise will help to lower your risk for many diseases. Start slowly and work your way up. The most important thing to remember is that no diet plan alone will help you reach and stay at the weight that is right for you without an exercise component to the plan.

Yet, almost three quarters of American women are still not getting enough exercise. Older women are particularly prone to be couch potatoes: 42 percent of those over sixty-five compared with 26 percent of those eighteen to thirty-four. Currently, as stated earlier, the Centers for Disease Control recommends twenty minutes of heavy-breathing aerobic activity three times a week or less strenuous thirty-minute sessions at least five times a week.

Keeping a Health Diary

Family history and personal history both pertain to your health and your risk factors for many diseases such as cancer, heart disease, osteoporosis, and diabetes. Yet many of us don't know much at all about our family health history except, perhaps, the health of our parents. Do you know what your grandparents died of? Or your great-aunt or -uncle? I didn't until I asked my mother. Now I keep a health diary, which includes who in the family has had breast cancer, heart disease, and anything else I know about—not just so that I can tell my doctor and take care of myself better, but also for my children. I want them to know as much as they can about the health of their family so they can protect themselves and take care of their own health in the future.

You may want to think of keeping a health notebook and adding to it as you find out more about which relatives have had what in your family and what was the cause of death for your grandparents and great-grandparents. Be particularly careful to include any first-degree and second-degree relatives on your mother's or your father's side who have had breast cancer, colon cancer, any other cancer, heart disease and diabetes. (A first-degree relative refers to a mother, sister, daughter, or father, brother, son.) Second-degree relatives include grandparents, aunts, and uncles.

Your health notebook should also record treatments or medications that have worked or failed for you or a family member in the past. It can include other health information you have uncovered. For example, if you're able to obtain your parent's HDL and LDL cholesterol levels, you will want to note these, since high cholesterol may be hereditary. And if you can pry out information about her menopause from your mother or grandmother, you will want to include this too.

Out Stress, Damn Stress

"I used to think stress is good for me, it keeps me moti-
vated. But now I know how stupid that is. Some stress
may be necessary but the excess I can do without."

Judy Mallenkrodt (age 49)

A S IF LIFE weren't hard enough just to get through, then there's stress—and boy, is there! We have stress at home, stress on the job, stress with our kids . . . stress, stress, stress.

Stress can be measured scientifically by monitoring the level of what was once simply called adrenaline in the body. Adrenaline is really two substances, epinephrine and norepinephrine that are released by the adrenal glands whenever a person perceives a situation to be dangerous or challenging. These hormones are now referred to as catecholamines or simply as stress hormones.

A Swedish study of male and female Volvo managerial employees came up with some interesting findings about the different ways men and women react to stress. Male managers were found to wind down from a stressful day more quickly than women. Their catecholamine levels began to fall at five o'clock on the dot, while those of women, which had risen almost as high as men's during the day, did not drop off nearly as quickly. Doctors interpreting the study hypothesized that this occurs because at the end of the workday, women aren't looking forward to the pipe and slippers—they're looking forward to the second shift.

I don't want to generalize, but most of us would probably say that we just don't have the same ability to "tune out" as our male mates do. Whether it's the child whose best friend was mean to him at school, the phone call for a car pool substitution tomorrow, or the empty toilet paper roll in the bathroom, we may take it in stride, but still we notice it, are affected by it, and must cope with it. The same Swedish study also showed the different ways men's and women's blood pressure levels varied with their emotions. The men's blood pressure tended to rise when they were angry. In the women, it was anxiety that caused the blood pressure to rise. However, there was no evidence that women's anger or anxiety levels raised their risk for heart disease.

Here are some of the stresses of working life that women report bother them the most:

- **Equity.** It comes as no surprise that women on every rung of the corporate ladder feel that they have to outperform men to even come close to being treated as equals. And it's a no-brainer that women also believe that they are paid less for the same work than men or—to put it another way—they do a man's job for a woman's wages. It's true: on average, we still make only $0.72 for every dollar a man makes for the same job!

- **Type of Job.** Women (and, in this case, men) experience frustration with jobs that offer little hope of advancement, require the performance of a repetitive task, or offer little or no intellectual stimulation in general.

- **Workload.** Most women report that running a household adds another component to the workload that makes it all that much harder.

- **Frustration.** Many women say that they seem unable to get their point across, make themselves heard, and, in general, stay in communication with managers and superiors.

- **Isolation.** While women in subordinate positions are often satisfied with the camaraderie they share with co-workers, women managers and executives usually report a sense of being left out of the loop and a feeling of being alone on the job.

> *"I think the hardest word to say in the English language is no. And even when you learn to say it, it's something else to stick to it."*
>
> Martha Snyderman (age 37)

WOMEN TEND to deal with these stresses in ways that may not be professionally strategic or personally satisfying. A 1990 Gallup poll reported that 35 percent of women reacted to chronic stress on the job by leaving their jobs. Even though this is certainly not an ideal solution, in some cases it may be the best one available. Nevertheless, I do have some suggestions that may make for a better solution for the woman who really wants to keep her job.

- *Setting priorities will help you say no and mean it.* "No" is a complete sentence. Yet it is a difficult one for most of us to say. I can say no. I know I can. I've heard myself say it. But once I say yes, that's it. I'm hooked. I can't tell you the number of times I have found my brain saying no while my lips were proceeding with an unqualified yes. But then I realized that the more I said yes, especially when I didn't mean it, the less time I had for myself and my family. One of my favorite professors once told me that time is our most valuable commodity and everyone will waste it for us if we let them. So, I no longer let them. Now I set priorities realistically and have a better chance of saying no when I really mean it.
- *Express yourself. Don't fume.* Don't tell yourself you have a better solution. Tell *them.* There have been countless studies done that show that women lose out in business settings because they're accustomed to avoiding conflict by keeping silent and yielding the floor to others (meaning men). Even if you need to seek help, such as assertiveness training, to do this, go ahead and try. You will not only alleviate your stress at work, you will also probably advance in your profession.
- *If you have a complaint, find someone to tell it to.* Many companies provide an ombudsperson to whom you can air your grievances and who may help you find ways to solve your problems.
- *Never underestimate a good shoulder to cry on.* To put it more professionally, find the support you need to lighten your stress load if you are going through a crisis at work.
- *Don't put all your emotional commitment into one basket.* Believe it or not, studies have shown that women who are balancing raising a family with having a career are better able to manage the stresses of the workplace.
- *Exercise.* I still think exercise is one of the best stress relievers around. When things get overwhelming or tense for me, nothing clears the air as well as getting my heart rate up and sweating. This is one time I will try to get out of the house and take a very brisk walk or a run. I think the fresh air and change in locale help clear the brain. I

have come up with some of my best solutions to problems when I have used this escape valve.

Alternative Medicine and Other Paths of Healing

"Open your mind and say 'ah.' "

James Suen, M.D.

I'M A SURGEON who's been trained by other Western-trained surgeons. I have been taught to treat disease by the best in their fields and I have always considered myself to be a good doctor. But I haven't always been so good at understanding the importance of preventing disease, and I haven't always understood the role that alternative medicine can play in treating patients. In fact, I have learned much of what I know about alternative medicine from my patients. Whether it's back pain or the pain of arthritis or chronic bladder infections, there are times when your doctor can help you just so much and no more. Add to this that more and more of us are growing very cautious about invasive medical techniques, excessive use of antibiotics, and the suspiciously high profits of the pharmaceutical and medical industries, and you will find people turning to natural and ancient healing techniques with greater frequency. Many people feel that they have been helped by alternative medicine while some feel their time and their money have been wasted. But the truth is that there are times when alternative medicine can be an excellent supplement to good medical care. In some cases, I believe that alternative medicine can even replace conventional treatments. Dr. Andrew Weil, a physician and noted expert in the field of alternative medicine, calls the wedding of modern medicine with ancient healing techniques "integrative medicine." He encourages young physicians to "first do no harm"—which has been a motto of medicine since Asclepiades. But Weil follows that with one other: "Believe in the healing power of nature."

Change is never easy, but it can be exciting and rewarding. That we are living in a time that may be called a watershed decade in the history of health care is nowhere more evident than in how we as a culture have begun to view alternatives to the traditional paths of medicine. Suddenly (or not so suddenly) we have begun to reject the notion that invasive procedures—from numerous tests to grueling surgeries—are the only curative measures worth considering, and we have started to embrace the overall concept of healing. In fact, a recent study published in the *New England Journal of Medicine* found that more than a third of a sample of the general population surveyed said they chose alternative medicine instead of conventional methods; they said they believed medicine should focus on the patient as a whole. But 71 percent of these patients don't tell their physicians about their use of alternative remedies because they fear disapproval.

There are also many situations involving your health that are not going to be emergencies and that you may be able to take care of without a long wait at the doctor's office and take care of just as well or even more efficiently on your own. But I balance that by saying I believe it prudent to always let your doctor know what you are doing and what you are taking. The treatments may complement each other.

As a doctor, I've seen patients embrace forms of alternative medicines as if they were cure-alls for deadly diseases and be hurt and disappointed, but I've also seen patients who were helped enormously by alternative therapies *in conjunction with responsible medical care*. I use alternative treatments in my own health care such as Echinacea and Golden Seal at the first sign of a respiratory infection and chamomile tea for cramps. I also believe in using stinging nettles for the alleviation of hay fever symptoms. Alternative medicine often includes modifications in diet, exercise, and vitamin therapy—which all of us are involved with to some degree on a daily basis. It also includes acupuncture, chiropractic medicine, and herbology, to name a few disciplines that I'll try to describe briefly here in the hopes of demystifying what may be very viable alternatives for health care.

Acupuncture

The practice of acupuncture originated in China over five thousand years ago and is based on the belief that health is determined by the balanced flow of qi (or ch'i). Qi is the vital life energy that is present in all organisms. In the theory of acupuncture, it is believed that there are twelve major energy pathways, or meridians, which are linked to specific internal organs and organ systems. There are considered to be more than a thousand acupoints on these meridians that can be stimulated to enhance the flow of qi.

According to the World Health Organization, acupuncture can have a positive effect in treating 104 different conditions, including:

- Addictions
- Asthma
- Back pain
- Chronic pain
- The common cold
- Duodenal ulcer
- Inflammation of the eyes
- Ménière's disease
- Myopia
- Obesity
- Osteoarthritis
- Pain
- Paralysis from stroke
- Sciatica
- Tennis elbow

Until more information is known, there are certain illnesses I cannot endorse this practice for—e.g., ear infections in children. I admit that this is my bias, but at this stage I am more comfortable with conventional treatment for most infectious processes. Ten years from now, I may be singing a different tune—but not yet.

A typical acupuncture treatment involves an interview with the practitioner, in which he or she will ask questions about just about everything from the color of your urine to your menstrual cycle, sleep habits, sensitivity to heat and cold, digestive problems and stress levels. You will also probably be asked to fill out a form regarding medical history.

As you've probably heard, acupuncture does involve needles. The good news is that no more than ten to twelve are used during a procedure, and acupuncture is essentially painless, except for a tiny pricking sensation when a needle punctures the skin. The needles are of different lengths and gauges, but they are essentially hair-thin. If you do feel any prolonged discomfort at an acupoint (where the needle has been placed), it's important that you tell your practitioner because the discomfort can probably be eliminated with a slight change of the needle's position. Needles are generally left in position for twenty to thirty minutes.

If you're feeling squeamish even though you think acupuncture may be helpful to you, just think of this. Much as you hate to have your blood drawn, you let your doctor do this with a needle deep in your arm, because you think it's for your own good. The insertion of acupuncture needles is not nearly as uncomfortable, so why not reorient yourself by reading up on acupuncture and interviewing those who've had it (who generally sing its praises). Talk to your friends. You'll probably be surprised just how many people you know who've had acupuncture.

Chiropractic

The relationship of the spinal column and the musculoskeletal structures of the body to the nervous system forms the basis for the philosophy of chiropractic. The spinal column acts as a type of switchboard for the nervous system.

There are three overlapping systems that constitute the nervous system:

- The central nervous system, including the brain and spinal cord
- The autonomic nervous system, responsible for controlling involuntary functions such as digestion, heart rate, and glandular function
- The peripheral nervous system, responsible for connecting the central nervous system to the voluntary muscles and the tissues of the body

The interbalance and equilibrium of these three interrelated systems determines to a great extent the health of the body. Doctors of chiropractic believe that when a vertebra gets out of alignment, there is pressure on the nerves in that area which can prohibit the nerves from carrying out their proper functions. This will lead to dysfunction and eventually abet the development of disease.

Years ago, some chiropractors thought that subluxations, the misalignment of vertebrae, were the cause of all disease. There was a sense that they could cure all. Now the chiropractic profession—a well-organized, well-monitored group of professionals—understands the multidimensional nature of illness and health and tries to respond with treatment that may work by itself to resolve a health situation or work in conjunction with other treatment to make that treatment more successful.

Since its introduction in 1895, chiropractic has slowly but surely become accepted worldwide, despite endless haranguing by the established medical profession. Among other things, chiropractic adjustments can be extremely beneficial in cutting down on the wear and tear of joints and ligaments.

Every year more than 15 million people in the United States consult chiropractic physicians. In many quarters of traditional Western medicine there is growing acceptance of this field—such that many sports medicine doctors who are orthopedic surgeons by training now work hand in hand (so to speak) with chiropractors.

Here are some of the conditions that chiropractic may be helpful in treating:

- Back pain
- Carpal tunnel syndrome
- Headaches
- Knee injuries
- Neck pain
- Sprains
- Tendinitis
- Tennis elbow

In addition, many people believe chiropractic helps maintain an overall sense of wellness.

When you see a chiropractor for the first time, he or she will take a health history and discuss it, your family history, eating habits, and general way of life. Then you will undergo a thorough physical exam, including palpation and a general analysis of your spine, which is done to determine any muscle imbalances or subluxations. You will also be queried regarding posture and work habits. If you are there because of a physical injury, you will be asked what position you were in when the injury occurred. Your visit will deal primarily with the problem that brought you to a chiropractor in the first place, but attention will also be paid to improving your coordination and general body motion as well. The proper functioning of the body is just as important to a good chiropractor as the relief of pain, since one has everything to do with the other.

Herbal medicine

Most of us practice some form of herbal medicine whether we know it or not. If you are saying, "No, not me. Nope. I just don't trust those plants and things," you may not be aware of how much herbs have to do with traditional medicine. In fact, about 25 percent of all prescription drugs are derived from trees, shrubs, or herbs. And the word "drug" comes from the middle English *drogge*, "to dry," as dried plants were often used as medicines. Ironically, as a culture we've been indoctrinated into believing in synthetic, prescription drugs, no matter what the side effects. You may not be aware of just how simple a medicinal herb may be. For example, even a cup of chamomile tea may qualify as an herbal remedy.

What is an herb? An herb is a flower, leaf, or stem, a seed or root, a fruit or the bark or any other part of a plant that is used for its flavor, medicinal, or odiferous properties. Interestingly, herbal medicines work in the same manner that pharmaceutical drugs work—that is, via their chemical makeup. Herbs contain naturally occurring chemicals such as morphine (from certain poppies) and digoxin (from foxglove) and many more. Herbs have many properties that make them useful in treating a variety of illnesses or physical problems. They may work to soothe inflammation or work to destroy or resist disease-causing microorganisms. They may also help increase the body's resistance to stress through supporting the adrenal glands. They may also work as astringents, diuretics, expectorants, or laxatives, as well as in many other ways.

Homeopathy

Homeopathy is based on the principle that "like cures like." The word itself is derived from the Greek *homoios* (similar) and *pathos* (suffering). Homeopathic remedies are created to match the symptoms or "profiles" of a particular illness. Homeopathy was founded in the late eighteenth century by Samuel Hahnemann, known for his contributions to pharmacology, public health, toxicology, and psychiatry. On observing the inhumane practices popular in the medicine of the day, such as blood-letting and highly toxic mercury-based laxatives, he thought, logically enough, that there must be a better way. After years of experimenting with numerous substances, he outlined the principles of homeopathy as follows:

- Like cures like or "the law of similars" (i.e., that which you have is that which I will give you in tiny doses; this, by the way, is the principle behind most vaccines—infecting you with a minute amount of virus helps your body's immune system defend against the virus).
- The more a remedy is diluted, the greater its potency, or "the law of the infinitesimal dose."
- Every illness is specific to the individual. This is a holistic approach to medicine based on the concept that each person is a distinct and integrated entity and more than the sum of her parts. Thus, any illness or condition you suffer from will have unique characteristics common only to you.

Those who believe in homeopathy believe homeopathic treatment can have a beneficial effect on almost any disease or health condition. However, a classic homeopath does not believe in immunizations for children; this is one area where I very much disagree, believing that conventional medicine has a very important role to play. Children should be immunized against communicable childhood diseases.

Does homeopathy work? In an article in the *British Medical Journal* in which 107 clinical studies of homeopathic remedies were reviewed, it was reported that 81 of these studies found that homeopathy was beneficial in treating such conditions as headaches (including migraines), digestive problems, respiratory infections, sprains, and post-operative infections. Studies reviewed in the *British Journal of Pharmacology* have also found homeopathic treatment effective in the relief of symptoms of rheumatoid arthritis.

In the United States homeopathy has had its ups and downs. But if sales of homeopathic remedies are any indication, homeopathy is alive and thriving in the United States. Annual sales of homeopathic medicines have now reached $150 million per year in this country.

408

Vitamin Therapy

"Nutrient density is the hallmark of good food."

Paul McTaggart, nutritionist

THE WORD "VITAMIN" was coined only at the beginning of the twentieth century and since that time doctors and scientists have relished debating what nutritional adequacy is and isn't. You listen to the news. One day, it's take this; the next day, it's don't bother. What's a self-respecting, intelligent person who wants to take care of herself to do? Here's what. Chart a nutritional course that is moderate and consistent. Such a course should include a healthy diet rich in fruits and vegetables, a general multivitamin (which you should not take on an empty stomach), and a calcium supplement, at the very minimum. There is, of course, no substitute for the nutrients you obtain directly from the food you eat, and if you are expecting to make up for a nutrient-poor diet of junk food and black coffee with a handful of vitamins, you might as well forget it.

These days the newest miracle cure is considered to be antioxidants—vitamins that may slow the production of destructive free radicals in the blood. We debate antioxidants and what they can or cannot do to prevent or cure cancer, as if vitamins were our new dream team or the next miracle cure. Well, vitamins are vitamins. They are good for some things and we don't know if they are or are not good for others. But while the debate rages, we can continue to use vitamins in a reasonable manner for those physical conditions they are known to help. Nonetheless, I believe there is more evidence to support the use of antioxidants than not. Just remember, vitamins can help in moderation, but too many may be toxic.

Here is a regimen I am comfortable with:

- **Calcium.** You should take a calcium supplement—1500 mg of elemental calcium per day.

- **Vitamin E.** 400–800 IU, taken with a meal.

- **Vitamin C.** 400 mg two or three times a day.

Whether or not to take them and how much to take already has us confused enough about vitamins. Then we must contend with the fact that there are two sets of dietary recommendations used in the United States.

The Recommended Dietary Allowances (RDAs) are determined by the Food and Nutrition Board of the National Academy of Sciences' National Research Council; they were last updated in 1989. The second set is what you will find on most food and vitamin labels; these are the United States Recommended Daily Allowances (USRDA) and these numbers are generally much older.

The two recommendations may differ in dosage, but also differ in the units used. RDAs are now given in micrograms (mcg) or milligrams (mg; 1 mg = 1,000 mcg). USRDAs are given in International Units (IUs). When dealing with either of these standards of measurement, it should be remembered that nutrition as a science is fairly new and definitely evolving. Remember, mainly, that you don't want to take too much of anything, and yet you do want to make sure you match a minimum standard for a vitamin supplement to do any good.

The Race Is to the Moderate

Hard as it may be to accept, the best medicine is moderation. And the older you get, the more this axiom applies. The trouble with moderation is that it's not a particularly dramatic or attractive or exciting concept. To put it mildly, moderation seems dull. But in this era of fanatical fads, fanatical exercise programs, fanatical diets, and work overload, moderation may finally be viewed as a beautiful thing and one of the greatest of indulgences.

All moderation really means is that you try not to treat yourself poorly, but well; and if you are in need of a lifestyle overhaul, you change your life little by little, not overnight. You do need to get enough sleep and eat a balanced diet most of the time, but not all the time. You don't need to exercise rigorously every day and you don't need to skip dessert every day. Moderation also means as long as you don't have a problem with alcohol, you may have that glass of wine with dinner. You may also have a cup of coffee in the morning. Moderation means learning to know your limits and taking time to relax,

YOUR HOME MEDICINE CHEST

A well-stocked medicine cabinet is an important part of any household. Being able to find basic medical supplies can make your life easier and more comfortable if you're talking about a headache; and it can literally save a life if you're faced with someone who has been cut or poisoned. Know what you have on hand and keep the area well organized. Run through the use for everything with your family members, but keep all out of the reach of children.

Medicine cabinets are best kept out of the bathroom. The humidity and swings in temperature can age medications prematurely. I keep mine in a separate area in a hall closet.

If you are on prescription medications, be sure to discard them after their expiration dates. Teach children at an early age to respect that this area is off-limits except for emergencies. Under no circumstances should a child ever be given medicine and told that it's candy.

If you don't have the storage space in a hall closet, you can still have a good first-aid kit that's mobile too! Just grab one of your old shoe boxes and arrange the essentials neatly inside. But remember: if you have children or grandchildren around your home, you must keep this box out of their reach.

I consider the following elements essential for a well-stocked first-aid kit:

- Ace bandages. For wrapping sprains or strains. If an injury is serious, however, you should see your physician. He or she may prescribe an air cast to immobilize the injured area.
- Acetaminophen. A must for reducing fever and pain.
- Adhesive bandages. To cover cuts and scrapes.
- Antibiotic ointment. A neomycin or multiple antibiotic ointment is always a good thing to have for minor scrapes and cuts.
- Aspirin. To relieve pain or reduce fever or inflammation.
- Baking soda. Baking soda can be mixed with water and used as an antacid as long as you don't have high blood pressure.
- Calamine lotion. To relieve skin irritations, from eczema to poison ivy and insect bites.
- Cotton gauze bandages and adhesive tape. To stop the flow of blood from a cut and to cover large scrapes or cuts.

continued

- Hydrogen peroxide. An antiseptic for cleaning scrapes and cuts.
- Ibuprofen. Good for headaches and cramps and relieving inflammation.
- Ipecac. Syrup of ipecac should be in every medicine cabinet and everyone in the house should know what the bottle looks like. It should be taken *only as directed by your local poison control unit* in the case of swallowing a possible poison.
- Penlight. Use to examine throat, mouth, and gums.
- Scissors. Use to cut cotton bandages and tape.
- Sunburn ointment. Invaluable in reducing discomfort after too much sun.
- Thermometers. Digital thermometers are now available at reasonable prices.
- Ziploc bags. Use to make an ice bag to apply to sprains.

whether this means watching a beautiful sunset, going to the symphony, or just putting your feet up. Relaxation is part of health care.

And while you may never fall for the old adage "you're not getting older, you're getting better," you may find that with a little age comes a little wisdom, and learning to take care of yourself may help you like this more mature you just a little bit better.

LIVING WITH YOUR LIVING WILL

"Please don't keep me alive in a futile situation. Use your common sense and preserve my dignity. And at my service, play the 'Evening Prayer' from Hansel and Gretel. It was the first real theater I saw as a little girl and I have always loved it."

Joy Snyderman (age 69)

We live in a time when people confess their most intimate problems and secrets publicly, and yet when it comes to the subject we must all face silence still abounds. Few of us speak with our parents about how they wish to die. Few of us speak with our children, spouses, or friends about how we wish to die. While this is changing, it is changing slowly— even though when people do discuss decisions about the end of life, they report feeling comforted by such discussions.

And then Camelot met Watergate in a place called Death with Dignity. In 1994, both Richard Nixon and Jacqueline Kennedy Onassis impressed America by having taken the steps to ensure that they would die on their own terms as much as was possible. Democrat and Republican watched as Nixon was not resuscitated, according to his own wishes, and Jackie went home to die, according to her own wishes. Each had filed living wills and each had had conversations with loved ones to make clear what his or her last wishes were and to make clear that these wishes be fulfilled. Because of their courage, then, in some way, dealing with how we die seemed to emerge from the closet as the last taboo subject.

I grew up in a family where no subject was taboo. In fact, some of our dinner conversations were rather wild—but as kids we loved talking about anything that we thought was important. Even the gross stuff. The desire to talk about sometimes unsavory subjects went both ways. My father, the surgeon, always stressed that death is a normal part of the human process and a topic that should not be avoided.

Although there is no way to make death a pleasant subject, it is possible to influence how and where we die. We have seen this in the two very public examples cited. By planning for the possibilities surrounding the end of our lives, we are really continuing to participate in

continued

413

life and to exert what control we are able to. We are not being morbid. We are continuing to care. Like most things in life, while there are no guarantees, it is still better to plan ahead.

One of the best and easiest steps toward participating in the closure of life is to file a living will. Living wills are available through many organizations, including Choice in Dying. Your doctor can help you with the process, and keeping him or her involved will help ensure that your wishes are ultimately followed. If you use a lawyer as well, you should make sure your living will is in your legal file.

But it is one thing to have a living will; it's another to have it enforced according to your wishes. There is some debate about how well the terms of living wills are enforced at the end of life. However, it should not be assumed that problems occur primarily because doctors are unwilling to heed patients' wishes regarding the withdrawal of various life support measures; indeed, studies show that in most cases it is the *family* who have difficulty giving permission to withdraw life support. This makes sense. No matter how dire the suffering and how hopeless the situation, it is difficult to let go of loved ones at the end of life. It's simply human nature not to want to lose those we love.

The living will should be viewed as the beginning of communication—not an end in itself, but the first step in the discussion among family members regarding mortality and end-of-life care. The purpose of a living will is to let your loved ones know your wishes. This cannot be done effectively unless you are willing to discuss your wishes with those who love you and with your doctor. If you simply file a living will with an attorney, there is no guarantee that your wishes will be respected. When used effectively, the living will is the beginning of a process and not an end in itself. And this process should be ongoing.

Granted, it's hard to discuss your own mortality or that of your parents. But the more you consider this discussion vital to your family and as a way of taking control of your own medical care, the more comfortable you will be with the conversation. In fact, you are doing your family a favor by opening these channels of communication. The more you make it clear to your loved ones that you wish to have this conversation and that it is helpful to you, the more this discussion will be seen as a positive one. If you have older parents, a spouse, or another family member who has not shared their wishes with you, you should also encourage him or her to do so.

DIRECTORY OF HEALTH RESOURCES

HEART DISEASE

American Heart Association
122 East 42 Street
New York, NY 10168
800-242-8721

Provides informational pamphlets on heart disease and prevention, including literature on heart disease and how it relates to women. Also publishes cookbooks on low-fat and low-cholesterol cooking. Local offices may provide physician and/or hospital references. Call for address of a local branch.

National Heart, Lung and Blood Institute
Information Center
P.O. Box 30105
Bethesda, MD 20824-0105

Provides informational pamphlets and fact sheets on various diseases. A very informative guide called *Healthy Heart Handbook for Women* can be ordered, free of charge.

The Difference in a Woman's Heart Hotline
800-866-0400

You may order a twenty-eight-page brochure that lists questions you should ask your doctor about symptoms and risk factors. Recorded message. Affiliated with the American Medical Women's Association.

National High Blood Pressure Education Program
Information Center
National Institutes of Health
7200 Wisconsin Avenue
Bethesda, MD 20814

Provides literature on high blood pressure.

National Hypertension Association
324 East 30th Street
New York, NY 10016
212-889-3557

Provides literature on hypertension.

415

American Institute of Stress
124 Park Avenue
Yonkers, NY 10703
914-963-1200
800-24-RELAX

Has a wide range of literature for women available, such as how stress relates to breast cancer. Publishes a newsletter.

Related Books

Preventing Heart Disease, by Rita Baron-Faust with the Physicians of New York University Medical Center Women's Health Service and Division of Cardiology. Hearst Books, 1995.

The American Heart Association Family Guide to Stroke Treatment, Recovery, Prevention, by Louis R. Caplan, M.D., Marl L. Dyken, M.D., and J. Donald Easton, M.D. Times Books/Random House, 1994.

The Mayo Clinic Heart Book, by the Mayo Clinic. William Morrow, 1993.

Dr. Dean Ornish's Program for Reducing Heart Disease, by Dean Ornish, M.D. Random House, 1990.

The Yale University School of Medicine Heart Book, edited by Barry L. Zaret, M.D., Marvin Moser, M.D., and Lawrence S. Cohen. Hearst Books, 1992.

The Female Heart: The Truth About Women and Heart Disease, by Marianne J. Legato, M.D., and Carol Colman. Avon, 1991.

FITNESS

President's Council on Physical Fitness and Sports
707 Pennsylvania Avenue, N.W.
Suite 250
Washington, DC 20004
202-272-3421

Provides literature on physical fitness, including *Nolan Ryan Fitness Program*, a guide to starting a fitness program for those over the age of forty.

The Melpomone Institute for Women's Health
c/o Judy Mahle Lutter
1010 University Avenue
St. Paul, MN 55104
612-642-1951

Membership organization whose mission is to educate women about the health benefits of physical fitness. It distributes literature and has a video library, which is accessible by mail. The yearly membership fee is approximately $32: this includes a subscription to *The Melpomene Journal*, published three times a year.

416

SMOKING

Action on Smoking and Health
2013 H Street, N.W.
Washington, DC 20006
202-659-4310

Lobbying group pushing for smoke-free workplaces and restaurants and a ban on tobacco advertizing. Also provides up-to-date information on the effects of smoking on health. Publishes a newsletter called the *ASH Smoking and Health Review*.

Smokenders
1430 East Indian School Road
Suite 102
Phoenix, AZ 85014
800-828-4357

Distributes brochures and sponsors six-week stop-smoking seminars throughout the country for about $325. Self-study audio tapes and interactive workbooks are also available for approximately $129.

Environmental Protection Agency
401 M Street, S.W.
Washington, DC 20460

Provides useful material on smoking and its hazards.

Related Book

Women Can Quit: A Different Approach, by Sue Delaney. Women's Healthcare Press, 1989.

WOMEN'S HEALTH (General)

National Women's Health Resource Center (NWHC)
2440 M Street, N.W.
Suite 201
Washington, DC 20037
202-293-60450

Membership organization. Publishes a bimonthly women's health report.

National Women's Health Network
1325 G Street, N.W.
Washington, DC 20005
202-347-1140

Membership organization whose purpose is to enlighten women about the latest developments in women's health care. Provides informational packets on women's health.

Related Books

The New Our Bodies, Ourselves, by the Boston Women's Health Book Collective. Touchstone/Simon and Schuster, 1992.

The Good Housekeeping Illustrated Guide to Women's Health, edited by Kathryn A. Cox, M.D. Hearst Books, 1995.

Our Health, Our Lives: A Revolutionary Approach to Total Health Care for Women, by Eileen Hoffman, M.D. Pocket Books, 1995.

Women's Health Alert, by Sidney M. Wolfe, M.D., and the Public Citizen Research Group, with Rhoda Donkin Jones. Addison-Wesley, 1991.

The New Ourselves, Growing Older, by Paula B. Doress-Worters and Diana Laskin Siegal. Touchstone/Simon and Schuster, 1994.

CANCER

American Cancer Society, Inc.
National Headquarters
1599 Clifton Road, NE
Atlanta, GA 30329
800-ACS-2345

Distributes literature on cancer. The Cancer Information Hotline provides up-to-date information on cancer research, treatment, and education. Call your local number for programs near you.

National Cancer Institute Information
National Institute of
Health
Bethesda, MD 20205
800-4-CANCER
Alaska: 800-638-6070
Hawaii: 800-524-1234

The helpline can help you find a treatment center near you, and will update you on developments in breast cancer research and the availability of clinical trials. Provides printed material on cancer education and community programs.

NABCO (National Alliance of Breast Cancer Organizations)
9 East 37 Street, 10th Floor
New York, NY 10016
212-719-0154
Emergency line: 212-889-0606

A network of breast cancer awareness that provides information and referral services. Recorded message.

Y-ME National Organization for Breast Cancer
Information and Support
National Office
18220 Harwood Avenue
Homewood, IL 60403
708-799-8338
Hotlines: 800-221-2141 (9 A.M. to 5 P.M. Central Time)
708-799-8228 (24 hours)

Distributes literature on breast cancer. The hotline faculty are breast cancer survivors. To find the mammography facilities nearest you, contact:

American College of Radiology
1891 Preston White Drive
Reston, VA 22091
800-227-5463, ext 4912

Related Books

Breast Cancer: What Every Woman Should Know, by Rita Baron-Faust with the Physicians of the New York University Medical Center Women's Health Service and the Kaplan Comprehensive Cancer Center. Hearst Books, 1995.
The Breast Cancer Companion, by Kathy LaTour. William Morrow, 1993.
Dr. Susan Love's Breast Book, by Dr. Susan Love, M.D. Addison-Wesley, 1995.
Cancer, by Robert M. McAllister, et al. Basic Books, 1994.
To Be Alive: A Woman's Guide to a Full Life After Cancer, by Carolyn D. Runowicz, M.D., and Donna Haupt. Henry Holt, 1995.

PREGNANCY AND CHILDBIRTH

Related Books

Dr. Kathryn Schrotenboer's Guide to Pregnancy over 35, by Kathryn Schrotenboer, M.D., and Joan Solomon Weiss. Ballantine, 1985.
What to Expect When You're Expecting, 2d ed., by Arlene Eisenberg, Heidi Eisenberg Murkoff, and Sandee Eisenberg Hathaway. Workman, 1991.
The Women's Encyclopedia of Health and Emotional Healing, by Denise Foley, Eileen Nechas, and the Editors of *Prevention*. Rodale Press, 1993.
The Tentative Pregnancy, by Barbara Katz Rothman. Penguin, 1987.
Surviving Pregnancy Loss: A Complete Sourcebook for Women and Their Families, by Rochelle Friedman, M.D., and Bonnie Gradstein. Little Brown, 1982.
Birth over Thirty, by Sheila Kitzinger. Viking Penguin, 1985.

ADOPTION

Holt International Children's Services
503-687-2202

Related Books

A Handful of Hope, by Suzanne Arms. Celestial Arts, 1990.
To Love and Let Go, by Suzanne Arms. Alfred A. Knopf, 1983.
Beating the Adoption Game, by Cynthia Martin. Harcourt Brace Jovanovich, 1988.
Adoption Choices, by Ellen Paul. Visible Ink Press, 1991.

OTHER GYNECOLOGICAL ISSUES

National Cancer Institute
Office of Cancer Communications
Building 21, Room 10A-24
Bethesda, MD 20892
Write to request a booklet entitled *Questions and Answers About DES Exposure Before Birth.*

DES Action
516-775-3450
A consumer group that publishes a quarterly newsletter about DES.

Related Books

Womancare, by Lynda Madaras and Jane Patterson, M.D. Avon, 1984.
A Woman's Book of Choices: Abortion, Menstrual Extraction, RU-486, by Rebecca Chalker and Carol Downer. Four Walls Eight Windows, 1992.
The Mismeasure of Woman, by Carol Tavris. Touchstone/Simon and Schuster, 1992.

SEXUALITY

Sex Information and Education Council of the United States
80 Fifth Avenue, Suite 801
New York, NY 10011
Write for literature on sex disorders and help in finding a sex therapist.

Related Books

Love and Sex After 60, by Robert N. Butler, M.D., and Myrna I. Lewis. Ballantine, 1993.
150 Most Asked Questions About Midlife Sex, Love and Intimacy, by Ruth S. Jacobowitz. Hearst Books, 1995.
Inhibited Sexual Desire, by Jennifer Knopf, M.D., and Michael Seiler, M.D. 1991.

AIDS

National AIDS Hotlines:
800-342-AIDS (English)
800-344-AIDS (Spanish)
800-AIDS-TTY (hearing-impaired access)

CDC National AIDS Clearinghouse
P.O Box 6003
Rockville, MD 20849-6003
Write to get information and statistics about HIV and AIDS.

Related Books

AIDS Care at Home, by Judith Greif and Beth Ann Golden. John Wiley & Sons, 1994.
The Woman's HIV Sourcebook, by Patricia Kloser, M.D., and Jane MacLean Craig. Taylor Publishing, 1994.

MENOPAUSE

North American Menopause Society
c/o University Hospitals of Cleveland
Department of OB/GYN
11100 Euclid Avenue
Cleveland, OH 44106
216-844-3334
Membership organization dedicated to improving care of menopausal women and promoting women's understanding of menopause.

Related Books

The Change, by Germaine Greer. Fawcett Books, 1993.
The Complete Book of Menopause: Every Woman's Guide to Good Health, by Carol Landau, Ph.D., Michele G. Cyr., M.D., and Anne W. Moulton, M.D. Grosset/Putnam, 1994.
150 Most Asked Questions About Menopause, by Ruth S. Jacobowitz. Hearst Books, 1992.
Estrogen: A Complete Guide to Reversing the Effects of Menopause Using Hormone Replacement Therapy, by Lila E. Nachtigall, M.D., and Joan Ratner Heilman, HarperPerennial, 1991.
Natural Menopause, by Susan Perry and Katherine O'Hanlan, M.D. Addison-Wesley, 1993.
The Silent Passage, by Gail Sheehy. Pocket Books, 1995.

HYSTERECTOMY

HERS (Hysterectomy Educational Resources and Services)
422 Bryn Mawr Avenue
Bala Cynwyd, PA 19004
610-667-7757
Counsels women in every state, all of Europe, and some of the Middle East. Provides information regarding alternatives to hysterectomies and coping with the consequences of the surgery and referrals to specialists. Publishes a newsletter, holds semiannual conferences, and provides copies of medical journal articles.

Related Book

The Hysterectomy Hoax, by Stanley West. Doubleday, 1994.

ASTHMA AND ALLERGY

American Lung Association
800-588-8686
Can provide helpful information on asthma.

National Institute of Allergy and Infectious Diseases
Office of Communications
Building 31, Room 7A-50
31 Center Drive MSC2520
Bethesda, MD 20892-2520
Write to request informational brochures.

Asthma and Allergy Foundation of America
1125 15th Street, N.W.
Suite 502
Washington, DC 20005
800-7-ASTHMA
This organization seeks to educate, funds research, and advocates for health care. Provides physician and/or treatment referrals and information on asthma support groups.

DIABETES

American Diabetes Association
National Service Center
1660 Duke Street
Alexandria, VA 22314
800-232-3472
Provides the public with the latest information on diabetes. Call to get local branch address for programs in your area.

Related Books

The New Diabetes Without Fear, by Dr. Joseph I. Goodman. Avon Books, 1995.
The Diabetic Woman, by Lois Jovanovic, June Bierman, and Barbara Toohy. Jeremy Tarcher, 1987.

SUBSTANCE ABUSE

Alcoholics Anonymous
475 Riverside Drive
New York, NY 10015
212-870-3400

Al-Anon Family Group Headquarters
1372 Broadway
New York, NY 10018
212-302-7240
800-356-9996

National Council on Alcoholism and Drug Dependence, Inc.
12 West 21 Street
New York, NY 10010
212-206-6770

This organization provides referral services and literature, including fact sheets on the treatment of alcoholism and the process of intervention.

Narcotics Anonymous
212-874-0700

Cocaine Abuse Hotline:
800-COCAINE
201-522-7055 (in Hawaii and Alaska)

ALZHEIMER'S DISEASE

Alzheimer's Disease and Related Disorders Association (ADRDA) National Headquarters
70 E. Lake Street
Chicago, IL 60601
800-621-0379 (outside Illinois)
800-572-6037 (Illinois)

Provides information on local support groups and organizations. Publishes a newsletter and provides informational brochures.

Related Books

The Vanishing Mind: A Practical Guide to Alzheimer's Disease and Other Dementias, by Leonard L. Heston and June A. White. Freeman & Co., 1991.

The 36-Hour Day: A Family Guide to Caring for Persons with Alzheimer's Disease, Related Dementing Illnesses, and Memory Loss in Later Life, by Nancy L. Mace and Peter V. Rabins. Johns Hopkins University Press, 1991.

Related Periodical

The American Journal of Alzheimer's Care and Related Disorders. 470 Boston Post Road, Weston, MA 02193. Published quarterly.

ANEMIA

National Sickle Cell Disease Branch
Division of Blood Disease and Resources

National Heart, Lung, and Blood Institute
Room 504, Federal Building
7550 Wisconsin Avenue
Bethesda, MD 20892
Write for literature on sickle-cell anemia.

EATING DISORDERS

Overeaters Anonymous
P.O. Box 44020
Rio Rancho, NM 87174-4020
505-891-2664
Their world service number will direct you to a local branch. Call between 8 A.M. and 5 P.M. Mountain Time.

American Anorexia/Bulimia Association
293 Central Park West
#1R
New York, NY 10024
Call for physician and hospital referrals. For an information packet, send a self-addressed stamped envelope and $3.

CHRONIC FATIGUE SYNDROME

Chronic Fatigue and Immune Dysfunction Syndrome Association of America
P.O. Box 220398
Charlotte, NC 28222-0398
800-442-3437
Literature and referrals to local support groups.

PAIN DISORDERS

American Chronic Pain Association
P.O. Box 850
Rocklin, CA 95677
916-632-0922
International membership organization that leads groups for chronic pain sufferers—led by persons afflicted with chronic pain. Offers pain management training, including exercise, nutrition, and better sleep. Publishes a quarterly newsletter, *The ACPA Chronicle*.

Related Book

Free Yourself from Chronic Back Ache, by Edmund Blair Bolles. Dell, 1990.

OSTEOPOROSIS

National Osteoporosis Foundation
1150 17th Street N.W.
Suite 500
Washington, DC 20036-4603
Publishes brochures and a quarterly newsletter, *The Osteoporosis Report.*

Osteoporosis Society of Canada
P.O. Box 280, Station Q
Toronto, Ontario M4T 2MI
800-463-6842
Publishes a free booklet, which provides answers to commonly asked questions, called *Building Better Bones: A Guide to Active Living,* and extends services to people living with osteoporosis.

Related Books

Healthy Bones: What You Should Know About Osteoporosis, by Nancy Appleton, Avery Publishing, 1991.
150 Most Asked Questions About Osteoporosis, by Ruth S. Jacobowitz. Hearst Books, 1993.

PARKINSON'S

Parkinson's Disease Foundation
710 West 168 Street
New York, NY 10032
800-457-6676
Provides informational literature and doctor referrals. Between 9 A.M. and 5 P.M. Eastern Time, a clinician is available to take questions.

AGING

National Council on the Aging (NCOA)
409 3rd Street, S.W.
Washington, DC 20024
800-424-9046
Call for recorded information on aging and instructions on how to purchase publications about aging.

SKIN

American Academy of Dermatology
930 N. Meacham Road
P.O. Box 4014
Schaumburg, IL 60168-4014

Distributes a wide range of literature on care of the epidermis, from melanoma to varicose veins and hair loss. Special fact sheets available on the perils of tanning.

National Psoriasis Foundation
6600 South West 92nd Street, Suite 300
Portland, OR 97223
800-723-9166
Provides informational brochures on psoriasis.

The Skin Cancer Foundation
245 Fifth Avenue
Suite 2404
New York, NY 10016
800-327-5786
Literature and information on latest developments in skin cancer research.

PLASTIC SURGERY

Breast Implant Hotline
800-532-4440
This information line has been set up by the FDA for questions about breast implants. Regular information updates. A seventy-page, free book can be ordered.

Related Book

The Complete Guide to Women's Health, 2d ed., by Bruce D. Shephard, M.D., and Carroll Shephard. Plume/Penguin, 1990.

DENTAL

American Dental Association
Department of Public Information and Education
211 East Chicago Avenue
Chicago, IL 60611
312-440-2500
For written information on oral health, send a self-addressed stamped envelope. Pamphlets available include *Tips for Older Adults*.

EYE CARE

National Eye Care Project
American Academy of Ophthalmology
P.O. Box 6988
San Francisco, CA 94120-6988
800-222-EYES
Provides literature to public. Send a self-addressed stamped envelope.

KIDNEY DISEASE

National Kidney and Urologic Diseases Information Clearinghouse
P.O. Box NKUDIC
Bethesda, MD 20892
301-654-4415

American Foundation for Urologic Disease
300 W. Pratt Street
Suite 401
Baltimore, MD 21205
800-242-2383
An information service for those with questions about incontinence, bladder problems, urinary track infections, prostate disease, and other urologic problems.

DIGESTIVE/BOWEL DISORDERS

National Digestive Disease Education and Information Clearinghouse
1555 Wilson Boulevard, Suite 600
Rosslyn, VA 22209
703-751-5763
Write for the latest information on the treatment of digestive disease.

MENTAL ILLNESS

American Psychiatric Association
Division of Public Information, Code WM
1400 K Street, N.W.
Washington, DC 20005
202-682-6000
Write to receive *Let's Talk Facts About Mental Illness*, a series of eighteen concise, comprehensive brochures covering a wide range of mental-health issues, including one about special mental-health concerns of the elderly.

American Suicide Foundation
1045 Park Avenue
New York, NY 10028
212-410-1111
Write for general information packet on depression and suicide.

American Association of Suicidology
2459 S. Ash Street
Denver, CO 80222
303-692-0985
Provides referrals to crisis intervention services throughout the United States.

427

Anxiety Disorders Association of America
Dept. B
P.O. Box 96505
Washington, DC 20077-7140
301-231-9350

Membership organization "that promotes the prevention and cure of anxiety disorders." Publishes the *Reporter*, a quarterly newsletter, and a directory of local self-help groups.

Related Book

Triumph over Fear: A Book of Help and Hope for People with Anxiety, Panic Attacks, and Phobias, by Jerilyn Ross. Bantam Books, 1995.

Women and Self-Esteem, by Linda Tschirhart Sanford and Mary Ellen Donovan. Penguin, 1985.

DOMESTIC VIOLENCE

National Center on Women and Family Law
799 Broadway, Room 402
New York, NY 10003
212-674-8200

Offers free publications on topics ranging from child support to child subsidy and domestic violence.

National Crime Prevention Council
1700 K Street N.W.
2nd Floor
Washington, DC 20006
202-466-6272

Provides literature on domestic violence.

NUTRITION

American Dietetic Association
800-366-1655

Between the hours of 9 A.M. and 4 P.M. Central Time, a dietician is on hand to answer questions about nutrition. They can also help you find a registered dietician in your area.

Food and Drug Administration
Office of Consumer Affairs
5600 Fishers Lane
Rockville, MD 20857
301-443-3170

The FDA's consumer information line answers your questions about all FDA-regulated products. Information about clinical trials of new drugs.

Related Books

Nutrition for Women: The Complete Guide, by Elizabeth Somer. Henry Holt, 1993.
A Woman's Guide to Vitamins and Minerals, by Sherry Wilson Sultenfuss and Thomas J. Sultenfuss, M.D. Contemporary Books, 1995.

ALTERNATIVE MEDICINE

National Commission for the Certification of Acupuncturists
1424 16th Street, N.W.
Suite 601
Washington, DC 20036
202-232-1404
This organization administers a national examination for the certification of acupuncturists. They distribute an information packet on acupuncture for $3.

American Chiropractic Association
1701 Clarendon Boulevard
Arlington, VA 22209
703-276-8800
Provides information packet and referrals.

National Center for Homeopathy
801 North Fairfax, Suite 306
Alexandria, VA 22314
703-548-7790
Membership organization. Provides a directory of pharmacies and practitioners specializing in homeopathic medicine.

American Association of Naturopathic Physicians
2366 Eastlake Ave East, Suite 322
Seattle, WA 98102
206-323-7610 (referral and information request line)
Provides brochure and referral directory for $5.

Related Books

The Healing Herbs, by Michael Castleman. Rodale Press, 1991.
Everybody's Guide to Homeopathic Medicines, by Stephen Cummings, M.D., and Dana Ullman. Jeremy Tarcher, 1991.
Discovering Homeopathy: Your Introduction to the Science and Art of Homeopathic Medicine, by Dana Ullman. North Atlantic Books, 1991.
Spontaneous Healing, by Andrew Weil. Alfred A. Knopf, 1995.

Related Periodicals

Foster's Botanical & Herbs Review, B&H Review, P.O. Box 106, Eureka Springs, AR 72632.
HerbalGram, American Botanical Council, P.O. Box 201660, Austin, TX 78720.

INDEX

abdomen, 118, 324
 cramps and pain in, 97, 121, 134, 141, 142, 145, 165, 173, 187, 330
 surgery on, 97, 146, 151–158, 163, 301
abortion, 183–187
 dilation and evacuation, 186
 prenatal testing and, 139–142
 therapeutic, 74
 timing of, 140–142, 184, 185, 186
 vacuum, 185
Accutane, 293–294
ACE inhibitors, 33
acetaminophen, 261, 263, 306–308, 318
acne, 215, 293–294
Acquired Immune Deficiency Syndrome (AIDS), 177–180
 death rates from, 62, 288
 gynecological symptoms of, 178
 prevention of, 171–173, 179–180
 testing for, 166, 178–179, 180, 329
acupuncture, 216, 259, 261, 403–405
adenocarcinomas, 70, 111
adenosine (Adenocard), 26, 28
adoption, 127, 158, 164, 167–170
adrenal glands, 18, 211, 212
adrenaline, 252, 399
Aesop, 201
agoraphobia, 351
Agriculture Department, U.S., 377
AIDS, see Acquired Immune Deficiency Syndrome
air pollution, 120, 121, 243, 244, 267
Al-Anon, 251, 355
alcohol, xx, 46, 197, 202, 227, 236, 250, 294, 335, 359
 abstaining from, 38, 129, 191, 233, 251, 335, 352
 guidelines for, 247–248
Alcoholics Anonymous (AA), 251, 355
alcoholism, 247–248, 251, 255, 340
Aliferis, Lisa, xxiv
allergies, 14, 244, 251–252
Altace (ramipril), 33
alteplase (t-PA), 14

alternative medicine, 402–410
 see also specific disciplines
Alzheimer's disease, 252–253
American College of Obstetrics and Gynecology, 135
American Diabetes Association, 246
American Heart Association, 377, 378, 379
American Psychiatric Association, 190
aminopterin, 92
amniocentesis, 137–138, 139
amniotic fluid, 135, 138, 141, 148, 153
amphetamine, 354
amputations, 245–246
anal fissures, 97, 100
analgesics, 244, 250, 261, 307, 309
anaphylaxis, 252
anemia, 97, 153, 233, 247, 253–256, 268, 373
 folic acid, 255
 hemolytic, 256
 iron-deficiency, 254
 pernicious, 254
 sickle-cell, 255
anencephaly, 130
anesthesia:
 epidural, 146, 150, 154
 general, 70, 120, 154, 185, 219, 264
 local, 29, 36–37, 70, 185
 spinal, 154
anesthesiologists, 39, 260
aneurysm, 280
anger, 51, 68, 140, 349
angina pectoris, 21–24, 36
 diagnosis of, 22, 24, 42–43
 heart disease and, 21–22, 23–24, 27
 men vs. women and, 21, 22, 23, 42
 microvascular, 42–43
 nitroglycerin treatment of, 12, 13, 24, 31–32
 symptoms of, 12, 13, 21–24, 42–43
 variant (Prinzmetal's), 23–24, 32
 see also chest pain
angiograms, 9, 28–30, 34–35, 42–43, 119
angioplasty, 31, 34–35, 36, 50
 candidates for, 35

431

437

447